ESSENTIALS OF FOOT AND ANKLE SURGERY

T0138824

ESSENTIALS OF FOOT AND ANKLE SURGERY

Edited by
Maneesh Bhatia, MBBS, MS (Orth), PG Dip (Tr & Orth), FRCS (Tr & Orth)
Consultant Orthopaedic Foot and Ankle Surgeon
University Hospitals of Leicester NHS Trust
Leicester, UK

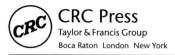

CRC Press
Taylor & Francis Group
Boca Raton London New York

CRC Press is an imprint of the
Taylor & Francis Group, an **informa** business

First edition published 2021
by CRC Press
6000 Broken Sound Parkway NW, Suite 300, Boca Raton, FL 33487-2742

and by CRC Press
2 Park Square, Milton Park, Abingdon, Oxon, OX14 4RN

© 2021 Taylor & Francis Group, LLC

CRC Press is an imprint of Taylor & Francis Group, LLC

This book contains information obtained from authentic and highly regarded sources. While all reasonable efforts have been made to publish reliable data and information, neither the author[s] nor the publisher can accept any legal responsibility or liability for any errors or omissions that may be made. The publishers wish to make clear that any views or opinions expressed in this book by individual editors, authors or contributors are personal to them and do not necessarily reflect the views/opinions of the publishers. The information or guidance contained in this book is intended for use by medical, scientific or health-care professionals and is provided strictly as a supplement to the medical or other professional's own judgement, their knowledge of the patient's medical history, relevant manufacturer's instructions and the appropriate best practice guidelines. Because of the rapid advances in medical science, any information or advice on dosages, procedures or diagnoses should be independently verified. The reader is strongly urged to consult the relevant national drug formulary and the drug companies' and device or material manufacturers' printed instructions, and their websites, before administering or utilizing any of the drugs, devices or materials mentioned in this book. This book does not indicate whether a particular treatment is appropriate or suitable for a particular individual. Ultimately it is the sole responsibility of the medical professional to make his or her own professional judgements, so as to advise and treat patients appropriately. The authors and publishers have also attempted to trace the copyright holders of all material reproduced in this publication and apologize to copyright holders if permission to publish in this form has not been obtained. If any copyright material has not been acknowledged please write and let us know so we may rectify in any future reprint.

Except as permitted under U.S. Copyright Law, no part of this book may be reprinted, reproduced, transmitted, or utilized in any form by any electronic, mechanical, or other means, now known or hereafter invented, including photocopying, microfilming, and recording, or in any information storage or retrieval system, without written permission from the publishers.

For permission to photocopy or use material electronically from this work, access www.copyright.com or contact the Copyright Clearance Center, Inc. (CCC), 222 Rosewood Drive, Danvers, MA 01923, 978-750-8400. For works that are not available on CCC please contact mpkbookspermissions@tandf.co.uk

Trademark notice: Product or corporate names may be trademarks or registered trademarks and are used only for identification and explanation without intent to infringe.

ISBN: 9780367486495 (hbk)
ISBN: 9780367464240 (pbk)
ISBN: 9781003042099 (ebk)

Typeset in Utopia
by KnowledgeWorks Global Ltd.

Dedication

The best way to learn is to teach. I would like to dedicate this book to my teachers and trainees who have inspired me.

My family has always been behind me as a rock, and I would like to convey my heartfelt thanks and dedication for the never-ending support and love from my dearest wife Sulaxni, my precious kids Juhi and Yash and my Mum and Dad for their countless blessings.

Maneesh Bhatia

Contents

Foreword

When I was asked to write a foreword by Maneesh Bhatia, the editor, for this important new book, I reflected on my own reading across the years from journals and, of course, from the many books of great pioneers in the world of Foot and Ankle Surgery. It made me realise how much our Surgical Specialty has progressed from the early split from General Surgery to Trauma and Orthopaedics to sub-specialisation. Foot and Ankle Surgery has developed so much, particularly over the past 50 years, with huge advances in our understanding of the anatomy, biomechanics (including gait analysis, prosthetics and orthotics), neurophysiology and, ultimately, the conservative and surgical treatment of Foot and Ankle pathology in our patients.

Basil Helal used the term "Cinderella" specialty in his famous book co-edited with Derek Wilson, a reference to "never quite being at the ball". He described that frequently our cases were on the end of elective orthopaedic lists and that this type of surgery was commonly performed by more junior surgeons. He went on to suggest that the Foot and Ankle was more complex anatomically and biomechanically than other weight-bearing joints and, therefore, deserved greater respect from the medical and scientific world. What has happened since those enlightened words is nothing short of remarkable. The British Orthopaedic Foot Surgery Society (now Foot and Ankle Society) has gone from a small number meeting in John Angel's kitchen to a large world renowned organisation, which contributes increasingly each year to the specialty. Many of the contributors to this book have held executive positions in BOFAS including president. I very much enjoyed reading all of the chapters. More recently, increasing links have developed across Europe with the European Foot and Ankle Society and globally with the International Federation of Foot and Ankle Surgeons. Long may this continue.

Finally, I should like to congratulate Maneesh Bhatia, an excellent editor, and the many contributors, well known in this field, for producing this impressive book adding to and assessing the current knowledge and practice in our developing specialty. Similar progress in the next 50 years is to be expected.

Don McBride
Past President BOFAS
Immediate Past President BOA
President EFAS
Council Member IFFAS

Preface

It is a proud moment to write the editorial note as the two-year journey is finally coming to an end. This mammoth task has been possible only because of the invaluable contribution by the 42 co-authors who have done a fantastic job. The lead authors of all the chapters are experts in their respective fields who have laid out pearls of wisdom from their vast experience.

Each of the 22 chapters contains a wealth of information that has been presented in a way that is easy to understand and is backed up by current evidence. One of the attractions of this book is that there are a number of excellent illustrations in each chapter (altogether over 500 in the book) that convey the information clearly helping to keep readers engaged. The book covers almost everything in the foot and ankle spectrum (trauma & elective, paediatric & adult, clinical examination & surgical approaches, orthotics & prosthetics, biomechanics & radiology, etc.).

Essentials of Foot and Ankle Surgery will not only help orthopaedic registrars and trainees to prepare for the examination, but it will also be a very useful tool for clinicians and surgeons to refer to this foot ankle comprehensive guide in their day-to-day practice. I have been practicing foot and ankle surgery for the last 12 years, and there is so much I have learned during the editing process of this book and I am confident that readers will feel the same.

Last but not least, I would like to convey my sincere thanks to two people who provided very useful input. *Nikhil Nanavati* is a bright young man who is ever so positive and very passionate. His enthusiasm and drive pushed me to go ahead to write this book. He advised me as to what orthopaedic trainees preparing for the exam need for their revision. *Anthony Sakellariou* is a well-respected and experienced senior colleague who I feel is one of the most knowledgeable critics in the world of foot and ankle surgery. He has been the quality check of this book during the editorial process.

Maneesh Bhatia
Editor: Essentials of Foot and Ankle Surgery

Contributors

Pilar Martínez de Albornoz
Consultant Orthopaedic Foot and Ankle Surgeon
Hospital Universitario Quironsalud
Madrid, Spain

Raju Ahluwalia MBBS BSc (Hons), MFSEM, FRCS (Tr & Orth)
Consultant Orthopaedic Foot and Ankle Surgeon
Department of Orthopaedics
King's College Hospital
London, UK
Executive Commitee Member Diabetic Foot Study
  Group of the EASD

Patricia Allen MB ChB, FRCS (Tr & Orth)
Consultant Orthopaedic Foot and Ankle Surgeon
University Hospitals of Leicester NHS Trust
Leicester, UK
Past President BOFAS

Maneesh Bhatia MBBS, MS (Orth), PG Dip (Tr & Orth), FRCS (Tr & Orth)
Consultant Orthopaedic Foot and Ankle Surgeon
University Hospitals of Leicester NHS Trust
Leicester, UK
Member of EFAS Scientific Committee

Raj Bhatt MD, FRCR
Consultant Musculoskeletal Radiologist
University Hospitals of Leicester NHS Trust
Leicester, UK

Rick Brown MA, MBBS, FRCS, FRCS (Tr & Orth)
Consultant Orthopaedic Surgeon
Nuffield Orthopaedic Centre
Oxford, UK
Honorary Senior Clinical Lecturer
University of Oxford
Chair Education Committee BOFAS

Basil Budair MBBS, MSc, FRCS (Tr & Orth)
Consultant Trauma & Orthopaedic Surgeon
  Foot & Ankle Surgery
University Hospitals Birmingham Foundation
  Trust
Birmingham, UK

Oliver Chan PGCert MedEd, MD(res), FRCS (Tr & Orth)
Post CCT Fellow, Guy's and St Thomas' NHS
  Foundation Trust
London, UK

Donatas Chlebinskas MBBS, FEBOT
Specialty Doctor, Trauma and Orthopaedics
Milton Keynes University Hospital NHS Trust
Milton Keynes, UK

Robert Anthony Emilius Clayton BSc (Hons Virology), MB ChB (Hons), MRCSEd, FRCSEd (Tr & Orth)
Consultant Orthopaedic Foot and Ankle Surgeon
Victoria Hospital
Kirkcaldy, UK
BOFAS Media and Communications Director

Nicholas Eastley MBChB, BMedSci, PhD, FRCS (Tr & Orth)
Specialist Registrar, Trauma and Orthopaedics
University Hospitals of Leicester NHS Trust
Leicester, UK

Nick Gallogly MSc, BEng, BSc, MBAPO
Consultant Orthotist
Royal Berkshire NHS Foundation Trust
Berkshire, UK

Jasdeep Giddie MBBS, MRCS, FRCS (Tr & Orth)
Consultant Orthopaedic Foot and Ankle Surgeon
Wexham Park and Heatherwood Hospitals
Slough, UK

Mansur Halai BSc (Hons), MBChB, MRCA, MRCS, FRCS (Tr & Orth)
Assistant Professor, University of Toronto
Orthopaedic Surgeon: Trauma, Foot & Ankle
St Michael's Hospital
Toronto, Canada

Rajiv S Hanspal, MBBS, DSc, FRCP, FRCS
Retd. Consultant in Rehabilitation Medicine, RNOH
  Stanmore, UK
Past President, International Society for Prosthetics
  and Orthotics

Kartik Hariharan MB, BcH, FRCS(I), FRCS
(Tr & Orth)
Consultant Orthopaedic and Foot & Ankle Surgeon
Aneurin Bevan University Health Board
Newport, South Wales, UK
Past President BOFAS

Rajesh Kakwani MS, DNB, MRCS Ed, Dip Sports
Medicine, PG Cert Clin Ed, MCh, FRCS (Tr & Orth)
Consultant Orthopaedic Foot and Ankle Surgeon
Northumbria Healthcare NHS Trust
Newcastle upon Tyne, UK

Venu Kavarthapu FRCS (Tr & Orth)
Associate Professor University of Southern
   Denmark
Consultant Orthopaedic Surgeon
Department of Orthopaedics
King's College Hospital
London, UK
Member of Education Committee BOFAS
President of Association of Diabetic Foot Surgeons

Chinnasamy Senthil Kumar FRCS (Tr & Orth)
Consultant Orthopaedic Foot and Ankle Surgeon
Glasgow Royal Infirmary
Glasgow, UK

Sangoh Lee MBBS, BSc, MRCP, FRCR
Consultant Musculoskeletal Radiologist
Imperial College Healthcare NHS Trust
London, UK

Zoe Lin BM, BSc, PgDip, FRCS (Tr & Orth)
Specialist Registrar, Trauma and Orthopaedics
Hampshire Hospitals NHS Foundation Trust
Hampshire, UK

Devendra Mahadevan BMedSci, BMBS, FRCS
(Tr & Orth)
Consultant Orthopaedic Foot and Ankle Surgeon
Royal Berkshire Hospital
Berkshire, UK

Nilesh Makwana MBBS, FRCS, FRCS (Tr & Orth),
PGCert Education
Consultant Trauma and Orthopaedic Surgeon
The Robert Jones and Agnes Hunt Hospital
   Foundation Trust
Oswestry, Shropshire, UK

Karan Malhotra MBChB (Hons), MRCS, FRCS (Tr & Orth)
Consultant Orthopaedic Foot & Ankle Surgeon at
   Royal National Orthopaedic Hospital
Stanmore, UK
Honorary Clinical Lecturer at University College
London, UK

Shahbaz S Malik BSc (Hons), MB BCh, MSc
(Orth Engin), LLM, FRCS (Tr & Orth)
Consultant Orthopaedic Surgeon
Worcestershire Acute Hospital NHS Turst
Worcester, UK

Sheraz S Malik MBBS, MSc (Orth Engin), LLM, FRCS
(Tr & Orth)
Senior Clinical Fellow, Trauma and Orthopaedics
Manchester University NHS Foundation Trust
England, UK

Daniel Marsland MSc (SEM), FRCS (Tr & Orth)
Consultant Orthopaedic Surgeon
Hampshire Hospitals NHS Foundation Trust
Hampshire, UK

Lyndon Mason MB BCh, MRCS (Eng), FRCS (Tr & Orth)
Hunterian Professor 2020, Royal College of Surgeons
   England
Trauma and Orthopaedic Consultant, Liverpool
   University Hospitals NHS Trust
Liverpool, UK

Manuel Monteagudo
Consultant Orthopaedic Foot & Ankle Surgeon
Hospital Universitario Quironsalud
Associate Professor and Director of Medical
   Education – Faculty Medicine UEM
Madrid, Spain
Chair Scientific Committee EFAS

Nikhil Nanavati MBBS, FRCS (Tr & Orth), MSc
Consultant Orthopaedic Foot and Ankle Surgeon
Rotherham Foundation Trust
Rotherham, UK

Shelain Patel BSc, DipSEM, FRCS (Tr & Orth)
Consultant Orthopaedic Foot & Ankle Surgeon
Royal National Orthopaedic Hospital
Stanmore, UK
Honorary Clinical Lecturer at University College
London, UK

Hari Prem MBBS, MS, FRCS (Tr & Orth)
Consultant Orthopaedic Surgeon
Royal Orthopaedic Hospital
Birmingham, UK

**Arul Ramasamy MA (Cantab), PhD, MFSEM, FRCS
(Tr & Orth)**
Consultant Orthopaedic Foot and Ankle Surgeon
Academic Department of Military Surgery and Trauma
Royal Centre of Defence Medicine, ICT Centre
Edgbaston, Birmingham, UK

Anthony Sakellariou BSc, MBBS, FRCS (Orth)
Consultant Orthopaedic Foot and Ankle Surgeon
Deputy Chief of Service for Orthopaedics & Plastics
Frimley Park Hospital
Surrey, UK
Past President BOFAS
Member of EFAS Education Committee

**Aabid Sanaullah MBBS, MRCS, MRCPS, PG Dip
(Trauma Surgery), FEBOT, FRCS (Tr & Orth)**
Consultant Trauma and Orthopaedics Surgeon
Milton Keynes University Hospital NHS Trust
Milton Keynes, UK

Avtar Singh MS (Orth), Dip (Orth)
Director and Chief Joint Replacement Surgeon
Amandeep Hospital
Amritsar, India

Dishan Singh FRCS (Orth)
Consultant Orthopaedic Foot and Ankle Surgeon
Royal National Orthopaedic Hospital
Stanmore, UK
Past President BOFAS
Past President Scientific Committee EFAS

John Sullivan MSc
HCPC Registered Prosthetist, NHS Lead
  Prosthetist
Royal National Orthopaedic Hospital
Stanmore, UK

Adam Sykes MBBS, BSc, FRCS (Tr & Orth)
Foot and Ankle Fellow
Royal Orthopaedic Hospital
Birmingham, UK

Hiro Tanaka
Consultant Foot and Ankle Surgeon
Aneurin Bevan University Health Board
Newport, UK
BOA Council Member and the Honorary Treasurer
  for BOFAS

Babaji Sitaram Thorat DNB (Orth), MNAMS
Arthroplasty Fellow
Amandeep Hospital
Amritsar, India

Rajeev Vohra MS (Orth), DNB (Orth), MNAMS
Senior Consultant, Foot and Ankle Surgeon
Amandeep Hospital
Amritsar, India
Immediate Past President, Indian Foot and Ankle
  Society
Executive Committee Member APOA Foot and Ankle
  Council

Companion Website

The following link will take you to the companion website for this book, featuring MCQs, videos and further information about the authors.

www.routledge.com/cw/Bhatia

Foot and ankle examination

Nikhil Nanavati, Nicholas Eastley, and Maneesh Bhatia

Introduction

The foot and ankle are composed of multiple bones, joints, ligaments and tendons, each of which may be a source of a patient's pathology and symptoms. A general foot and ankle examination consists of seven components – inspection, gait analysis, palpation, joint range of movement, neurovascular (NV) status, key muscle strength and special tests.

History

A focussed, structured history can be a valuable tool to guide clinical examination. Begin by determining the patient's age and occupation. The most common presenting complaints in the foot and ankle are pain, stiffness, deformity, swelling, instability and difficulty with ambulation. The history should be used to characterise each of these symptoms, in particular their duration and impact on a patient's function. It is important to establish any history of trauma or any neurological changes. A significant past medical history, smoking and drinking in excess may have a major influence on a patient's fitness and outcome following surgery. It is important to determine any known history of diabetes, peripheral neuropathy, inflammatory arthropathy or peripheral vascular disease. Past or family history of deep vein thrombosis (DVT) or pulmonary embolism and other risk factors for thromboembolism are important if the patient needs plaster cast immobilisation or Achilles tendon surgery. A detailed history of current medications, especially warfarin or the newer direct oral anticoagulants (DOAC), is essential for perioperative planning. It is also key to get an idea of the expectations of every patient. Towards the end of the history taking session, the question "Is there anything I might have missed that you would like me to know?" can pay dividends.

General inspection

Inspection is a key component and will guide the remainder of the examination to provide a good idea of what clinical signs to expect moving forwards. Start by inspecting the patient's footwear, noting the distribution of any sole wear (remembering to ask when the shoes were bought) and any orthotic modifications or insoles. Take note of any walking aids nearby. Adequate exposure above the knees is required, and patients should be inspected from the front, side and back. Ask the patient to stand facing you and inspect their knees, noting any malalignment. Moving in a proximal to distal direction, note any scars (Figure 1.1), swellings (synovitis, osteoarthritis, ganglion) or skin abnormalities (colour changes, callosities, ulcer, nail changes). Also note any deformity involving the ankle, hindfoot, midfoot or toes. Ask the patient to turn 90° so that the medial border of the foot can be inspected. Look for swellings around the heel or Achilles tendon (Haglund's deformity or Achilles tendinopathy) or any flattening or accentuation of the medial longitudinal arch (pes planus or pes cavus, respectively). Next, ask the patient to turn a further 90° allowing you to inspect the back of the foot and ankle. Note any calf asymmetry (wasting or hypertrophy) or hindfoot valgus/varus which may be subtle (Figure 1.2). If deformity is identified in the coronal plane, the next step is to perform either the heel raise test (valgus deformity) or Coleman block test (varus deformity) (see in section "Special tests"). From behind the ankle, the little toe and half of the 4th toe should normally be visible. More toes will be visible in cases of severe planovalgus due to midfoot abduction (the 'too many toes' sign). Beware, however, that more toes will also become visible in any external rotational abnormality involving the leg or ankle. Finally, ask the patient to rotate another 90° to allow you to inspect the lateral border of the foot. A callosity at the base of 5th metatarsal is usually present when the patient walks on the lateral border of foot which can be seen in a cavovarus deformity.

Inspection of the plantar aspect of the foot is important in order to check for callosities under the metatarsal heads (indicating overload) or infection between toes. This can be performed by asking the patient to sit (with feet over the edge) or lying on a couch.

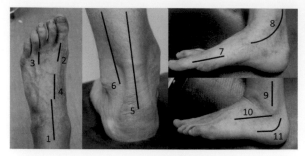

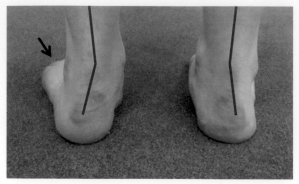

Figure 1.1 The most common surgical scars seen in the foot and ankle. 1: Anterior approach to ankle; 2: Dorsal approach to 1st MTPJ; 3: Dorsal intermetatarsal longitudinal incision (Morton's neuroma excision from 3rd intermetatarsal space); 4: Approach for TMTJ fusion or ORIF for Lisfranc injury; 5: Posterior longitudinal approach Achilles tendon; 6: Posterolateral approach ankle; 7: Medial approach 1st MTPJ; 8: Posteromedial approach ankle/tibialis posterior reconstruction; 9: Lateral approach fibula; 10: Ollier's approach hindfoot/subtalar joint; 11: Lateral approach calcaneum.

Figure 1.2 A subtle pes planovalgus deformity of the left foot. Increased hindfoot valgus can be seen (red lines superimposed for comparison) with the 'Too many toes' sign (black arrow).

Gait

Human gait is the cyclical forward progression of the body (Figure 1.3). A single gait cycle is defined as one heel strike to the next heel strike of the same leg. This cycle can be divided into the 'stance' and 'swing' phases. The swing phase comprises 35% of the gait cycle and occurs whilst the leg is progressing forwards in the air, i.e., between toe-off and heel strike of the same foot. During the swing phase, the ankle dorsiflexors bring the ankle to a neutral position to facilitate ground clearance. The stance phase comprises the remaining 65% of the gait cycle, and occurs whilst the foot is in contact with the ground, i.e., between heel strike and toe-off of the same foot. The stance phase is further subdivided into three 'rockers' (1):

First Rocker: Period between heel strike and foot flat. Eccentric tibialis anterior contraction controls foot drop and the plantarflexion moment occurring about the ankle. The heel ground reaction force (GRF) occurs behind the ankle joint, resulting in ankle movement from neutral to 10° plantarflexion.

Second Rocker: Period between foot-flat and heel-off. The ankle acts as fulcrum whilst the gastrocsoleus complex contracts eccentrically to control progression of tibia over talus. The ankle joint moves from 10° plantarflexion to 10° dorsiflexion as the GRF moves anterior to the ankle.

Third Rocker: Period between heel-off and toe-off. Tibial progression continues over the talus, and ankle rapidly shifts from 10° dorsiflexion to 20° plantarflexion. Strong concentric contraction of the gastrocsoleus complex produces this ankle plantarflexion.

Gait analysis

Ask the patient to walk back and forth across the available space. Look for any obvious pain, instability or stiffness. The common gait patterns seen in relation to foot and ankle problems include:

Pronation gait: This is characterised by feet rolling inward resulting in more pressure on the medial column and is usually seen in pes planovalgus.

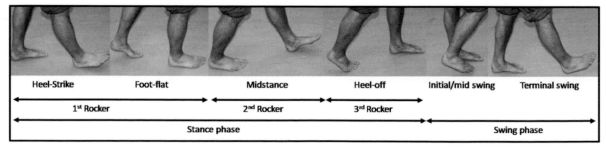

| Heel-Strike | Foot-flat | Midstance | Heel-off | Initial/mid swing | Terminal swing |

| 1st Rocker | 2nd Rocker | 3rd Rocker |

| Stance phase | Swing phase |

Figure 1.3 Diagrammatic representation of a full gait cycle of the right foot.

Supination gait: This is characterised by excessive pressure on the lateral border of the foot. It is usually seen in pes cavovarus.

Equinus gait: In the presence of severe equinus deformity the patient walks on the toes with heel not touching the ground.

Antalgic gait: This is characterised by a shortened stance phase of the affected side. This is usually seen in arthritis of ankle or foot.

High-steppage gait: A patient with a foot drop will present with an absent heel strike and uncontrolled 2nd rocker (foot 'slaps' to the floor). This is seen with weakness of ankle dorsiflexors.

Weak 'push-off' (apropulsive) gait: The 'push-off' (also known as the 'toe-off' phase of gait cycle) is predominantly produced by the gastrocsoleus complex. When weakness is present in this muscle complex or the Achilles tendon, the stride length is reduced and the gait velocity falls. Achilles rupture, lengthened Achilles tendons and neurological disease are the more common causes for this type of gait abnormality.

Palpation

Based on history and examination so far, focus on structures thought to be the cause of symptoms. It is better to palpate the area of suspected maximum tenderness towards the end of the examination. A suggested approach is to begin at the anterolateral ankle joint followed by the medial ankle, tibialis posterior tendon, Achilles tendon and peroneal tendons. Palpate the sinus tarsi 2 cm anterior and 1 cm inferior to the lateral malleolus, where tenderness may represent subtalar joint (STJ) arthritis. Palpate the calcaneocuboid joint (CCJ), which is located midway between the sinus tarsi and the base of the 5th metatarsal. The talonavicular joint (TNJ) is approximately 2 cm distal to the tip of medial malleolus. If midfoot pathology is suspected, palpate the tarsometatarsal joints (TMTJs), using the metatarsal shafts for orientation. Palpate the 1st metatarsophalangeal joint (MTPJ) if any hallux pathology is suspected, and the lesser toe interphalangeal joint (IPJ) in the presence of any lesser toe deformities. Palpation of intermetatarsal space (2nd and/or 3rd) is recommended to elicit tenderness if a Morton's neuroma is suspected. It is important to differentiate tenderness in the 2nd MTPJ (which feels hard due to solid structures of the joint) as compared to intermetatarsal tenderness (which feels soft due to the tissue). A useful guide is to notice splaying of toes which can be seen with intermetatarsal palpation of a Morton's neuroma. Finally, palpate the plantar aspect of the foot as tenderness at the medial or central origin of the plantar fascia is typical of plantar fasciitis.

Range of movement

A comparison of bilateral active range of ankle and toe joint movements provides useful information and can be performed before starting passive range of motion examination.

Ankle joint (tibiotalar joint): Whilst checking ankle range of motion, the hindfoot should be inverted to lock the neighbouring STJ. Check ankle dorsiflexion (normal = 20°) and plantarflexion (normal = 40°), and if any evidence of equinus, perform Silfverskiöld test (see in section "Special tests").

Hindfoot

Subtalar joint (STJ): Grasp the heel with one hand and fix the talus by holding the talar neck between the thumb and middle finger of the other hand (Figure 1.4). Using the hand grasping the heel, assess inversion and eversion at the STJ (normal = 5° varus and 5° valgus).

Talonavicular joint (TNJ) and Calcaneocuboid joint (CCJ): Identify the prominent navicular tuberosity and

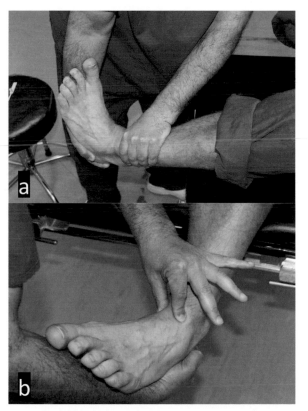

Figure 1.4 Assessment of ankle and subtalar joint range of movement. (a) Note inversion of the hindfoot to lock the subtalar joint and use of the forearm to dorsiflex the ankle joint. (b) The examiner's left thumb and index finger are used to fix the patient's talus/talar neck whilst their right grasps and inverts/everts the patient's heel.

use this as a landmark. Move the midfoot on the hind-foot (adduction and abduction). Remember to note any uncovering of the talar head, which is seen in talona-vicular abduction deformity associated with pes planus.

Midfoot

Tarsometatarsal joints (TMTJs): Small amounts of abduction, adduction, plantarflexion and dorsiflexion all occur at the TMTJs (medial < lateral). In patients with midfoot pain, passive plantarflexion and dorsiflex-ion should be assessed at each TMTJ. In cases of hallux valgus, any 1st TMTJ laxity must also be identified as this requires special surgical consideration.

Forefoot

First metatarsophalangeal joint (MTPJ): Assess 1st MTPJ plantarflexion (normal = 30°) and dorsiflexion. A wide range of passive dorsiflexion has been reported in literature ranging between 60–90°.

 Lesser toe MTPJs: Assess lesser toe MTPJ plantarflex-ion and dorsiflexion in the presence of any lesser toe deformities. Describe any deformities and whether these are flexible (correctable) or not.

Neurovascular status and key muscle strength

Power: It is useful to check the power of tibialis posterior (tibial nerve), tibialis anterior (deep peroneal nerve) and the peronei (superficial peroneal nerve). This is partic-ularly important for any pathology where neurological involvement is suspected.

 Tibialis posterior: Tibialis posterior's function is to plantarflex and invert the foot. To test, place the patient's foot into maximum plantarflexion and inver-sion. Next, try to move the foot from this position asking the patient to resist, whilst simultaneously palpating the tibialis posterior tendon behind the medial malleolus (Figure 1.5a).

 Tibialis anterior: Tibialis anterior's function is to dorsiflex and invert the foot. To test, move the patient's foot into maximum dorsiflexion and inversion and, by applying direct pressure onto the top of the 1st meta-tarsal head, attempt to move the foot from this position. Ask the patient to resist whilst palpating the tibialis anterior tendon anterior to the ankle joint (Figure 1.5b).

 Peronei: Eversion of the ankle is mainly attributed to Peroneus brevis. Peroneus longus in addition to ever-sion, plantar flexes the 1st metatarsal. Both tendons are secondary plantar flexors of the ankle. There are incon-sistencies in literature regarding testing of the Peronei. Since both tendons cross the ankle joint posteriorly, it is best to test them in plantarflexion of the ankle joint. Resisted plantarflexion of the first ray is good way of testing peroneus longus, whereas peroneus brevis is

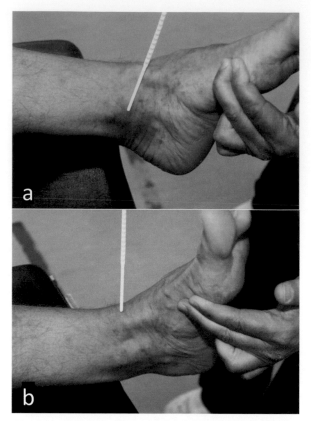

Figure 1.5 An assessment of tibialis posterior and tibialis anterior power. (a) It highlights where tibialis posterior should be palpated. (b) It highlights where tibialis ante-rior should be palpated.

best tested by resisted eversion of the foot (Figure 1.6). If instability of peroneal tendons is suspected, then active circumduction of the ankle is helpful to reveal this.

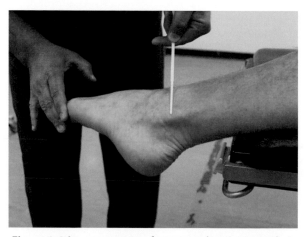

Figure 1.6 An assessment of peroneus brevis strength. It shows the peroneal brevis (yellow pointer) being tested with resisted eversion of ankle in plantarflexion.

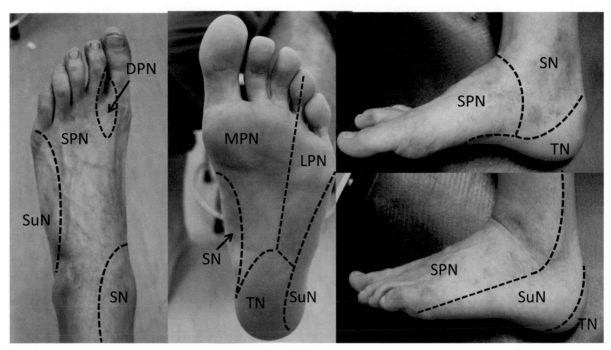

Figure 1.7 Cutaneous distribution of the sensory nerves of the foot. (Abbreviations: DPN, deep peroneal nerve; SN, saphenous nerve; SPN, superficial peroneal nerve; SuN, sural nerve; TN, tibial nerve.)

Sensation: To perform a complete assessment of sensation, the saphenous nerve (medial border of the foot), deep peroneal nerve (1st web space), superficial peroneal nerve (dorsum of the foot), sural nerve (lateral border of hindfoot) and tibial nerve (plantar aspect of heel and foot) should all be tested (Figure 1.7). Medial plantar nerve is the main sensory nerve of the plantar aspect of the foot. Lateral plantar nerve supplies sensation to plantar surface of 5th toe, plantar lateral half of 4th toe and strip of skin on lateral plantar area of the foot.

Vascularity: The dorsalis pedis pulse can be felt on the dorsum of the foot in the 1st intermetatarsal space just lateral to the extensor hallucis longus tendon. The posterior tibial pulse can be felt 1 cm posterior and inferior to the medial malleolus. If either pulse is absent or diminished, the contralateral side should be assessed, and a vascular opinion may be required.

Special tests

Heel raise test

Aim: To check if valgus deformity is flexible (bilateral heel raise) and to check strength of plantar flexors (tibialis posterior and Achilles) (single heel raise).

Ask the patient to face a nearby wall and place both hands against it for support. Next, ask them to rise onto their tiptoes. In normal feet, the action of tibialis posterior on the naviculum will lead to varus tilt of the hindfoot

(Figure 1.8). In cases of hindfoot stiffness, arthritis, coalition or tibialis posterior weakness, this will not occur and the hindfoot will remain in valgus. Note that in cases of severe ankle, subtalar or 1st MTPJ arthritis, patients may not be able to rise onto their tip toes due to pain. In cases of suspected pes planovalgus due to tibialis posterior insufficiency, ask the patient to perform repeated single heel raises. An inability to perform this 'single stance' test will highlight any subtle weakness in ankle plantar flexors (particularly tibialis posterior).

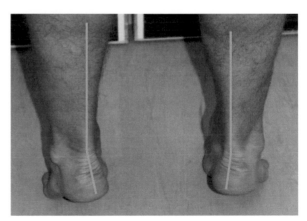

Figure 1.8 Normal hindfoot alignment during the heel raise test. The expected hindfoot varus is highlighted by superimposed blue lines.

Coleman block test (2)

Aim: To determine whether a pes cavovarus deformity is flexible or fixed.

The test is performed by placing the heel and lateral border of the foot on a raised surface (block or book), 2–4 cm thick, with the first ray unsupported (Figure 1.9). Flexible 'forefoot driven' cavovarus deformity occurs as a result of compensatory hindfoot supination in response to a pronated forefoot/plantar flexed first ray. During Coleman block test with a flexible hindfoot, the heel will correct to a neutral or valgus position. In contrast, a rigid 'hindfoot driven' cavovarus deformity will not correct and the heel will remain in varus. Performing Coleman block test is essential in any case of hindfoot varus, as a flexible deformity can be addressed by correcting the first ray in isolation (e.g., with a dorsi-flexion osteotomy of the 1st metatarsal or cuneiform), whilst a fixed deformity requires surgery to both the hindfoot and forefoot.

Simmonds-Thompson test (3)

Aim: To diagnose Achilles tendon rupture.

This is performed prone (Figure 1.10) or with patient kneeling on the examination couch whilst facing away from examiner. In the prone position, the first step is to flex the knees to 90 degrees and observe the position of feet (not required in kneeling position with ankle dependent over end of couch). In cases with an Achilles rupture, the affected foot will fall into neutral or dorsiflexion position as the 'resting tension' from the Achilles tendon is lost (Matles Test). The next step is to squeeze the calf with knee extended and compare the effect this has on both ankles – plantarflexion will be weaker or absent in a positive test.

Silfverskiöld test (4)

Aim: To identify gastrocnemius tightness.

Extend the knee and invert the hindfoot. Record maximum ankle dorsiflexion in this position. Next, flex

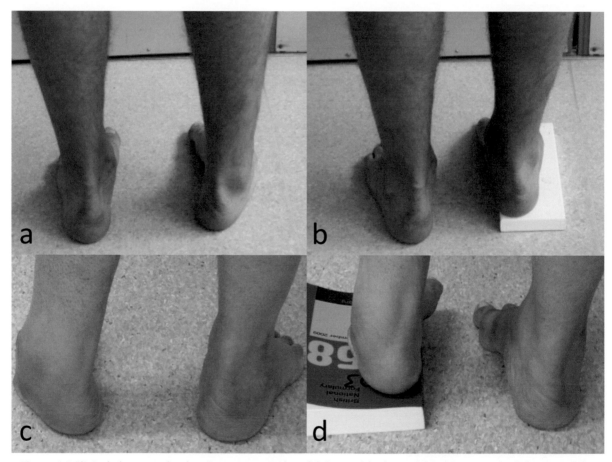

Figure 1.9 Clinical photographs showing two examples of Coleman block test. (a) It shows a varus deformity of the right hindfoot. (b) It shows the Coleman block being performed on the same patient, during which the varus deformity corrects, confirming it is flexible (forefoot driven). (c) It shows a rigid (hindfoot driven) varus deformity of the left hindfoot, which as shown in (d), fails to correct during Coleman block test.

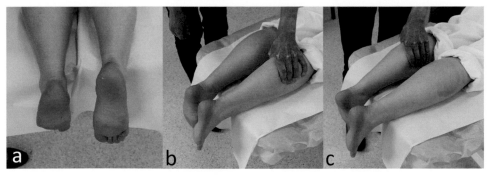

Figure 1.10 The Simmonds-Thompson test highlighting a ruptured left Achilles tendon rupture. As shown in (a) the affected foot (left side) will rest in less plantarflexion as compared to the normal side due to loss of resting tension. This becomes more pronounced when the knees are flexed to 90 degrees and the affected foot falls into neutral or dorsiflexion position – (Matles Test). On compression of the calf on the normal side there is plantarflexion of the foot (b). The affected side displays reduced or no ankle plantarflexion on calf squeeze (c).

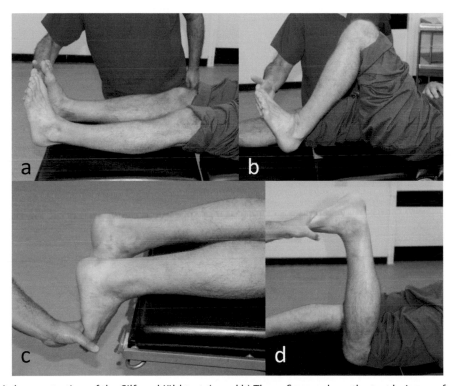

Figure 1.11 A demonstration of the Silfverskiöld test. (a and b) These figures show the test being performing in the traditional way with the patient supine. Note the increased passive ankle dorsiflexion seen with knee flexion (b). (c and d) These figures show the test being performed with the patient prone. This is particularly useful in those with severe ipsilateral hip pathology preventing any significant movement.

the knee to 90° (to relieve tension on the gastrocnemius) and repeat the procedure, again recording maximum ankle dorsiflexion (Figure 1.11). If reduced dorsiflexion is seen with the knee extended, equinus is secondary to gastrocnemius tightness. If dorsiflexion is limited with the knee both extended and flexed, equinus is secondary to gastrocsoleus complex or Achilles tightness.

Ankle ligament instability tests

Aim: To identify ankle ligament (Deltoid/ATFL/CFL) insufficiency.

Deltoid ligament: The deltoid ligament is the primary stabiliser of the medial ankle, resisting excessive hindfoot eversion and external rotation. It is assessed using the *eversion stress test.* The patient is positioned in a sitting position with the ankle plantigrade. The examiner uses one hand to stabilise the tibia and the other to evert and abduct the heel. Any pain or excessive eversion compared to the contralateral side is suggestive of a deltoid ligament injury.

Anterior talofibular ligament (ATFL): The ATFL is the weakest of the ankle ligaments and the most commonly injured. Its primary function is to resist inversion and internal rotation in the plantar flexed foot. The ATFL can be assessed by either the *anterior drawer test* or the *inversion stress test*:

- *Anterior drawer test:* The patient is placed in a sitting position with the knee flexed to relieve tension in the calf muscles, and the ankle in 20° plantarflexion (Figure 1.12). The examiner uses one hand to stabilise the lower leg, and the other hand to grasp the heel. Simultaneously, an anterior pressure is applied to the heel and a posterior pressure is applied to the lower leg. An anterior talar translation of >4–5 mm at the ankle joint is highly suggestive of an ATFL rupture. In reality this is often difficult to quantify, making comparison to the contralateral ankle important.
- *Inversion stress test:* Position the patient in a sitting position, flex the knee and position the ankle in 20° plantarflexion (Figure 1.12). The examiner uses one hand to stabilise the lower leg, and the other to hold the heel and invert and adduct the ankle. Any excessive inversion compared to the contralateral ankle suggests ATFL insufficiency.

Calcaneofibular ligament (CFL): The CFL is an extra-articular ligament that resists internal rotation and inversion in a plantigrade or dorsiflexed foot. It is assessed using the anterior drawer test and inversion stress test with the ankle in a *plantigrade* position.

Mulder's click test (5), thumb index finger squeeze test (6) and plantar percussion test

Aim: For clinical diagnosis of Morton's neuroma.

Mulder's click test: This is performed by manually compressing the medial and lateral forefoot at the level of the metatarsal heads. The examiner may also simultaneously palpate the symptomatic interdigital web space (Figure 1.13). In a positive test, compression results in a palpable painful 'click.' Be careful not to confuse the Mulder's click test with Mulder's sign, the latter of which describes paraesthesia over the ball of the foot +/− toes caused by digital plantar nerve irritation.

Thumb index finger squeeze test: The symptomatic interdigital space is squeezed between the tips of the index finger (dorsal) and thumb (plantar). Splaying of the involved toes is a guide for correct positioning and pressure of the thumb and index finger. The test is considered positive if the patient experiences pain (Figure 1.13).

Plantar percussion test: This is performed by percussing the plantar aspect of each web space. Patient describes paraesthesia or discomfort following percussion of affected web space.

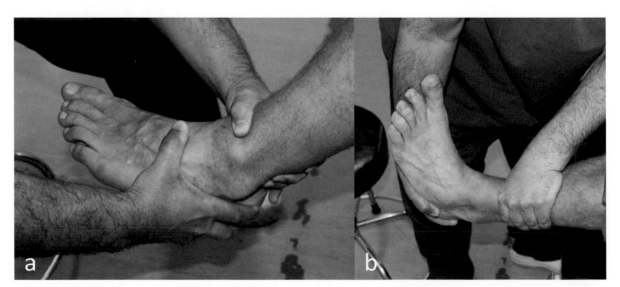

Figure 1.12 Special tests used to assess the anterior talofibular ligament (ATFL). (a) It shows the anterior draw test. (b) It shows the inversion stress test. Note the ankle's position in 20° of plantarflexion during the inversion stress test. To perform the talar tilt test and test the calcaneofibular ligament, the ankle should instead be in a plantigrade position.

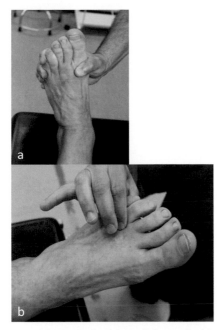

Figure 1.13 (a) It is the Mulder's click test for Morton's neuroma. In a positive test the examiner will feel a palpable (painful) click during compression of the metatarsal heads. Simultaneous palpation of the symptomatic web space may help identify this click. (b) It represents the thumb index finger squeeze test.

Grind test

Aim: To identify and characterise hallux rigidus.

The examiner uses the index fingers and thumbs to grasp the patient's 1st metatarsal neck and hallux proximal phalanx (Figure 1.14). An axial compression force

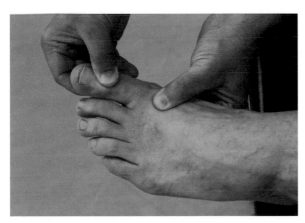

Figure 1.14 Demonstration of the Grind test used to identify first MTPJ osteoarthritis. In this example the examiner is using his right hand to apply axial compression through the 1st MTPJ whilst simultaneously plantarflexing and dorsiflexing the toe.

is then applied through the joint in a distal to proximal direction, whilst the toe is passively plantar flexed and dorsiflexed. Pain throughout this range of motion suggests severe 1st MTPJ arthritis distributed throughout the joint. Pain at the end range of dorsiflexion or a limited range of dorsiflexion suggests predominantly dorsal MTPJ involvement.

Windlass test (7)

Aim: To identify plantar fasciitis.

The foot and its ligaments were originally described by Hicks et al., 1954, as a triangular arch in the sagittal plane (8). The windlass test applies this principal to test for plantar fasciitis by using passive MTPJ dorsiflexion to stretch the plantar fascia (Figure 1.15a). A positive test is defined as reproducible heel pain upon passive toe MTPJ dorsiflexion.

Drawer test

Aim: To identify plantar plate insufficiency of a lesser toe (commonly 2nd toe).

The examiner stabilises the metatarsal head between the thumb and index finger of one hand and grasps the proximal phalanx between the thumb and index finger of the other hand. A dorsally directed force is applied to the proximal phalanx whilst the metatarsal shaft is stabilised (Figure 1.15b). Any pain or excessive translation is likely due to a plantar plate insufficiency (9).

Dorsiflexion-eversion test (10)

Aim: To identify tarsal tunnel syndrome.

The examiner dorsiflexes the ankle, everts the foot and dorsiflexes all toes for 10 seconds (Figure 1.15c). By performing this manoeuvre, the tibial nerve is compressed under the flexor retinaculum to reproduce symptoms of sensory disturbance in the tibial nerve distribution.

High ankle sprain and syndesmotic injury

Aim: To identify injury to the syndesmosis.

Squeeze test (11): The examiner compresses the fibula to the tibia above the midpoint of the calf (Figure 1.16a). The test is positive when proximal compression produces pain in the area of the distal tibiofibular and interosseous ligaments.

External rotation stress test (12): The examiner applies an external rotation stress to the involved foot and ankle in a plantigrade position whilst simultaneously stabilising the lower leg (Figure 1.16b). A positive test produces pain over the anterior or posterior tibiofibular ligament(s) and over the interosseous membrane.

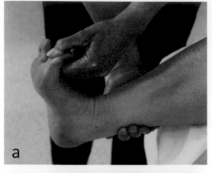

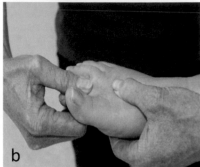

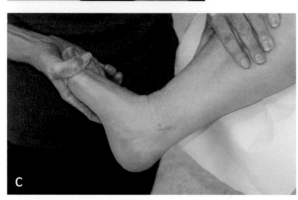

Figure 1.15 (a) Windlass test with passive dorsiflexion of the MTPJs. (b) Drawer test for plantar plate injury. (c) Dorsiflexion-eversion stress test for tarsal tunnel syndrome.

The fibula translation test (13): The examiner applies an anterior and posterior drawer force to the fibula with the tibia stabilised. Syndesmotic injury is associated with pain and increased translation of the fibula.

Ankle impingement tests

Aim: To identify lesions that may restrict or cause pain at the anterior or posterior aspects of the ankle.

Anterior ankle impingement: Ask the patient to squat noting any pain, restriction and asymmetry in dorsiflexion around the ankle joint. This is commonly due to dorsal tibiotalar soft tissue impingement (Figure 1.17a).

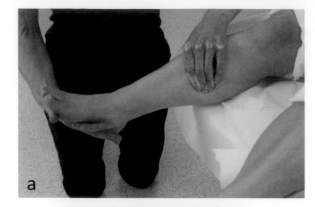

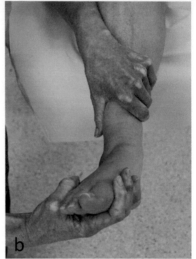

Figure 1.16 Squeeze test (a) and external rotation stress test (b) for a high ankle sprain and syndesmotic injury.

Posterior ankle impingement: Passive forced plantarflexion of the ankle results in pain and a 'grinding' sensation as the posterolateral talar process is compressed between the posterior tibia and the calcaneus (Figure 1.17b).

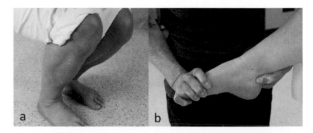

Figure 1.17 Demonstration of clinical tests used for ankle impingement. (a) It shows the squatting position used to identify anterior impingement. Note the reduced ankle dorsiflexion seen on the right side suggesting impingement. (b) It shows the clinical test for posterior ankle impingement – forced passive plantarflexion.

Table 1.1 Common conditions encountered in postgraduate exit exams. The salient special tests and key questions to address are shown for each scenario

Pathology	Deformity	Key test(s)	Key points in assessment
Tibialis posterior (TP) dysfunction	• Pes planovalgus • Forefoot abduction	• TP strength • Tip toe test (double/single stance)	• Is TP weak? • Is hindfoot deformity flexible? • Is there any ankle/hindfoot OA?
CMT, CP, Friedreich's ataxia, Spinal cord lesion, Polio	• Hindfoot varus • Pes cavus	• Coleman block test • Inspect spine for dysraphism • Inspect hands for small muscle wasting	• Is hindfoot deformity flexible (forefoot driven) or fixed?
Hallux valgus	• Lateral deviation/pronation 1st MTPJ • May be associated deformity of lesser toes or Morton's neuroma	• Plantar callosity underneath 2nd metatarsal head on inspection • Passive overcorrection of deformity • Grind test • Assess 1st TMTJ laxity	• Is there transfer lesion under 2nd metatarsal head? • Is deformity correctable? • Is the 1st MTPJ arthritic? • Is the 1st TMTJ lax and so requires fusion?
Lesser toe deformities	***Hammer toe:*** • DIPJ extension • PIPJ flexion • MTPJ normal/extended	• Assess if the deformity can be corrected	• Is the deformity flexible or fixed?
	Claw toe: • DIPJ/PIPJ flexion • MTPJ hyperextension	• Assess if the deformity can be corrected	• Is the deformity flexible or fixed? • Is MTPJs subluxed/dislocated (plantar callosity)?
	Mallet toe: • DIPJ flexion • PIPJ/MTPJ normal	• Assess if the deformity can be corrected	• Are deformities flexible, correctable or fixed?
Hallux rigidus	• Swelling of 1st MTPJ	• Range of movements • Grind test	• Is pain present throughout 1st MTPJ passive range of movement or predominantly DF?
Morton's neuroma	• Usually no findings on inspection • There might be increased gap between lesser toes (enlarged intermetatarsal bursa) • Could be secondary to hallux valgus	• Mulder's squeeze test • Thumb index finger squeeze test • Sensation at tip of toes and plantar aspect • Tenderness in MTPJ (usually 2nd)	• Which interdigital space is involved? • Rule out lesser MTPJ synovitis
Achilles tendinopathy (insertional or non-insertional)	• Swelling at AT insertion (insertional) or 5–7 cm proximal (non-insertional)	• Silfverskiöld test • Arc sign (non-insertional)	• Is tendinopathy insertional or non-insertional? • Is there any associated gastrocnemius/AT tightness?
Chronic Achilles tendon rupture	• Visible/Palpable gap • Loss of normal Achilles contour	• Simmonds-Thompson test • Single heel raise • Excessive ankle dorsiflexion	• Size of gap

Abbreviations: CMT, Charcot-Marie-Tooth; CP, Cerebral palsy.

Take home messages

- There are 7 key components to the general foot and ankle examination – inspection, gait analysis, palpation, joint range of movement, NV status, key muscle strength and special tests.
- Coleman block test must be performed and accurately interpreted for any hindfoot varus.
- The heel raise test must be performed and accurately interpreted for any case of hindfoot valgus.
- Ensure joints, ligaments and tendons are adequately isolated when tested.
- Have a clear understanding of the nerve supply to the foot and ankle.
- Special tests should be used on the basis of history, initial clinical findings and suspected pathology.

References

1. Perry J, Burnfield JM. Gait analysis: Normal and pathological function. J Sports Sci Med. 2010; 9(2):353.
2. Coleman SS, Chesnut WJ. A simple test for hindfoot flexibility in the cavovarus foot. Clin Orthop Relat Res. 1977; 123:60–2.
3. Thompson TC, Doherty JH. Spontaneous rupture of tendon of Achilles: A new clinical diagnostic test. J Trauma. 1962; 2:126–9.
4. Silfverskiöld N. Reduction of the uncrossed two-joints muscles of the leg to one-joint muscles in spastic conditions. Acta Chirurgica Scandinavica. 1924; 56:315–30.
5. Mulder JD. The causative mechanism in Morton's metatarsalgia. J Bone Joint Surg Br. 1951; 33-B(1):94–5.
6. Mahadevan D, Venkatesan M, Bhatt R, Bhatia M. Diagnostic accuracy of clinical tests for Morton's neuroma compared with ultrasonography. J Foot Ankle Surg. 2015; 54(4): 549–53.
7. Brown C. A review of subcalcaneal heel pain and plantar fasciitis. Aust Fam Phys. 1996; 25:875–85.
8. Hicks JH. The mechanics of the foot, II: The plantar aponeurosis and the arch. J Anat. 1954; 88(1):25–30.
9. Thompson FM, Hamilton WG. Problems of the second metatarsophalangeal joint. Orthopedics. 1987; 10(1):83–9.
10. Kinoshita M, Okuda R, Morikawa J, Jotoku T, Abe M. The dorsiflexion-eversion test for diagnosis of tarsal tunnel syndrome. J Bone Joint Surg Am. 2001; 83(12):1835–9.
11. Hopkinson WJ, St Pierre P, Ryan JB, Wheeler JH. Syndesmosis sprains of the ankle. Foot Ankle. 1990; 10(6):325–30.
12. Boytim MJ, Fischer DA, Neumann L. Syndesmotic ankle sprains. Am J Sports Med. 1991; 19(3):294–8.
13. Ogilvie-Harris DJ, Reed SC. Disruption of the ankle syndesmosis: Diagnosis and treatment by arthroscopic surgery. Arthroscopy. 1994; 10(5):561–8.

Applied anatomy and surgical approaches

Rajeev Vohra, Babaji Sitaram Thorat, and Avtar Singh

Introduction

An appropriate selection and execution of a surgical approach is essential for the success of any surgical procedure done for foot and ankle injuries and ailments. A number of anatomical structures are at risk while performing these approaches, and their anatomy needs to be understood to avoid injury to these structures. The anatomical course of the relevant nerves, blood vessels and muscle tendon units are discussed in the first part of the chapter on applied anatomy, followed by discussion of surgical approaches used commonly in foot and ankle trauma and elective surgery.

Applied anatomy

Nerves

Superficial peroneal nerve (SPN)

It is the terminal branch of the common peroneal nerve (CPN) and pierces the deep fascia over the anterior compartment at different levels (Figure 2.1). It divides into medial and intermediate dorsal cutaneous nerves of the dorsum of the foot at different levels, and these branches supply dorsal areas of the foot and toes except for the web space between the great and second toe and the lateral side of the little toe (1). SPN and its branches must be isolated, protected and avoided during *anterior* (2), *anterolateral* (3), *lateral and transfibular approaches to the ankle* (3, 4), *anterolateral approach to the talus* (5) *and dorsal approach to the tarsometatarsal (TMT) joints* (6). Its terminal dorsal digital branches need to be protected while performing *Morton's neuroma (MN) excision* (7) *and medial part of the distal soft issue release (DSTR) for hallux valgus (HV) correction* (8).

Sural nerve (SN)

It is formed by the union of the medial sural nerve and a communicating branch from the lateral sural nerve or CPN. In the lower third of the leg it courses between the posterior border of the fibula and the lateral border of the Achilles tendon (AT), accompanied by the lesser saphenous vein draining lateral surface of leg (Figure 2.2). Both structures need to be isolated or protected while performing the *posterolateral approach to the posterior malleolus (PM) and fibula* (9), and when making the vertical component of the L-shaped incision in the *extensile approach for calcaneus fractures* (10). It turns around the posterior border of the lateral malleolus (LM) towards the tuberosity of the fifth metatarsal (MT) to divide into terminal medial and lateral branches. In some cases, there is an anastomotic branch going medially towards the sinus tarsi, either arborising in the sinus tarsi region or joining the lateral branch of SPN.

Deep peroneal nerve (DPN)

It is one of the terminal branches of the CPN which lies deep to extensor digitorum longus (EDL) in the anterior compartment of the leg and accompanies the anterior tibial artery (ATA) distally, and injury to it should be avoided during the *anterior approach to the ankle and dorsal approaches to the medial TMT joints* (2, 6) (Figure 2.17a). It divides into a lateral branch, and a medial branch which is a continuation of the DPN and lies lateral to the dorsalis pedis artery (DPA) to divide into two dorsal digital nerves which supply the adjacent sides of the great and second toes, which need to be protected during the *DSTR* (8) (Figure 2.1).

Tibial nerve (TN)

In lower third of the leg TN it is located in the posterior compartment between flexor digitorum longus (FDL) and flexor hallucis longus (FHL) (Figure 2.3). In this region it can be easily confused with the FHL tendon during *posteromedial and posterolateral approaches to the ankle* (9). The nerve courses behind the medial malleolus (MM) and divides into its terminal branches, the medial and lateral plantar nerves before entering the tarsal tunnel. In the tarsal tunnel, it lies between FHL and FDL along with the posterior tibial artery (PTA), and both structures should be protected during *tarsal tunnel release*. The lateral plantar nerve supplies all but 4 intrinsic muscles of

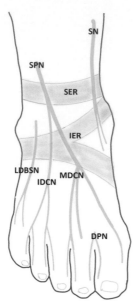

Figure 2.1 Nerve supply of the foot. (Abbreviations: **DPN** – Deep peroneal nerve, **IDCN** – Intermediate dorsal cutaneous nerve, **IER** – Inferior extensor retinaculum, **LCBSN** – Lateral cutaneous branch of sural nerve, **MDCN** – Medial dorsal cutaneous nerve, **SER** – Superior extensor retinaculum, **SN** – Saphenous nerve, **SPN** – Superficial peroneal nerve.)

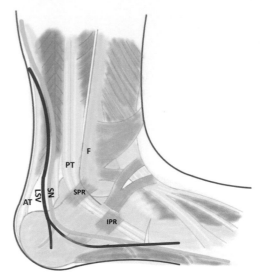

Figure 2.2 Important lateral structures of the foot and ankle. (Abbreviations: **AT** – Achilles tendon, **F** – Fibula, **IPR** – Inferior peroneal retinaculum, **LSV** – Lesser saphenous vein, **PT** – Peroneal tendons, **SN** – Sural nerve, **SPR** – Superior peroneal retinaculum.)

the foot and the medial plantar nerve is the main sensory nerve of the plantar aspect of the foot.

Saphenous nerve

The saphenous nerve descends in the leg along with the great saphenous vein. Its anterior branch is in front of the MM and close to the posterior aspect of the great saphenous vein, and both need to be protected if undertaking an anteromedial approach to the distal tibia (Figure 2.3).

Arteries of the foot

Anterior tibial artery (ATA) lies between extensor hallucis longus (EHL) and tibialis anterior (TA) in front of the interosseous membrane and becomes the DPA as it crosses the foot. The DPA extends to the proximal end of the first MT space, where it slopes downwards between the two heads of the first dorsal interosseous muscle to enter the sole of the foot where it anastomoses with the lateral plantar artery (Figure 2.4). It is accompanied by the DPN, and the neurovascular bundle should be protected during *anterior and anterolateral approaches to the ankle and the dorsal approach to the medial two TMT joints* (3, 6).

Posterior tibial artery (PTA)

The PTA enters the foot through the tarsal tunnel where it lies between the tendons of FHL posteriorly and FDL anteriorly, under the flexor retinaculum (Figure 2.3). At

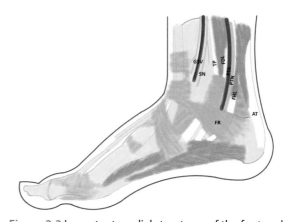

Figure 2.3 Important medial structures of the foot and ankle. (Abbreviations: **AT** – Achilles tendon, **FDL** – Flexor digitorum longus, **FHL** – Flexor hallucis longus, **FR** – Flexor retinaculum, **GSV** – Greater saphenous vein, **PTA** – Posterior tibial artery, **SN** – Saphenous nerve, **TN** – Tibial nerve, **TP** – Tibialis posterior.)

this location it should be protected when performing a *posteromedial approach to the ankle and tarsal tunnel release* (9). It splits into medial and lateral plantar arteries.

The lateral plantar artery passes deep to abductor hallucis and flexor digitorum brevis towards the base of fifth MT and then curves medially to create the deep plantar arch. At the proximal end of the first intermetatarsal space it anastomoses with the deep plantar artery which is a branch of the DPA (Figure 2.5). Four MT arteries arise from the convexity of the arch, which divides

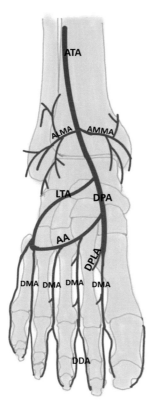

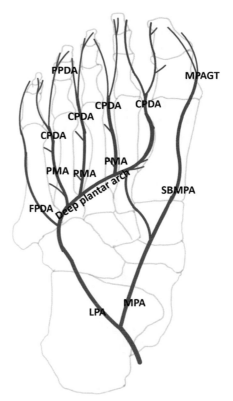

Figure 2.4 Arterial supply on the dorsal aspect of the foot. (Abbreviations: **AA** – Arcuate artery, **ALMA** – Anterior lateral malleolar artery, **AMMA** – Anterior medial malleolar artery, **ATA** – Anterior tibial artery, **DDA** – Dorsal digital artery, **DMA** – Dorsal metatarsal artery, **DPA** – Dorsalis pedis artery, **DPLA** – Deep plantar artery.)

Figure 2.5 Arterial supply on the plantar aspect of the foot. (Abbreviations: **CPDA** – Common plantar digital artery, **FFPDA** – Fifth plantar digital artery, **LPA** – Lateral plantar artery, **MPA** – Medial plantar artery, **MPAGT** Medial plantar artery of great toe, **PMA** – Plantar metatarsal artery, **PPDA** – Proper plantar digital artery, **SBMPA** – Superficial branch of medial plantar artery.)

further into a pair of plantar digital arteries supplying the foot webs and adjacent toes. The medial plantar artery runs deep to abductor hallucis and then between it and flexor digitorum brevis to reach the medial border of the hallux. It supplies muscles of the hallux and skin on the medial aspect of the sole (Figure 2.5).

Peroneal artery (PA)

The PA courses along the medial side of the fibula and bifurcates distally into the anterior perforating and lateral calcaneal branch. The PA may bifurcate and perforate through the interosseous membrane as little as 41 mm from the tibial plafond (11). Due to wide variation in vascular anatomy in this region, a careful dissection is suggested while performing *anterolateral, posterolateral and transfibular approaches to the ankle* (3, 4, 9).

The lateral calcaneal branch of the PA is the source vessel to the angiosome of the lateral heel flap raised during a *lateral extensile approach to the calcaneum* (Figure 2.15a). In calcaneal fractures, the lateral calcaneal branch of the PA may be directly injured or

secondarily thrombosed due to massive oedema. Some studies have suggested evaluation of the patency of this branch by ultrasound Doppler before selecting a lateral extensile approach to the calcaneum (12).

Muscles and tendons around the foot

Lateral compartment muscles

Peroneus longus (PL) and Peroneus brevis (PB) are muscles of the lateral compartment. Injury to their tendons should be avoided *during the posterolateral and lateral approaches to the ankle* (3, 9), where they course in the retromalleolar groove posterior to the LM and deep to the superior peroneal retinaculum (Figure 2.2). If the superior peroneal retinaculum has to be incised, it should be repaired meticulously to avoid postoperative subluxation of the tendons. The tendons swing forward to descend obliquely, lateral to the calcaneum to lie in their respective sheaths near the peroneal tubercle. The tendons should be identified and protected during a *lateral extensile approach to the calcaneum and/or sinus tarsi* (10, 13) (Figures 2.15c and 2.16d), and the sheaths should be preferably left intact. The PB insertion on the tuberosity of the fifth MT, and the PL swinging medially under the cuboid groove should also be protected during deep dissection in the distal part of the *lateral extensile approach to the calcaneum* (10, 13).

Anterior compartment muscles

Four anterior compartment muscles – TA, EHL, EDL and peroneus tertius (PT) cross the anterior aspect of the ankle coursing towards the dorsum of the foot deep to the superior and inferior extensor retinacula at the ankle and dorsum of foot, respectively (Figure 2.17a). These retinacula prevent bowstringing of the anterior tendons and should be repaired after any approach that involves incision of the retinacula. TA is an important land mark for both the *anterior approach to the ankle and the anteromedial approach to the distal tibia and ankle* (2, 3). Opening of the sheath of TA should be avoided in both approaches. The relationship between the anterior neurovascular bundle and the dorsal tendons needs to be appreciated so as to avoid injury to the neurovascular bundle during an *anterior approach to the ankle* (2). The neurovascular bundle lies between TA and EHL proximally and crosses under EHL from lateral to medial at the ankle joint to lie between EHL and EDL distal to the joint (Figure 2.17a).

Posterior compartment muscles

Tibialis posterior (TP), FDL and FHL descend in the posterior compartment and their tendons course behind the MM under the flexor retinaculum (Figure 2.3). In the lower third of the leg the neurovascular bundle lying between FHL and FDL should be protected during a *posteromedial approach to the PM and if performing a medial malleolar osteotomy for talar body fractures* (5, 9). Behind the MM, TP is closest to the MM with FDL behind it and FHL the most posterior (Figure 2.3). The tendoachilles (AT) is the strongest muscle of the posterior compartment and an important land mark for *posterolateral and posteromedial approaches to posterior malleolar fractures* (9).

Muscles of the dorsum of the foot

Two sets of muscles comprising of EHL and extensor hallucis brevis (EHB), and EDL and extensor digitorum brevis (EDB) are present on the dorsum of the foot (Figure 2.17a,e). The interval between EHL and EHB is used during the *dorsal approach to the medial two TMT joints*. EHB serves as an important landmark as the neurovascular bundle lies beneath it. *In the anterolateral approach to the talus and the dorsal approach to the lateral three TMT joints*, EDL is retracted medially (5, 6). EDB, which originates from a roughened area on the superolateral surface of the calcaneum, lateral

to the sinus tarsi, is reflected as a flap for exposure of the anterior calcaneal process and the calcaneocuboid joint (CCJ) during the *sinus tarsi approach* (13).

Muscles of the sole of the foot

The muscles of the sole of the foot are divided into four layers. From medial to lateral, abductor hallucis, flexor digitorum brevis and abductor digiti minimi form the first layer. The second muscle layer consists of tendons of FDL, quadratus plantae and four lumbrical muscles. Lumbricals originate from the tendons of FDL and pass dorsally to insert into the free medial margins of the extensor hoods of the four lateral toes, and may be mistaken for nerves during *Morton's neuroma excision*. The third layer is formed by flexor hallucis brevis and adductor hallucis and the flexor digiti minimi brevis. Dorsal and plantar interossei comprise the fourth and the deepest layer of the sole.

Surgical approaches

Anterior approach to the ankle (2)

Indications

The anterior approach to the ankle is commonly used for arthrodesis and arthroplasty of the ankle and for fixation of Pilon fractures.

Technique

The malleoli and the TA tendon are palpated and marked. A 10–15 cm incision, depending on the requirement, is centred over the ankle joint, just lateral to the TA tendon (Figure 2.6a,b).

The incision is deepened through the skin and subcutaneous tissues and undermining of the skin is kept to minimum. The cutaneous branch of SPN, which is quite superficial, is preferably traced in the distal part of the incision and freed up sufficiently, and may be highlighted with a marker to avoid damage during further dissection (Figure 2.6c).

The extensor retinaculum is incised longitudinally over EHL, which is identified in the distal part of the incision by palpation, and by moving the great toe into plantarflexion and dorsiflexion (Figure 2.6c). The sheath of EHL is then opened, avoiding violation of the TA sheath (Figure 2.6d). The anterior neurovascular bundle is found distally next to EHL, traced proximally and gently teased off of the TA muscle belly by blunt dissection (Figure 2.6e).

The neurovascular bundle and EHL tendon are retracted laterally and the TA tendon in its sheath is retracted medially (Figure 2.6f,g). The soft tissue and capsule anterior to the ankle joint is incised longitudinally. The joint is exposed by detaching the anterior ankle capsule from the tibia or the talus by sharp dissection. Some periosteal stripping of the distal tibia is often

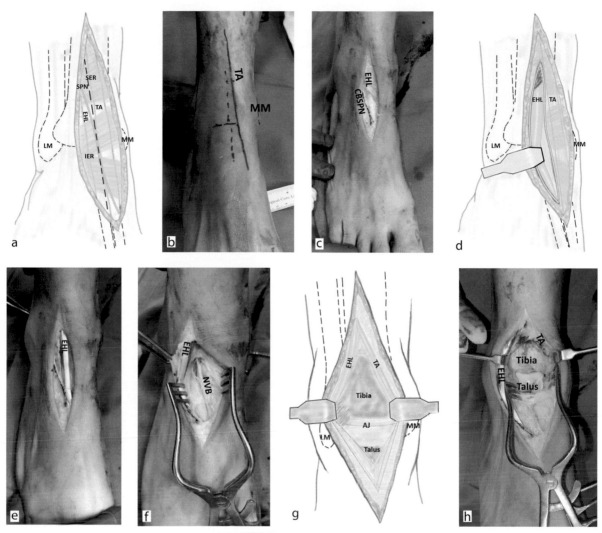

Figure 2.6 (a–h) Anterior approach to the ankle. (Abbreviations: **AJ** – Ankle joint, **CBPN** – Cutaneous branch of superficial peroneal nerve, **EHL** – Extensor hallucis longus, **IER** – Inferior extensor retinaculum, **LM** – Lateral malleolus, **MM** – Medial malleolus, **NVB** – Neuro Vascular Bundle, **SER** – Superior extensor retinaculum, **SPN** – Superficial peroneal nerve, **TA** – Tibialis anterior.)

required (Figure 2.6g,h). To expose the posterior part of the ankle joint and malleoli, the joint may be distracted with a laminar spreader or Hintermann retractor.

Anterolateral approach to the ankle (3)

Indications

The anterolateral approach provides excellent visualisation of distal tibia up to the medial shoulder and distal fibula, and is useful for fixation of intra-articular fractures of the distal tibia or osteochondral fracture of talus.

Technique

The patient is placed in the supine position. The ipsilateral hip is elevated with a sandbag so as to position the leg in a neutral position. The MM, LM, fibula, anterior tibial crest and base of fourth MT are palpated and marked.

The incision begins at least 5 cm proximal to the ankle joint, between the anterior border of the fibula and the anterior tibial crest, and extends distally to the base of the fourth MT (Figure 2.7a,b). Isolate and protect SPN which mostly crosses proximal to the ankle (Figure 2.7c), and then identify and incise the extensor retinaculum (Figure 2.7d,e).

Using blunt dissection, a plane between the interosseous membrane and the overlying contents of the anterior compartment is developed. The muscles and tendons of the anterior compartment, DPA, and DPN are mobilised from the underlying anterior tibiofibular

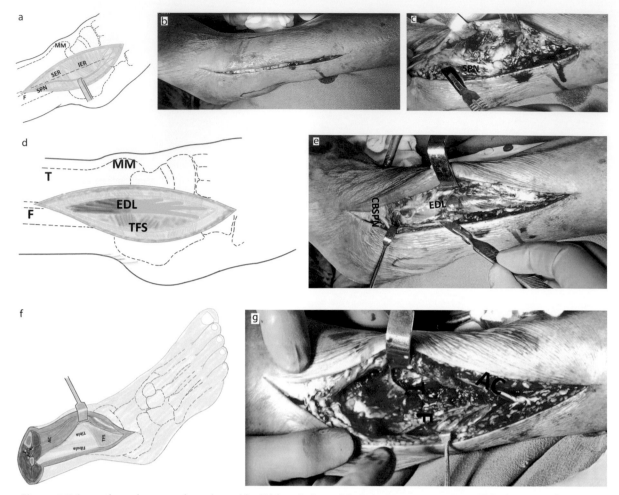

Figure 2.7 Anterolateral approach to the ankle. (Abbreviations: **AC**- Anterior compartment, **ELD**- Extensor digitorum longus, **IER**- Inferior extensor retinaculum, **CBSPN**- Cutaneous branch of Superficial Peroneal Nerve, **F**- Fibula, **SER**- Superior extensor retinaculum, **SPN**- Superficial peroneal nerve, **T**- Tibia, **TFS**- Tibiofibular syndesmosis.)

ligament, periosteum of the distal tibia and joint capsule, so as to expose the anterolateral aspect of the distal tibia and plafond (Figure 2.7f,g). If an arthrotomy is required, it is performed at or close to the fracture line to prevent devascularisation of the distal tibia.

Lateral approach to fibula (3)

Indications

Fractures of the LM and distal half of fibula.

Technique

The patient is placed in a supine position with a sandbag under the buttock of the affected limb – a manoeuvre which internally rotates the lower extremity and which results in better access to the fibula and LM. Tilting the table away can also help to internally rotate the

leg. Placing a bolster (or rolled gown) behind the ankle helps ensure that the heel is not directly on the operating table, thereby avoiding the talus being 'pushed forward' in the ankle mortise.

Palpate the subcutaneous surface of the fibula and LM. Make a 10–15 cm incision along the posterior margin of the fibula and not directly over the fibula. Avoid injury to the short saphenous vein and sural nerve posteriorly, and SPN proximally, where it may be exiting the lateral compartment.

The periosteum over the subcutaneous surface of the fibula is incised and gently elevated where required. Avoid extensive elevation of the periosteum to avoid damage to the vascularity of the bone (Figure 2.8a,b). If a more proximal exposure of the fibula is required, an interval between PT and PB is used and the peronei are retracted posteriorly.

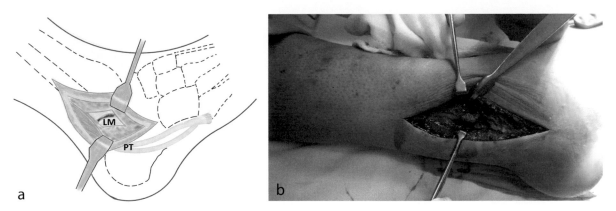

Figure 2.8 Lateral approach to fibula. (a) **LM** – Lateral malleolus, **PT** – Peroneal tendon.

Anteromedial approach to the distal tibia and ankle (3)

Indications

This approach provides access to the middle and medial aspects of the tibiotalar joint, and medial side of tibia. Only the lower part of the approach can be used to clear the medial gutter in anteromedial ankle impingement, reduce some medial malleolar fractures with joint impaction, and to perform minimally invasive ankle arthrodesis (Figure 2.9e).

Technique

The patient is in a supine position, and the anterior crest of the tibia and MM are palpated and marked. The incision begins about 1 cm lateral to the tibial crest and follows the course of TA to the ankle, and is then curved distally and medially to end just distal to the tip of the MM (Figure 2.9a,b). Protect the great saphenous nerve and saphenous vein in the subcutaneous plane in the distal part of the incision.

TA is identified after making the incision. Then, a full thickness incision is made, directly down to bone, medial to the TA tendon but without breaching its paratenon. The anteromedial skin and subcutaneous tissue and periosteum are elevated en-bloc, as a full thickness flap. Anterior compartment muscles can be retracted laterally for limited access to the lateral distal tibia (Figure 2.9c,d). For intra-articular exposure, the capsule is incised in line with the fracture or just medial to the MM (Figure 2.9e).

Posterolateral approach to the ankle (9)

Indications

This approach is used for fixation of the PM and posterior plating of fibula.

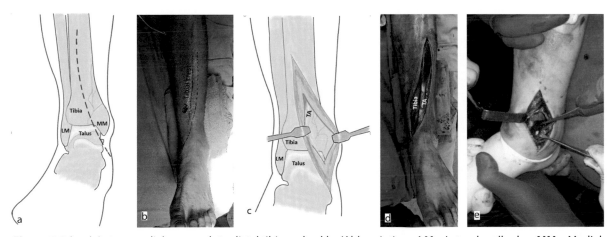

Figure 2.9 (a–e) Anteromedial approach to distal tibia and ankle. (Abbreviations: **LM** – Lateral malleolus, **MM** – Medial malleolus, **TA** – Tibialis anterior.)

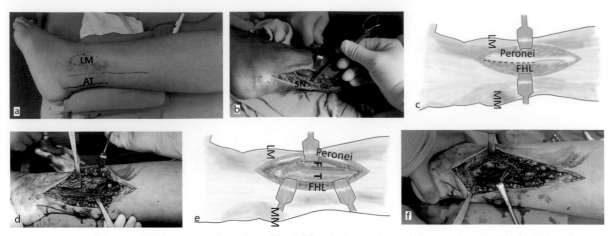

Figure 2.10 (a–f) Posterolateral approach to the ankle. (Abbreviations: **AT** – Achilles tendon, **F** – Fibula, **FHL** – Flexor hallucis longus, **LM** – Lateral malleolus, **MM** – Medial malleolus, **SN** – Sural nerve, **T** – Tibia.)

Technique

The posterolateral approach can be performed with patient in either the lateral or prone or recovery (sloppy lateral) position (14). The posterior border of the fibula and AT are palpated and marked.

Only a skin deep incision is made midway between posterior border of fibula and lateral border of AT and runs distally to end below the LM (Figure 2.10a). Avoid injury to the SN and lesser saphenous vein (Figure 2.10b). The fascia over the peroneal tendons is incised and the peronei are then retracted laterally (Figure 2.10c). Then plane is developed medial to the peroneal tendons and lateral to the FHL. FHL is elevated off the back of the fibula, interosseous membrane, and posterior tibia (Figure 2.10d,e,f).

Retraction of the FHL should be performed carefully to avoid injury to the TN and PTA lying medial to FHL. The posterior tibia and PM are now visible. The periosteum and posterior inferior tibiofibular ligament (PITFL) are almost always attached to the PM fractured fragment. The periosteum should be incised only at the proximal level to expose and reduce the fracture.

Posteromedial approach to the ankle (9)

Indications

This approach is used for PM fractures extending far medially and sometimes involving the posterior MM in trauma. In elective surgery this approach is used for TP reconstruction.

Technique

The patient can be placed supine (with sandbag under the contralateral buttock to externally rotate the limb) or prone. The AT and posteromedial border of tibia and MM are palpated and marked. An incision

is made between AT posteriorly and posteromedial border of the tibia anteriorly, and the proximal extension is along the course of the posterior tibial tendon, just behind the posteromedial border of the tibia (Figure 2.11a,b).

The incision is deepened through subcutaneous fat to expose the flexor retinaculum which is carefully incised to expose TP, FDL, the posterior tibial neurovascular bundle and FHL (Figure 2.11c). In order to access the posteromedial fragment, incise the deep fascia proximally, to protect the neurovascular bundle.

The interval used for deep dissection depends upon the location of the major fracture fragments. It may be developed between posterior border of tibia and TP, or between TP and FDL, or both TP and FDL can be retracted anteriorly (Figure 2.11d,e,f) which may require direct exposure of the neurovascular bundle. The posterior tibial tendon lies on top of a layer of fibrocartilage, which may be sharply incised to expose the posteromedial fragment. The posterior ankle capsule is opened sharply and the fracture is exposed. Minimal traction should be applied while retracting the tibial neurovascular bundle. Relaxing the retractor intermittently helps to prevent neurovascular injury.

Transfibular approach to the ankle (4)

Indications

This approach is used for ankle fusion and tibio-talo-calcaneal (TTC) fusion.

Technique

An incision is made along the posterior border of the fibula, extending to the tip of the fibula and then angled anteriorly towards the base of the fourth MT (Figure 2.12a). Protect branch of SPN if visible. Dissect

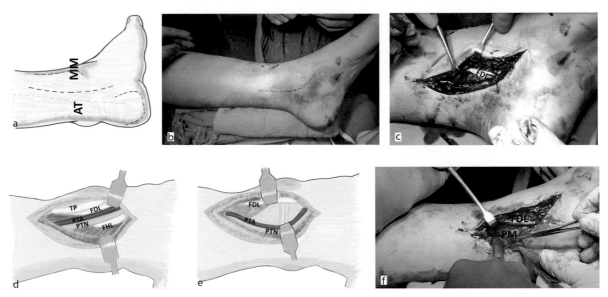

Figure 2.11 (a–f) Posteromedial approach to the ankle. (Abbreviations: **AT** – Achilles tendon, **FDL** – Flexor digitorum longus, **FHL** – Flexor hallucis longus, **MM** – Medial malleolus, **PM** – Posterior malleolus, **PTA** – Posterior tibial artery, **PTN** – Posterior tibial nerve, **TP** – Tibialis posterior.)

sharply to bone and divide AITFL, CFL, ATFL, and intraosseous ligaments inserted on LM (Figure 2.12b). An oblique osteotomy of the fibula is made under fluoroscopic guidance 2 cm above the ankle joint using an oscillating saw or osteotome (Figure 2.12c). Elevate the

EDB muscle from the calcaneum if exposure of the subtalar joint is needed (Figure 2.12g).

The osteotomised fibula is rotated posteriorly and then removed after stripping its soft issue attachments, to be later used as a graft (Figure 2.12d). This exposes

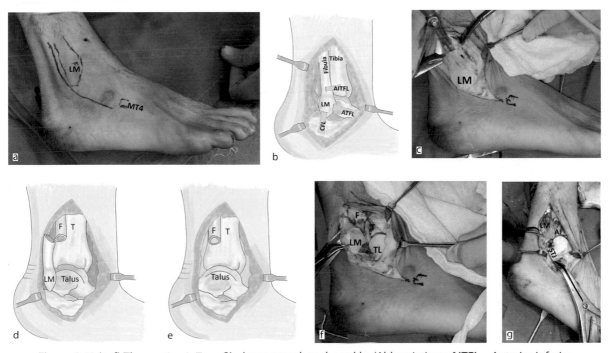

Figure 2.12 (a–f) The caption is Transfibular approach to the ankle. (Abbreviations: **AITFL** – Anterior inferior tibiofibular ligament, **AJ** – Ankle joint, **ATFL** – Anterior talofibular ligament, **CFL** – Calcaneofibular ligament, **F** – Fibula, **LM** – Lateral malleolus, **ST** – Subtalar joint, **T** –Tibia, **TL** – Talus.)

both tibiotalar and subtalar joints. To optimise visualisation of these joints, a Hintermann distractor or laminar spreader may be used. Another option is not to excise but instead, to rotate the distal fibula posteriorly on its preserved posterior inferior soft tissues, and to then remove its medial third with a saw, which exposes the cancellous bone of the fibula (Figure 2.12e,f). The rotated fragment is slightly shortened proximally and used as a vascularised onlay bone graft to the arthrodesis construct. The excised medial third fibula is used as bone graft.

Approaches to the talus

Indications

Anteromedial and anterolateral approaches are commonly used for talar head and neck fractures and talonavicular joint fusion.

Anteromedial approach (5)

Technique

The MM, TA and tuberosity of the naviculum are palpated and marked. The incision is midway between the TA and TP tendons starting distal to the talonavicular joint and extends proximally about 1–2 cm proximal to the MM (Figure 2.13a). The saphenous vein and nerve are protected in the proximal part and TA is identified within its sheath and protected. The capsule is incised directly over the neck and capsular tissue flaps are raised from the anteromedial aspect of the tibia to the talonavicular joint to facilitate exposure of the talar neck (Figure 2.13b,c). Dissection of the inferior aspect of the talar neck is avoided to protect the remaining blood supply.

Most talar body fractures require a medial malleolar osteotomy for adequate exposure and fixation,

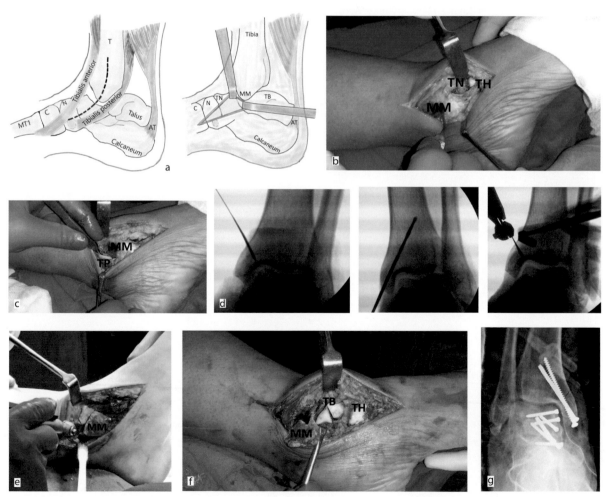

Figure 2.13 (a–g) Anteromedial approach to the talus. (Abbreviations: **AT** – Achilles tendon, **C** – Calcaneus, **MM** – Medial malleolus, **T** – Tibia, **TB** – Talar body, **TH** – Talar head, **TN** – Talar neck, **TP** – Tibialis posterior.)

which is done by extending the anteromedial approach proximally to expose the MM. The PT tendon is exposed and protected with a retractor during the osteotomy (Figure 2.13d). An oblique osteotomy running to the medial angle of the ankle joint is planned under fluoroscopy (Figure 2.13e). The holes for refixation of the MM with two screws are predrilled perpendicular to the proposed osteotomy (Figure 2.13f). The osteotomy is guided by fluoroscopy and the exposed medial aspect of the ankle joint (Figure 2.13g,h). The MM is reflected distally taking care not to violate the deltoid ligament (Figure 2.13i). After fixation of the fractures the medial malleolar osteotomy is fixed with couple of screws (Figure 2.13j).

Anterolateral approach (6)

The anterolateral approach starts from the anterior ankle syndesmosis and proceeds distally towards the base of the fourth MT. Protect the lateral branch of the intermediate dorsal cutaneous nerve during the superficial dissection. Further dissection is between EDL and PT. The capsule over the lateral neck is sharply incised to expose the fracture. Exposure of the lateral aspect of the talus and the subtalar joint requires extra caution to avoid injury to the blood vessels of the sinus tarsi (Figure 2.14).

Lateral extensile approach (10, 13)

Indications

The lateral extensile approach is used for open reduction and internal fixation of displaced intra-articular fractures of the calcaneum, and distraction arthrodesis or arthrodesis with realignment osteotomy for malunited calcaneal fractures. This approach provides access to the lateral wall, tuberosity, posterior and middle facets, and the calcaneocuboid joint (CCJ).

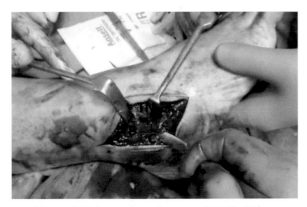

Figure 2.14 Anterolateral approach to the Talus.
(Abbreviations: **C** – Calcaneus, **TB** – Talar body
TN – Talar neck.)

Technique

It is essential to wait until soft tissue swelling and blisters resolve, which is demonstrated by the return of skin wrinkling. The patient is placed in a lateral position with a sandbag beneath the involved hindfoot that provides a stable platform for imaging and better leverage and access to the heel.

The landmarks for the incision are the posterior border of the distal fibula, lateral border of AT and base of the fifth MT (Figure 2.15a).

The incision begins laterally, 3–4 cm superior to the calcaneal tuberosity and just 1 cm anterior to the AT. The incision is continued downwards towards the junction of the dorsal and plantar skin, where a smooth curve is made, curving the incision anteriorly towards the CCJ and the fifth MT base (Figure 2.15a). It is important to note that the incision should form an open angle of approximately 100–110 degrees so as to avoid damaging the PA which results in skin flap necrosis. At the distal end, the incision may be curved upwards if CCJ exposure is required.

Over the central third of the incision (apex) incision should be taken "straight to bone" and care is taken not to undermine the skin (Figure 2.15a, green part). A subperiosteal, full-thickness flap is raised by sharp dissection using a blade (Figure 2.15b). The surgeon should refrain from using retractors at this stage, and "no-touch technique" retraction is often used to minimise trauma to the tissue flap. At the distal and proximal one-third of the incision, the incision is made through skin and only gentle dissection is utilised. If the SN is not encountered in the proximal and distal parts of the incision, then a full thickness incision is completed through the subcutaneous fat and deep fascia. Distally find the fascia over the abductor digiti minimi and go above it without cutting the muscle belly of abductor digiti minimi.

The peroneal tendons are identified and dissected off the peroneal tubercle avoiding their laceration (Figure 2.15c). The tendons are freed from the anterior calcaneum, using a periosteal elevator and retracted anterosuperiorly within the sheath. The calcaneofibular ligament is then identified and peeled off the calcaneum. Then anterior end of calcaneum is exposed by working anteriorly over the calcaneum and releasing the bifurcate ligament.

Once the entire lateral side of the calcaneum is exposed, one k wire is driven into the talar neck at the level of crucial angle and one in the cuboid to retract the flap. Another wire may be placed in the fibula so as to retract the peroneal tendons out of the field, and one more wire may be inserted into the talar body to visualise the posterior corner of the posterior facet (Figure 2.15d). This approach provides access to the lateral wall, tuberosity, posterior and middle facets, and CCJ.

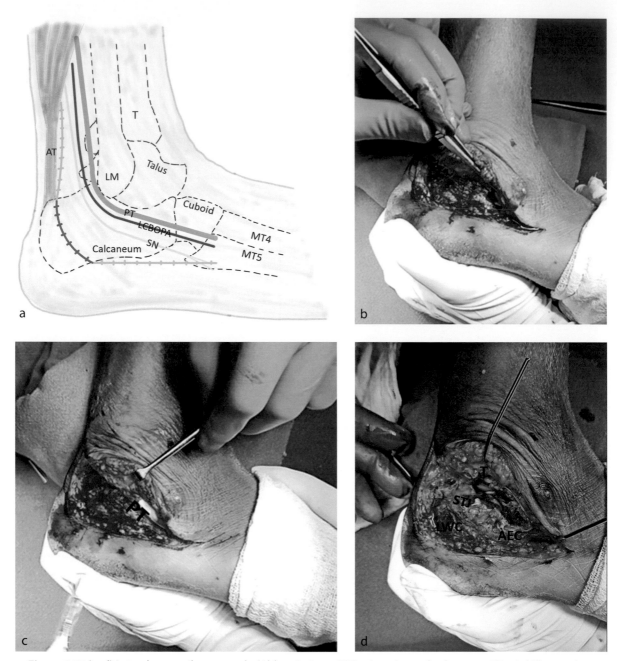

Figure 2.15 (a–d) Lateral expansile approach. (Abbreviations: **AEC** – Anterior end calcaneus, **AT** – Achilles tendon, **LCBOPA** – Lateral calcaneal branch of peroneal artery, **LM** – Lateral malleolus, **LWC** – Lateral wall calcaneus, **MT** – Metatarsal, **PT** – Peroneal tendon, **SN** – Sural nerve, **STJ** – Subtalar joint, **T** – Tibia.)

Sinus tarsi approach and lateral approach to subtalar and calcaneocuboid joints (10, 13)

Indications

The sinus tarsi approach is used for minimally invasive fixation of calcaneal fractures and subtalar arthrodesis.

It may be extended distally for arthrodesis of the subtalar and CC joints.

Technique

The patient is placed in the lateral decubitus position and a small sandbag is placed under the foot. Mark tip of the fibula, base of fourth MT and make a 3-cm incision from just below the tip of the fibula, through the sinus

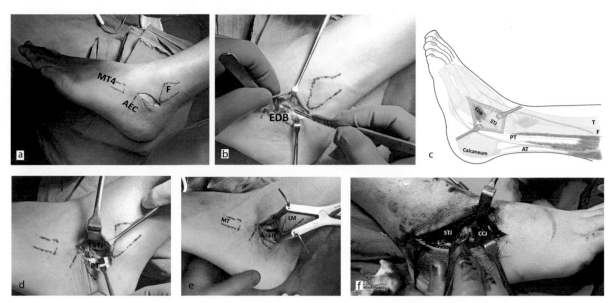

Figure 2.16 (a–e) Sinus tarsi approach. (f) Lateral approach to subtalar and calcaneocuboid joints. (Abbreviations: **AEC** – Anterior end calcaneus, **AT** – Achilles tendon, **CCJ** – Calcaneocuboid joint, **EDB** – Extensor digitorum brevis, **LM** – Lateral malleolus, **MT** – Metatarsal, **PT** – Peroneal tendons, **STJ** – Subtalar joint.)

tarsi towards the fourth MT base (Figure 2.16a). It can be extended to the cuboid when exposure of the anterior end of the calcaneum and CCJ is required for fixation of fractures involving the anterior calcaneal tuberosity or, for arthrodesis of both subtalar and CC joints (Figure 2.16f). Avoid injury to the lateral sural cutaneous nerve, PL and brevis tendons in the distal part of the incision. If the landmarks are obscured by swelling, the incision is marked under image intensifier by placing a wire over the proposed incision.

Use blunt dissection to avoid injury to the SN and branches of the SPN if anatomic variations are present. Typically, these nerves are not encountered during the exposure. Then, the peroneal tendons are identified in the inferior and posterior parts of the dissection (Figure 2.16b), but may be displaced superiorly due to widening of the calcaneum caused by the fracture. The retinaculum covering the peroneal tendons is incised and the tendons are retracted downwards and maintained within their sheath. At the anterior margin of the incision, the belly of the EDB muscle is subperiosteally elevated to allow for exposure of the anterior end of the calcaneum and CCJ (Figure 2.16d,e). Then, a gentle subperiosteal dissection of the lateral wall is completed.

Then, the sandbag is moved slightly proximally towards the ankle, which allows the foot to fall into inversion, and opens the subtalar joint. After completion of dissection, this approach allows easy visualisation of the anterior, middle, and posterior facets of the subtalar joint, anterior calcaneal tuberosity, CCJ and some parts of lateral wall of the calcaneum (Figure 2.16f).

Approaches to the tarsometatarsal (TMT) joints (6)

Indications

Open reduction and internal fixation of Lisfranc dislocations and fracture dislocations, and arthrodesis of TMT joints.

Technique

In acute injuries it is essential to be sure that the soft tissue envelope has recovered from the initial trauma and that the swelling has subsided. Two incisions with a skin bridge at least 4 cm are required to expose all TMT joints. The patient is positioned supine.

The dorsomedial incision is centred between the first and second rays (Figure 2.17a, marked green, Figure 2.17b). This incision should be long enough to allow exposure of the intercuneiform joint proximally, and at least 2–3 cm distal to the first and second TMT joints. Care is taken to identify and protect sensory branches of the SPN as they cross EHL in the proximal part of the incision. EHL and EHB and the neurovascular bundle comprising the DPA and vein and DPN are identified (Figure 2.17c). The neurovascular bundle is mobilised laterally and protected. The dissection is carried out sharply down to the bone in the interval between EHB and EHL. Subperiosteal flaps are developed both medially and laterally to expose the first and second TMT joints (Figure 2.17d).

The dorsolateral incision is centred over the fourth MT and can help visualise the lateral aspect of the

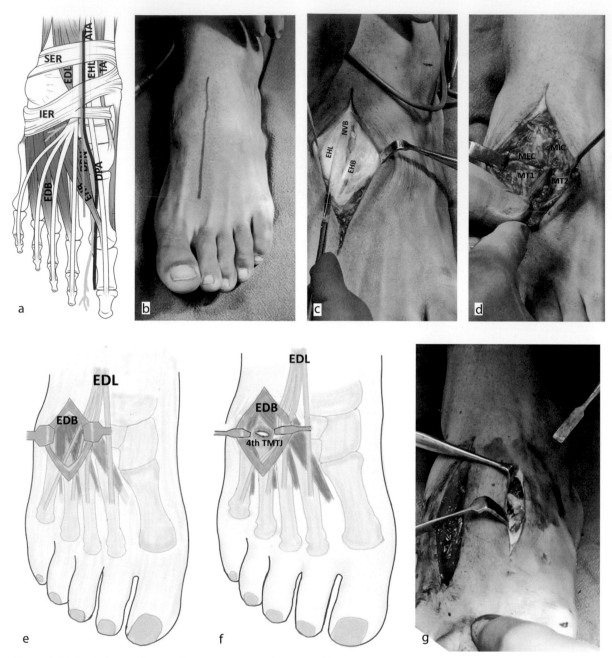

Figure 2.17 (a–g) Aprroaches to the tarsometatarsal joints. (Abbreviations: **ATA** – Anterior tibial artery, **DPA** – Dorsalis pedis artery, **DPN** – Deep peroneal nerve, **EDB** – Extensor digitorum brevis, **EDL** – Extensor digitorum longus, **EHB** – Extensor hallucis brevis, **EHL** – Extensor hallucis longus, **IER** – Inferior extensor retinaculum, **MEC** – Medial cuneiform, **MIC** – Middle cuneiform, **MT** – Metatarsal, **NVB** – Neuro vascular bundle, **SER** – Superior extensor retinaculum, **TA** – Tibialis anterior.)

second TMT joint, as well as to access the third, fourth and fifth TMT joints. The common extensor tendons are mobilised medially, and the muscle belly of EDB is split in line with its fibres to gain exposure of the affected joints (Figure 2.17e–g).

Distal soft tissue release for hallux valgus (8)

Make a 2–3 cm long incision over the first web space, and continue deep dissection bluntly to expose the adductor

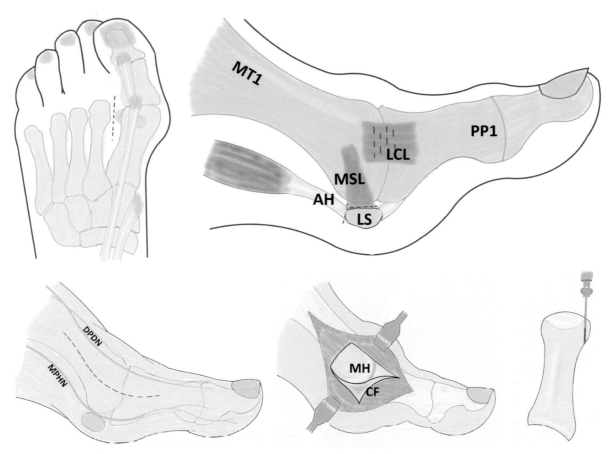

Figure 2.18 Surgical approach for hallux valgus surgery. (Abbreviations: **AH** – Adductor hallucis, **CF** – Capsular flap, **DPDN** – Dorsal proper digital nerve, **LCL** – Lateral collateral ligament, **LS** – Lateral sesamoid, **MH** – Metatarsal head, **MPHN** – Medial plantar hallucal nerve, **MSL** – Metatarso-sesamoid suspensory ligament, **MT1** – First metatarsal, **PP1** – Proximal phalanx.)

hallucis muscle and tendon (Figure 2.18a). The dissection is made in the midline to protect the superficial branches of the DPN, which pass on either side of the web space.

The adductor tendon is released from it is insertion onto the lateral aspect of fibular sesamoid and plantar base of proximal phalanx. Then, the lateral metatarso-sesamoid suspensory ligament running from the lateral tubercle of the MT head to the lateral border of the lateral sesamoid, is divided sharply in a proximal to distal direction. (Figure 2.18b). A gentle, medially directed force is then applied, and the hallux is brought into varus, completing the lateral release.

In the last few years single incision surgery for HV has evolved. The lateral soft tissue release can be performed by medial incision for HV followed by retracting EHL tendon medially and releasing the suspensory ligament between MT head and lateral sesamoid (15).

Medial approach for hallux valgus

The first MT is approached through a medial longitudinal incision extending from 1 cm proximal to the medial eminence, to the medial flare of the proximal phalanx (Figure 2.18c). Dorsal and plantar flaps to the level of the capsule are raised, protecting both the capsule and also the dorsal medial cutaneous nerve. 'T' or 'L' shaped or, longitudinal capsulotomies of the MTP capsule is performed and a full thickness well defined capsular flap is raised to expose the medial eminence (Figure 2.18d), which is resected 1 mm medial to the medial sulcus (Figure 2.18e). The plantar capsular release should not extend beyond the MT head flare as the vascularity of the MT head could be compromised by an extensive dissection.

Excision of Morton's neuroma (7)

Technique

Palpate the metatarsophalangeal joint of the two adjacent toes and make a dorsal longitudinal incision, in the centre of the relevant web space, so as to avoid injury to the dorsal digital nerves, starting at the distal end of the web space and extending proximally to the level of

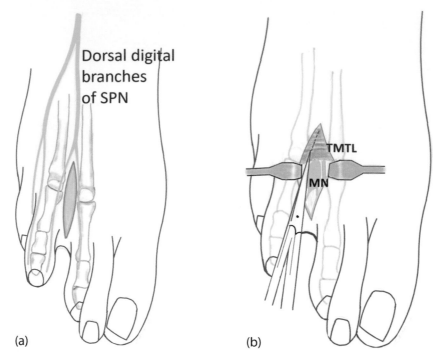

Figure 2.19 (a–b) Dorsal approach for Morton's neuroma excision. (Abbreviations: **MN** – Morton's neuroma, **SPN** – Superficial peroneal nerve, **TMTL** – Transverse intermetatarsal ligament.)

MT neck (Figure 2.19a). A laminar spreader is placed between the two adjacent heads. Digital pressure from the plantar surface, distal to MT heads, helps to identify the neuroma. A Freer elevator is placed under the intermetatarsal ligament to protect the underlying structures, and then the ligament is divided (Figure 2.19b). Division of the deep transverse MT ligament will expose the neurovascular bundle, which is dissected away from the common digital nerve. Gentle traction is placed on the common digital nerve and its two terminal branches are identified and resected first, before resecting the proximal trunk under tension (so as to allow retraction of the proximal stump).

Take home messages

- Soft tissues around foot and ankle are very tenuous. It is extremely important to wait for swelling to subside and blisters to heal before any open surgery is done in acute fractures.
- EHL is an important landmark for dorsal approaches to the ankle and foot. Its relationship to the neurovascular bundle, i.e., ATA and DPN proximally, and DPA and DPN distally, is crucial to avoid iatrogenic injury to these structures.
- The understanding of location of posterior compartment muscles and posterior tibial neurovascular structures is very important for the posteromedial approach to the ankle. These are in following order from anteromedial to posterolateral: TP, FDL, PTA and vein, Tibial nerve, FHL.
- While using a lateral extensile approach to the calcaneum, the incision should be open angled (not 90°), taken straight to bone over the central third or apex of the incision and a full thickness subperiosteal flap should be raised by using sharp dissection with a blade.
- During lateral and posterolateral approaches to the ankle, the superficial peroneal nerve and its branches and the sural nerve can be injured. Understanding of the anatomy of these superficial nerves is very important.

References

1. Rosson GD, Dellon AL. Superficial peroneal nerve anatomic variability changes surgical technique. Clin Orthop Relat Res. 2005; 438:248–252.
2. DeHeer PA, Catoire SM, Taulman J, et al. Ankle arthrodesis: A literature review. Clin Podiatr Med Surg. 2012; 29:509–527.
3. Assal M, Ray A, Stern R. Strategies for surgical approaches in open reduction internal fixation of pilon fractures. J Orthop Trauma. 2015; 29:69–79.
4. Hess MC, Abyar E, McKissack HM, et al. Applications of the transfibular approach to the hindfoot: A systematic review and description of a preferred technique. Foot Ankle Surg. 2020; https://doi.org/10.1016/j.fas.2020.01.006

5. Schwartz AM, Runge WO, Hsu AR, et al. Fractures of the talus: Current concepts. Foot & Ankle Orthopaedics. 2020; 5(1):1–10.

6. Weatherford BM, Anderson JG, Bohay DR. Management of tarsometatarsal joint injuries. J Am Acad Orthop Surg. 2017; 25:469–479.

7. Lee KT, Kim JB, Young KW, et al. Long-term results of neurectomy in the treatment of Morton's neuroma: More than 10 years' follow-up. Foot Ankle Spl. 2011; 4(6):349–353.

8. Wolfgang Schneider W. Distal soft tissue procedure in hallux valgus surgery: Biomechanical background and technique. Int Orthop (SICOT). 2013; 37:1669–1675.

9. Greisberg J, Sonnenfeld JJ. The posterior approaches to the posterior pilon fracture. Tech Foot & Ankle. 2018; 17:179–184.

10. Kiewiet NJ, Sangeorzan BJ. Calcaneal fracture management extensile lateral approach versus small incision technique. Foot Ankle Clin N Am. 2017; 22:77–91.

11. Lidder S, Masterson S, Dreu M, et al. The risk of injury to the peroneal artery in the posterolateral approach to the distal tibia: A cadaver study. J Orthop Trauma. 2014; 28:534–537.

12. Bibbo C, Ehrlich DA, Nguyen HM, et al. Low wound complication rates for the lateral extensile approach for calcaneal ORIF when the lateral calcaneal artery is patent. Foot Ankle Int. 2014; 35(7):650–656.

13. Fuentes EM, Staub RF, Cataldo MM, et al. Surgical technique and algorithm for the treatment of closed and displaced intra-articular calcaneal fractures by the sinus tarsi approach and plate fixation. Tech Foot & Ankle. 2014; 13:150–157.

14. Gougoulias N, Dawe EJ, Sakellariou A. The recovery position for posterior surgery of the ankle and hindfoot. Bone Joint J. 2013; 95-B:1317–1319.

15. Qasim SN, Elzubeir L, Bhatia M. Are two incisions necessary for hallux valgus correction? Foot Ankle Surg. 2018; 24(2): 128–130.

3 Biomechanics of the foot and ankle

Sheraz S Malik and Shahbaz S Malik

Introduction

The foot has been described as the 'root' between the body and earth. It provides a base of support that transmits force between the lower limb and ground, cushions the body, adapts to uneven surfaces and offers traction for movement and leverage for propulsion. This chapter provides an overview of the biomechanics of the foot and ankle as a basis for treating its disorders. The chapter is divided into three main sections: (1) Biomechanics of the ankle; (2) biomechanics of the midfoot and forefoot and (3) the gait cycle.

Definitions of motion

The three cardinal planes of motion of the body are sagittal, coronal and transverse, and rotation in each plane occurs about an axis perpendicular to the plane. Hence, flexion-extension in the sagittal plane occurs about a mediolateral axis, abduction-adduction in the coronal plane occurs about an anterior-posterior axis and internal-external rotation in the transverse plane occurs about a longitudinal axis. In regard to the foot, rotation in sagittal plane is referred to as dorsiflexion-plantarflexion, rotation in coronal plane is termed inversion-eversion and rotation in transverse plane is called abduction-adduction. The motions in coronal and transverse planes are different to the rest of the appendicular skeleton because foot is oriented 90° to the leg.[1] It is customary to describe hind foot motion with standard nomenclature and forefoot motion with the amended terms (Figure 3.1).

The mechanical axes of the joints of the foot are not aligned with the cardinal planes but instead pass through all three cardinal planes. The more a joint axis of motion diverges from a cardinal plane, the greater the coupled rotations in two planes. When the joint axis is oblique in all three planes, the resulting triplanar motion, pronation-supination, is a combination of three separate rotations in the cardinal planes.[1] Supination consists of inversion, adduction and plantarflexion, whereas pronation is a composite of eversion, abduction and dorsiflexion.

Biomechanics of the ankle

The ankle joint complex consists of three articulations: tibiotalar (talocrural), subtalar and transverse tarsal joints.

Tibiotalar joint

The ankle is functionally a simple hinge joint formed by the articulation of tibial plafond, talus and medial and lateral malleoli. The body of talus is shaped like a truncated cone, called frustum, with the apex directed medially (Figure 3.2). The load-bearing aspect of the joint is the tibiotalar interface. Experimental studies indicate that the talar dome, medial talar facet and lateral talar facet/fibula interface transmit up to 90%, 22% and 18% of the load, respectively.[2] Medial and lateral facets are loaded more in dorsiflexion with inversion and eversion, respectively, due to increased contact area.

The normal external torsion of distal tibia (and fibula) in relation to tibial plateau means that the ankle joint axis is externally rotated 20–25° in relation to the knee joint axis, although the foot is slightly internally rotated in relation to the ankle. The more posterior position of lateral malleolus is also a result of external tibial torsion.[3] The joint axis is laterally tilted 14° in the coronal plane, and 6° in the transverse plane (Figure 3.3). Inman[4] described the axis as passing just distal to medial and lateral malleoli. The joint movements mostly consist of dorsiflexion and plantarflexion. The normal range of motion of ankle is 10–20° of dorsiflexion and 25–30° plantarflexion, but usually only 10° of dorsiflexion and 20° of plantarflexion is required for normal locomotion. The varus tilt of the axis causes the talus to also rotate in the coronal plane, with dorsiflexion producing external rotation up to 10° and plantarflexion producing internal rotation up to 7°. Thus, dorsiflexion results in a lateral forefoot position and plantarflexion leads to medial forefoot position. When the foot is planted on the ground, dorsiflexion causes internal rotation of tibia and plantarflexion produces external rotation of tibia.

Plane	Sagittal	Coronal	Tranverse
Axis of motion	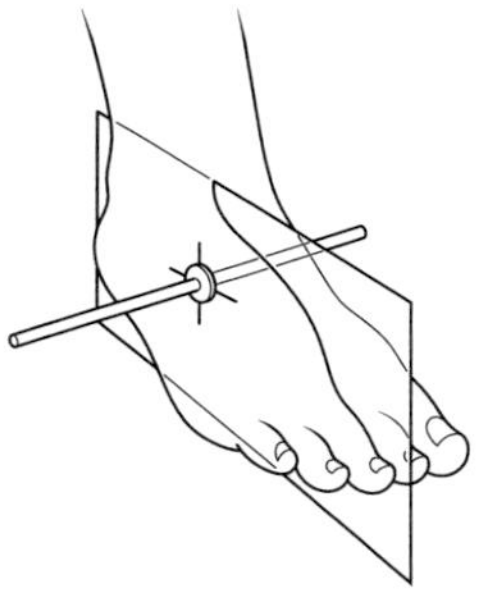	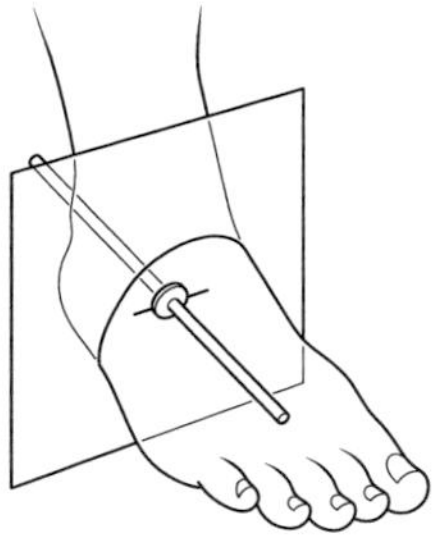	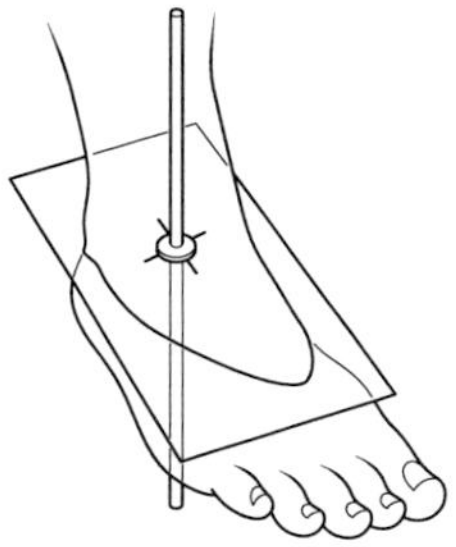
Ankle motion	Dorsiflexion- plantarflexion	Abduction-adduction	Internal rotation-external rotation
Foot motion	Dorsiflexion- plantarflexion	Inversion-eversion	Abduction-adduction

Figure 3.1 Planes and axes of motion of the ankle and foot.

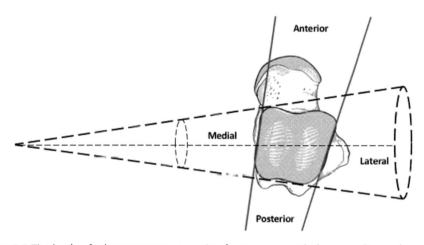

Figure 3.2 The body of talus represents a section from a cone, with the apex directed medially.

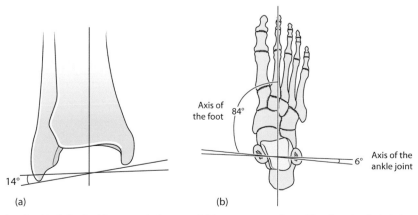

Figure 3.3 The axis of ankle joint in (a) coronal plane and (b) transverse plane. The foot is slightly internally rotated in relation to the ankle.

The joint is stabilised by congruent articular surfaces, joint capsule and ligaments. The talus is 4.2 mm wider anteriorly than posteriorly, and in dorsiflexion the ankle is in a 'closed packed' position of maximum stability.[5] The ligamentous support is critical in plantarflexion and when the ankle is unloaded. Lateral stability is provided by lateral ligament complex, which resists anterior draw of talus, inversion and internal rotation. The tensile strengths of anterior talofibular, calcaneofibular, and posterior talofibular ligaments are 139N, 346N and 261N, respectively. The anterior talofibular ligament is the weakest and most commonly injured ankle ligament. Medial stability is provided by superficial and deep deltoid ligaments, which resist eversion and external rotation stresses. The deep deltoid ligament has a tensile strength of 714N, and is the least frequently completely disrupted ankle ligament.[6] The syndesmotic ligaments maintain stability between distal tibia and fibula and support distal fibula loading.

Kinetics of the ankle joint

A static analysis with a free-body diagram can be used to estimate the loads acting at the ankle joint when a person stands on the tiptoes on one leg (Figure 3.4). This is an example of a class two lever system, with three coplanar forces acting on the foot:

1. Ground reaction force (Force W) – It is acting at the metatarsal heads, directed vertically upward and its magnitude is equal to body weight, W.
2. Muscle force through Achilles tendon (Force A) – This is acting at the point where tendon is inserted onto calcaneus,[7] taken to act vertically upward (although if the knee is flexed, it would be acting at an angle from vertical), and its magnitude is unknown. Due to its extension posterior to the ankle joint, the calcaneus acts as a lever arm for Achilles tendon, so that it acts at a short distance from centre of rotation of the ankle joint.
3. Joint reaction force (Force J) – This is the reaction (contact) force of tibia on the talar dome. It is taken to act vertically downward and its magnitude is unknown.

Dynamic analyses suggest that the ankle joint experiences a force of approximately five times body weight during stance in normal walking and up to thirteen times body weight when running.[5]

Subtalar joint

This triplane, uniaxial joint is formed by the articulation between talus, calcaneus and navicular. The subtalar joint has the largest surface area of all the joints in the ankle and foot. The posterior talocalcaneal articulation, between talus and posterior facet of calcaneus, comprises approximately 70% of the total joint surface area. The anterior talocalcaneonavicular articulation, between the head of talus, middle and anterior facets of calcaneus, navicular and spring ligament complex, comprises the remaining joint surface area. The two articulations move as one joint and have a common axis of motion.

Manter[8] described the axis of subtalar joint as inclined 42° upward from posterior to anterior and 16° medial to the longitudinal axis of the foot (Figure 3.5). The 42° obliquity of axis creates the component motions of inversion-eversion in the coronal plane and abduction-adduction in transverse plane. The subtalar joint is normally able to invert to 20° and evert to 5°. In the clinical setting this motion is assessed by measuring degree of calcaneal inversion and eversion with respect to longitudinal axis of the leg. Normal locomotion requires an average minimum 5° of calcaneal inversion and eversion. The 16° medial tilt of axis creates a very small component of dorsiflexion and plantarflexion in sagittal plane. All three component motions occur simultaneously in a single plane perpendicular to the axis, and the resulting triplanar movement is referred to as pronation and supination. However, only the inversion-eversion component of subtalar joint pronation-supination can be measured in the clinical setting.[9]

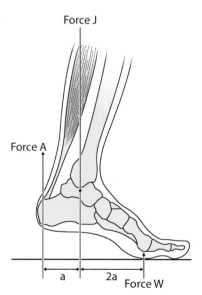

Figure 3.4 Free body diagram of the ankle. Newton's first law and the conditions of equilibrium are applied to determine the magnitude of forces A and J. The moment arm of Force W is approximately twice the moment arm of Force A. Hence, Force A $\cong$ 2W. As Forces W and A are acting upward, Force J is equal and opposite them. Hence, Force J $\cong$ –3W, i.e., tibiotalar joint reaction force is three times body weight, acting downward on the talar dome. (Force W = Ground reaction force; Force A = Muscle force through Achilles tendon; Force J = Joint reaction force).

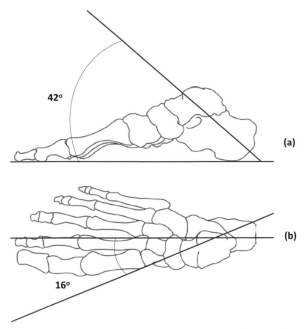

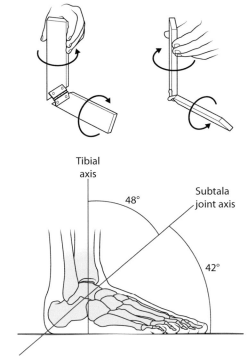

Figure 3.5 The axis of the subtalar joint in (a) sagittal plane and (b) transverse plane.

Figure 3.6 A mitred hinge is a joint where both sides are bevelled at 45° to form a 90° corner. Because of the obliquity of the joint axis, rotation of the vertical segment is translated to the horizontal segment, and vice versa. The subtalar joint functions like a mitred hinge.

The subtalar joint functions as a torque converter, or a mitred hinge, translating tibial rotation about the vertical axis, into inversion and eversion of calcaneus (Figure 3.6).[10] As the joint axis in the sagittal plane is 42°, 1° of tibial rotation generates approximately 1° of horizontal rotation. External tibial rotation results in subtalar supination and internal tibial rotation results in foot pronation, i.e., rotations of tibia and subtalar joint are in opposite directions.[11] A combination of movements at tibiotalar and subtalar articulations affords freedom of motion in all three planes, and the coordinated function of the two joints has been likened to a universal joint.

The subtalar joint receives support from components of lateral ligament complex and deltoid ligament of tibiotalar joint, as well as ligaments of sinus tarsi. The cervical ligament is the strongest of all ligaments stabilising this joint. It is located in anterior sinus tarsi and connects neck of talus to neck of calcaneus (hence the name). Kapandji,[12] however, regarded the interosseous talcocalcaneal ligament as the most important ligament of talocalcaneal articulation. It consists of two thick bands which occupy the sinus tarsi centrally and resist joint eversion.

Transverse tarsal joint

The transverse tarsal joint (Chopart's joint) separates hindfoot from midfoot, and consists of two articulations: talonavicular joint, which is a section of talocalcaneonavicular complex, and calcaneocuboid joint. The talonavicular joint is a ball and socket type – acetabulum pedis – and has a much greater range of motion than the saddle shaped calcaneocuboid joint. Both articulations are oriented towards a vertical plane and their motions are highly coupled with the actions of ankle and subtalar joints. However, unlike ankle and subtalar joints, transverse tarsal joint has considerable motion in all three planes and has two axes of motion.[13]

The transverse tarsal joint has a longitudinal axis and an oblique axis (Figure 3.7). The longitudinal axis is similar to longitudinal component of subtalar joint axis. Inversion-eversion and adduction-abduction occur about this axis, mainly at the talonavicular joint. The oblique axis is close to tibiotalar joint axis. Flexion-extension takes place primarily about this axis. Thus, the transverse tarsal joint acts to amplify the motions of tibiotalar and subtalar joints, and a loss of movement at these joints can be compensated, at least partially, by motion at the transverse tarsal joint.[1] It also acts as a break between hindfoot and midfoot, allowing the hindfoot to rotate while the midfoot and forefoot remain stationary, and vice versa.

Astion et al.[14] found that talonavicular joint is the key to subtalar, talonavicular and calcaneocuboid joint complex. In their cadaveric study, fusion of talonavicular joint limited the motion of other joints to less than

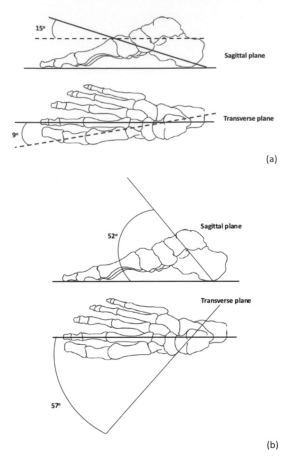

(a)

(b)

Figure 3.7 The orientation of (a) longitudinal axis (b) transverse axis of transverse tarsal joint in sagittal and transverse planes.

8% of normal values. In contrast, fusion of calcaneocuboid joint reduced talonavicular joint motion to 67% but had little effect on the motion of subtalar joint, and arthrodesis of subtalar joint limited calcaneocuboid joint motion to 56% and talonavicular joint motion to 46%. The talonavicular joint is supported inferiorly by spring (plantar calcaneonavicular) ligament, medially by the deltoid and laterally by bifurcate ligaments. The calcaneocuboid joint is stabilised inferiorly by short and long plantar ligaments, laterally by lateral band of bifurcate ligament and dorsally by dorsal calcaneocuboid ligament.

The main function of transverse tarsal joint is to 'unlock' the midfoot into a flexible structure for energy absorption and 'lock' it into a rigid lever to transmit force during gait. This is achieved through a change in the alignment of talonavicular joint and calcaneocuboid joint in the coronal plane. Elftman[15] showed that when calcaneus is everted, talonavicular and calcaneocuboid joints are parallel, and transverse tarsal joint has freedom of motion to adapt to various terrains. As the calcaneus inverts, the joints diverge and transverse tarsal joint motion is restricted. The midfoot becomes rigid and gives more stability to the longitudinal arch (Figure 3.8).

The posterior tibial tendon is the key to performing a heel rise at push-off. It has a broad insertion on the navicular, tarsal bones and metatarsals. It acts to rotate navicular medially over the head of talus, which adducts transverse tarsal joint and inverts the heel. Hence, the posterior tibial tendon action initiates heel rise and brings the hindfoot in varus position, and the powerful Achilles tendon then takes over and holds the heel

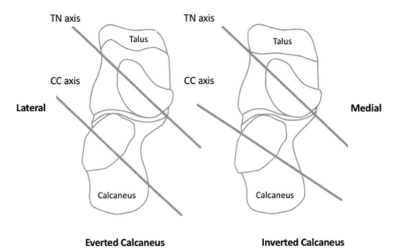

Figure 3.8 A coronal view of talonavicular (TN) and calcaneocuboid (CC) joints with navicular and cuboid removed. When the heel is everted, the joints are parallel and allow motion at transverse tarsal joint. As the heel is inverted, the joints diverge and transverse tarsal joint becomes stiffer (TN axis and CC axis show the relative orientation of joints in coronal plane. These are *not* axes of motion and are *not* related to longitudinal and oblique axes of motion of transverse tarsal joint).

in inverted position. In posterior tibial tendon dysfunction the foot remains in a position of excessive pronation during weight-bearing, leading to adult-acquired flatfoot deformity. As the tendon loses function, increased stress is placed on supporting structures of medial longitudinal arch. The subsequent rupture of spring ligament and then failure of talonavicular joint results in collapse of the longitudinal arch and progressive abduction of the forefoot through transverse tarsal joint and progressive valgus deformity of the subtalar joint.[16]

Biomechanics of the midfoot and forefoot

Whereas the hindfoot comprises a few major joints with large surface areas, the midfoot and forefoot comprise multiple relatively narrow joints.[17]

Midfoot

The midfoot provides an important bridge between hindfoot and forefoot and gives flexibility for energy absorption and stability for push-off.[18] It consists of intertarsal joints and tarsometatarsal joints (Lisfranc's joint). The tarsal bones – navicular, three cuneiforms and cuboid – form a transverse arch as well as support the medial and longitudinal arches of the foot. The three arches allow the foot to carry considerable loads and at the same time adapt to uneven surfaces.

The intertarsal joints – the naviculocuboid, three naviculocuneiform, intercuneiform and cuneocuboid joints – have limited motion due to a network of longitudinal and transverse dorsal and, stronger, plantar ligaments supporting the bones. The combined gliding (i.e., translation) motion of all the intertarsal joints ranges from a few degrees of dorsiflexion to about 15° of plantarflexion, which allows the transverse arch to rise and flatten with hindfoot supination and pronation, respectively.[19]

The tarsometatarsal joint complex consists of articulations of distal surfaces of three cuneiforms and cuboid with the bases of five metatarsals. It is inherently stable due to its configuration as a 'roman arch' and support from strong ligaments. As a result, only very little gliding motion occurs at these joints.

A ray describes the functional (movement) unit of each metatarsal. The first three rays are formed by a metatarsal and its articulating cuneiform bone, and the fourth and fifth rays are formed by the metatarsal alone as they both articulate with the cuboid bone. The second metatarsal is keyed into the midfoot and forms the most stable articulation and is considered the cornerstone of transverse arch. Lisfranc's ligament runs between medial cuneiform and base of second metatarsal. It is the largest and strongest of all the ligaments and a key stabiliser of the whole joint complex. Fourth and fifth

rays are the most mobile, followed by the first ray, then third and the second ray is the stiffest. The rigidity of the second ray allows for a rigid lever arm during push-off.

The tarsometatarsal joints assist transverse tarsal joint to rotationally position the forefoot (metatarsals) during weight-bearing. When the subtalar and transverse tarsal joints supinate, the forefoot tends to lift off the ground on the medial aspect and presses down on its lateral side. The muscles controlling the first ray plantarflex the first tarsometatarsal joint to maintain contact with the ground, whereas the fourth and fifth rays are forced into dorsiflexion due to ground reaction force, and the forefoot as a whole undergoes a 'pronator twist'. This acts to generate sufficient push-off from the medial border of the foot. Conversely, when the subtalar joint pronates substantially in weight-bearing, the transverse tarsal joint supinates to keep the foot in contact with the ground. If transverse tarsal joint supination is insufficient, the medial forefoot presses into ground, and the lateral side tends to lift off. The first ray is pushed into dorsiflexion by ground reaction force, and muscles controlling fourth and fifth rays plantarflex those tarsometatarsal joints to maintain contact with the ground. The accompanying rotation of the forefoot is referred to as 'supinator twist' of tarsometatarsal joints. This gives the foot flexibility to adapt to variable terrain. Pronator and supinator twists occur only when transverse tarsal joint motion is inadequate to align the forefoot.[3]

Forefoot

The forefoot comprises metatarsophalangeal and interphalangeal joints. The first metatarsal is the broadest and shortest of all metatarsals and bears 50% of weight acting on the foot. The second metatarsal is usually the longest and as a part of the rigid second ray experiences high stresses, and consequently stress fractures are more common in this metatarsal.[5]

The metatarsophalangeal joints are formed by convex metatarsal heads and concave bases of proximal phalanges. They are biaxial and allow dorsiflexion-plantarflexion and, to a much lesser degree, adduction-abduction. The first metatarsophalangeal joint has the most range of motion, from 85° dorsiflexion to 30° plantarflexion. Toe-off during normal gait requires approximately 60° of passive dorsiflexion. Metatarsal head contact area moves dorsally and compressive force between articulating surfaces increases with joint extension. This predisposes to formation of dorsal osteophytes in hallux rigidus.[5] The sesamoid bones function as pulleys for flexor hallucis brevis and protect the tendon of flexor hallucis longus from injury from body weight. The lesser metatarsophalangeal joints have an arc of motion from 65° dorsiflexion to 30° plantarflexion.

The metatarsophalangeal joints enable the weight-bearing foot to rotate over the toes when rising during

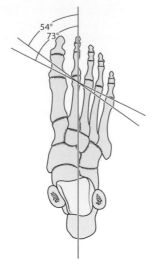

Figure 3.9 The metatarsal break is a hinge that forms at metatarsophalangeal joints as the heel rises and forefoot remains weight-bearing. It results from metatarsophalangeal joints extending around a single oblique axis that passes through the heads of four lesser metatarsals. The angle of the axis has a range of 54°–73° with respect to long axis of the foot in the transverse plane.

gait. The metatarsal break is the oblique axis that lies through the second to fifth metatarsal heads (Figure 3.9), around which dorsiflexion of metatarsophalangeal joints occurs. The obliquity of the axis allows the weight to be distributed evenly across the metatarsal heads and toes, as an axis orthogonal to the longitudinal axis of the foot would lead to disproportionate loading of first and second metatarsals. The metatarsal break also facilitates external rotation of the leg at toe-off.[3] The metatarsophalangeal joints are stabilised mainly by plantar plates, collateral ligaments, as well as by the joint capsule and deep transverse metatarsal ligament.

The intermetatarsal joints are hinge joints that allow simple flexion-extension; generally, flexion is greater than extension and proximal joints have a little more motion than distal joints. The toes function to smooth the weight shift to the opposite foot during gait and help maintain stability by pressing into ground in standing.

Arches of the foot

Kapandji[12] compared foot to a vault, which is supported by three arches: medial, lateral and transverse. These dynamic arches protect the foot by redistributing pressure and by creating a base that is both rigid and flexible. They are not present at birth but develop with progression in weight-bearing. The medial longitudinal arch has bony components composed of talus, calcaneus, navicular, the three cuneiforms and first three metatarsals, whereas the lateral longitudinal arch comprises calcaneus, cuboid and lateral two metatarsals. The transverse arch gives the 'vaulted' appearance to the foot. It is most easily appreciated at the level of tarsometatarsal joints.

The medial arch is higher, more mobile and resilient than its lateral counterpart, and is commonly regarded as the longitudinal arch. The talus sits at the top of the vault and is considered the 'keystone' of the arch. All weight transferred between the body to foot must pass through talus. The longitudinal arch transfers load between hindfoot and forefoot. The elements between calcaneus and heads of metatarsals do not usually transmit weight directly to the ground.[20] The longitudinal arch can therefore be considered to form a beam. In static weight-bearing, a bending load is applied to the longitudinal arch which produces compressive stress on the dorsal surface and tensile stress on the plantar aspect of the beam (Figure 3.10a).

The primary stabilisers of the longitudinal arch are interosseous ligaments and plantar fascia. The plantar fascia originates from medial aspect of calcaneus and passes distally under all the metatarsophalangeal joints to insert onto the bases of proximal phalanges of the toes. It supports the arch by forming a triangular tie-rod and truss connection with the bones. In this

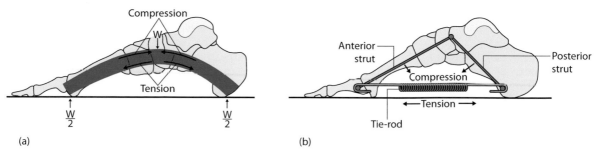

Figure 3.10 The beam and truss models of longitudinal arch. (a) A beam is a structure that supports bending loads. The longitudinal arch can be considered to function as a beam. (b) A truss is a constrained (unyielding) framework that supports applied loads. The plantar fascia acts as a cable connecting the ends of longitudinal arch. As the ends of the longitudinal arch are unable to move apart, the arch height is maintained under load.

arrangement, the talus and calcaneus form the posterior strut, tarsals and metatarsal form the anterior strut and plantar fascia forms a cable connecting them. When the body weight is applied, the bones are under compression and the plantar fascia is subjected to tension (Figure 3.10b).[21] As a result, bending moments that can cause injury to the components of the arch are minimised.

The plantar fascia is the most significant stabiliser of the longitudinal arch between heel rise and toe-off. As the heel rises and metatarsophalages joints extend during gait, plantar fascia is pulled distally around the metatarsal heads and tightens. This 'windlass mechanism', as first described by Hicks,[22] shortens the cable segment of truss and draws together the heel and metatarsophalangeal joints. This raises the longitudinal arch and holds midfoot joints in flexion in order to create a rigid lever arm (Figure 3.11).

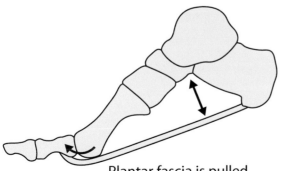

Toes neutral

Plantar fascia

Extension of metatarsophalangeal joints

Plantar fascia is pulled
distally around metatarsal heads

Figure 3.11 The increase in the height of medial longitudinal arch during push-off is not a result of muscular action, but generation of passive tension in plantar fascia through 'windlass mechanism'.

The gait cycle

The gait cycle extends from one heel strike to next heel strike of the same leg. It is divided into stance and swing phases, which comprise 62% and 38% of gait cycle, respectively. The stance phase extends from heel strike to toe-off on the same foot, and swing phase extends from toe-off to heel strike on the same foot.

Rockers of the normal gait

Perry[23] considered the stance phase as three rockers (intervals):

First (heel) rocker: This is the interval between heel strike and flatfoot in which the landing foot prepares to receive load. It comprises 15% of gait cycle (25% of stance phase) and includes a period of double limb stance. At heel strike, the ground reaction force is acting posterior to the ankle joint and causes the ankle to plantarflex until foot flat is achieved. The tibialis anterior and extensor hallucis longus (ankle dorsiflexors) contract eccentrically to decelerate the rate of plantarflexion and prevent the foot from rapidly hitting the ground.[24]

The tibia, along with the entire lower extremity, undergoes internal rotation during the first third of stance phase and external rotation in the latter two-thirds of stance. The internal rotation of tibia during first rocker produces pronation of subtalar joint, i.e., the heel everts. At the transverse tarsal joint, talonavicular and calcaneocuboid joints are parallel, so the forefoot is flexible and adapts to the ground absorbing energy.

Second (ankle) rocker: This is the period between foot flat and heel-off, when the firmly placed foot allows the supporting leg and the rest of the body to move forward. It consists of single limb stance and comprises 25% of gait cycle (40% of stance phase). The ankle dorsiflexes due to ground reaction force (i.e., body weight) moving anterior to the joint. The tibialis posterior, soleus and gastrocnemius (ankle plantar flexors) contract eccentrically to decelerate the rate of ankle dorsiflexion. At midstance, the tibia starts to externally rotate. The heel begins to rise just before maximum ankle dorsiflexion.

Third (forefoot) rocker: This push-off phase lasts from heel-off to toe-off, where the supporting foot prepares to take off. It comprises 22% of gait cycle (35% of stance phase) and includes a period of double limb stance. The ankle position rapidly changes from dorsiflexion to plantarflexion due to plantar flexors contracting concentrically, i.e., this is an acceleration rocker.

The accompanying external rotation of tibia is translated by subtalar joint into supination, i.e., the heel inverts.

The talonavicular and calcaneocuboid joints diverge, and the transverse tarsal joint is locked. This provides stability to the midfoot and converts the foot to a rigid lever for toe-off. Shortly after heel-off, the lateral side of the foot lifts from the ground, transferring the weight to the medial forefoot.[19] The toes undergo progressive extension, to a maximum just before toe-off, and the windlass mechanism tightens the plantar fascia, which provides stability to the medial longitudinal arch.

In early swing phase, the ankle is in plantarflexion. The motion reverses towards dorsiflexion in the mid-swing (foot clearance) and reverts again to slight plantarflexion and pre-positioning in terminal swing for initial contact.

Ankle motion during normal walking averages about 10° dorsiflexion and 14° plantarflexion. Maximum dorsiflexion occurs at 70% stance and maximum plantarflexion occurs at toe-off. The subtalar joint is in 2° supination at heel strike, and undergoes pronation up to foot flat, achieving 2° pronation, then it moves towards supination, achieving maximum supination of 6° at toe-off.[5] Most of transverse plane motion of the foot occurs in the last 20% of stance phase, when the joints are adducting.[17]

Kinetics of the foot

Studies measuring forces acting on the foot show that the vertical element of ground reaction force reaches 120% body weight at heel strike, then drops to 80% body weight during midstance and, due to acceleration of centre of mass, rises again to exceed body weight towards toe-off. During static weight-bearing, load distribution across the foot is as follows: heel 60%, midfoot 8%, forefoot 28% and toes 4%. The highest parts of the longitudinal arch, talonavicular and naviculocuneiform joints, bear most of the load through the tarsal joints.[5]

During the stance phase of gait, the ground reaction force vector progresses along the bottom of foot in a consistent pattern. It is initially located in the centre of the heel but shifts rapidly across the midfoot to reach the forefoot. In the forefoot, it lies under the second metatarsal head for half of the stance phase then passes distally to the hallux at toe-off. In a patient with hallux valgus deformity and significant metatarsalgia, the centre of pressure remains in the posterior aspect of the foot, and then rapidly passes over the metatarsal heads along the middle of the foot. In patients with amputation of great toe, the centre of pressure passes along a more lateral path.[25]

Take home messages

- Ankle joint force can be nearly five times the body weight between heel-off and toe-off. About 1/5 of the load acting on the ankle joint is borne by fibula, and the remainder passes through the tibia.

- The calcaneus is normally the first bone to contact the ground in the stance phase, and its position during weight-bearing often determines how to rest of the foot functions until toe-off.
- Motions of talonavicular and subtalar joints are highly coupled.
- Fusion of talonavicular joint leaves 8% of normal subtalar motion, whereas fusion of subtalar joint leaves 46% of normal talonavicular motion.
- A loss of motion from tibiotalar, subtalar or transverse tarsal joints overloads the others as they attempt to compensate for the lost motion. Hence, patients with ankle fusion inevitably develop hindfoot arthritis.
- The first metatarsal bears approximately 50% of weight acting on the foot, with the remainder distributed across lesser metatarsal heads. Resection of any metatarsal head should be avoided in general.

References

1. Oatis CA. Biomechanics of the foot and ankle under static conditions. Phys Ther. 1988; 68(12):1815–21.
2. Calhoun JH, Li F, Ledbetter BR, Viegas SF. A comprehensive study of pressure distribution in the ankle joint with inversion and eversion. Foot Ankle Int. 1994; 15(3):125–33.
3. Martin RL. The ankle and foot complex. In: Levangie PK, Norkin CC (Eds.). Joint structure and function – A comprehensive analysis (5th ed). Philadelphia: FA Davis Company 2005; pp 440–81.
4. Inman VT. The joints of the ankle. Baltimore: Williams & Wilkins. 1976.
5. Hagins M, Pappas E. Biomechanics of foot and ankle. In: Nordin M, Frankel VH (Eds.). Basic biomechanics of the musculoskeletal system (4th ed). London: Lippincott Williams & Wilkins. 2012. pp 224–53.
6. Attarian DE, McCrackin HJ, Devito DP, McElhaney JH, Garrett Jr WE. Biomechanical characteristics of human ankle ligaments. Foot Ankle. 1985; 6(2):54–8.
7. Greisberg JK, Baranek ES. Anatomy and biomechanics. In: Greisberg J, Vosseller JT (Eds.). Core knowledge in orthopaedics – Foot and ankle (2nd ed). Philadelphia: Elsevier. 2019. pp 2–9.
8. Manter JT. Movements of the subtalar and transverse tarsal joints. Anat Rec. 1941; 80:397–410.
9. Rockar PA. The subtalar joint: Anatomy and joint motion. JOSPT. 1995; 21(6):361–72.
10. Madhav R, Eastwood D, Singh D. Biomechanics and joint replacement of the foot and ankle. In: Ramachandran M (Ed). Basic orthopaedic sciences: The Stanmore Guide. London: Hodder Arnold. 2006. pp 210–8.
11. Monk AP, Simpson DJ, Riley ND, Murray DW, Gill HS. Biomechanics in orthopaedics: Considerations of the lower limb. Surgery. 2013; 31(9):445–51.
12. Kapandji IA. The physiology of the joints (2nd ed). New York: Churchill Livingstone Inc. 1970.
13. de Asia RJ, Deland JT. Anatomy and biomechanics of the foot and ankle. In: Thordarson DB (Ed). Orthopaedic surgery

essentials – Foot and ankle. London: Lippincott Williams & Wilkins. 2004. pp 1–23.

14. Astion DJ, Deland JT, Otis JC, Kenneally S. Motion of the hindfoot after simulated arthrodesis. J Bone Joint Surg Am. 1997; 79(2):241–6.

15. Elftman H. The transverse tarsal joint and its control. Clinic Orthop. 1960; 16:41–6.

16. Sammarco VJ. The talonavicular and calcaneocuboid joints: Anatomy, biomechanics, and clinical management of the transverse tarsal joint. Foot Ankle Clin N Am. 2004; 9:127–45.

17. Ledoux WR, Hahn ME. Lower limb structure, function and locomotion biomechanics. In: Winkelstein BA (Ed). Orthopaedic biomechanics. London: CRC Press. 2013. pp 265–300.

18. Kadakia AR, Seybold JD. Disorders of the foot and ankle. In: Miller DM, Thompson SR (Eds). Miller's review of orthopaedics (7th ed). Philadelphia: Elsevier. 2016. pp 482–575.

19. Harrold F, Abboud RJ. Biomechanics of the foot and ankle. In: Robinson A, Brodsky JW, Negrine JP (Eds). Core topics in foot and ankle surgery. Cambridge: CUP. 2018. pp 22–43.

20. Chan CW, Rudins A. Foot biomechanics during walking and running. Mayo Clin Proc. 1994; 69:448–61.

21. Dawe EJ, Davis J. Anatomy and biomechanics of the foot and ankle. Orthopaedic and trauma. 2011; 25(4):279–86.

22. Hicks JH. The mechanics of the foot II. The plantar aponeurosis and the arch. J Anat. 1954; 88(1):25–30.

23. Perry J. Gait analysis: Normal and pathological function thorofare. New Jersey: Slack Incorporated. 1992.

24. Malik SS, Malik SS. Orthopaedic biomechanics made easy. Cambridge: CUP. 2015. pp 150–7.

25. Haskell A, Mann RA. Biomechanics of the foot and ankle. In: Coughlin MJ, Saltzman CL, Anderson RB (Eds). Mann's surgery of the foot and ankle Vol I (9th ed). Philadelphia: Saunders. 2013. pp 3–36.

4

Principles of foot and ankle orthoses

Nick Gallogly

Introduction

An orthosis (orthoses – plural) is a medical device that is applied to an external part of the body with the aim of reducing load upon pathological soft tissue, preventing deformity, reducing pain and improving mobility. Every orthosis applies force with the aim of influencing a limb segment. These forces must be applied over a large surface area, where possible, to improve comfort and to minimise any pressure being exerted on the skin. If the forces are too high and not distributed well enough, this is likely to result in discomfort and rejection by the patient. The name of the orthosis is usually derived from the joints that it spans, e.g., functional foot orthosis (FFO), ankle foot orthosis (AFO), knee ankle foot orthosis (KAFO), etc.

Non-surgical treatment of foot and ankle disorders using orthotics is well recognised. The basic engineering principles behind their design have not changed much in 100 years. However, with advances in material science and manufacturing methodologies, the quality of orthoses has improved greatly. A thorough clinical examination and good communication (between the surgeon, patient and orthotist) is key to the success of orthotics.

Functional anatomy

An in-depth understanding of foot and ankle anatomy and gait is essential.

Eccentric and concentric muscle function should be understood in conjunction with the phases of recruitment within the gait cycle. In the context of functional anatomy, an eccentric muscle contraction is the lengthening of a muscle under load, and a concentric contraction is the shortening of a muscle whilst it applies force (1). All muscles have lever arms, some of similar length but it is their cross-sectional area that determines their functional capacity. Whilst there are seven muscles that help in plantarflexion of the ankle, due to their cross-sectional area, it is the soleus and the gastrocnemius that provide 93% of power which is why an

Achilles tendon rupture has such a negative impact on a patient's gait (2).

Material selection

The material choices available to those prescribing orthoses have changed considerably since the use of metal, leather and fabric in the early part of the 20th century (Figure 4.1). With material science advances, the materials that are designed to be strong can now also be lightweight. Composite material advances also mean that devices can be built to give both maximum strength and flexibility where it is needed within the gait cycle.

When choosing the most appropriate material, the clinician must understand important characteristics of the individual material including strength, stiffness durability, density and ease of fabrication (3).

FFOs can be made in a wide variety of expanded foams of different densities offering comfort, support and flexibility. These devices tend to be quite bulky in order to achieve the desired level of strength. Other materials include polypropylene and composites which offer greater strength and stiffness and are thinner. Some patients can struggle to tolerate the forces and pressure due to stronger materials, reporting a sensation of "hardness". All material choices can be covered with softer top layers of sponge rubber, but this can run the risk of making a bulky device that is not used.

AFOs are generally made from polypropylene due to their cost effectiveness and positive clinical outcomes. The thickness of the material is dictated by the size of the patient and the force being applied by the AFO, e.g., 4 mm polypropylene for a child or less active adult and 6 mm for an active adult. Disadvantages are that they can be bulky and difficultly to fit within footwear and, for this reason, the use of an AFO made from carbon fibre has become increasingly common practice. Carbon fibre can be expensive and generally there is little scope for adjustment of fit.

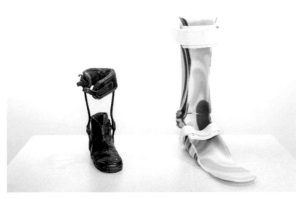

Figure 4.1 Advances in material. The conventional hinged AFO on the left is from 1884 compared with a present day hinged AFO prescribed to a child.

The importance of footwear

Whilst the presenting pathology determines the choice of orthosis, it is the patient's footwear that dictates the orthosis design and, ultimately, its effectiveness. For the orthosis to interact with the foot as it was originally prescribed, the foot must be securely positioned on the device (3). For this reason, a closed fastened shoe is recommended for best results. The ideal shoe characteristics should include a heel pitch of at least 1 cm, a heel stiffener, a stable sole unit, a secure fastening and a removable inlay to be able to accommodate an FFO. Trainers used to be the only footwear type that met these criteria, but as orthotic intervention has become more widely accepted, so too has the range of footwear options to accommodate them. For some patients with a foot pathology, in the presence of poor footwear selection, footwear advice is the only intervention required to achieve change (Figure 4.2).

It is important to understand the patient's use of footwear and the reasons behind their choice. Some of these choices can be due to fashion preferences, but other reasons could be as a result of other factors such as foot size, a large bunion, a high instep with sensitive exostosis or work dress code. For this reason, in some cases, a more minimalistic orthosis may have to be prescribed based on concordance, which may result in failure of non-surgical treatment.

Functional foot orthoses

An FFO is a device that applies deliberate forces to the foot, changing the way in which the foot interacts with the ground, and therefore the pathological load upon the foot and ankle.

FFOs are a common non-surgical treatment for many musculoskeletal problems, intended to alleviate pain and improve function (4, 5). They can be prefabricated, modular or custom-made. A custom-made orthosis does not always guarantee a better outcome.

FFOs can be three quarter, sulcus, or full length. Three quarter length devices are more suitable for hindfoot and midfoot pathologies, whilst sulcus and full-length devices can be more beneficial for forefoot disorders. A three-quarter length FFO may still be chosen for forefoot pathology due to a patient's footwear choice, as this design has a better chance of fitting into a wider variety of footwear. This decision lies at the end of a process of shared decision-making with the patient, so as to ensure that the device is worn.

Whilst the shell of the orthosis controls and influences the ground reaction forces, and therefore the load being exerted on the soft tissue, there are other aspects of orthotic design that are commonly employed to add further offloading or relief (Figure 4.3).

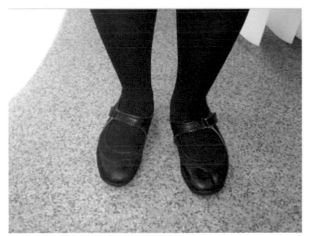
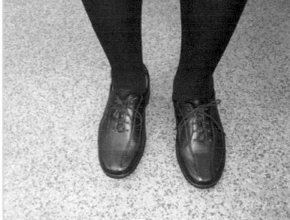

Figure 4.2 Effect of using appropriate footwear. The patient is wearing the same pair of FFO in both pictures. This demonstrates the difference that appropriate footwear can make.

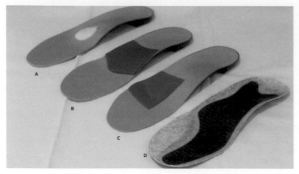

Figure 4.3 Functional foot orthoses. (A) Metatarsal dome, (B) Metatarsal bar, (C) Reverse Morton's extension, (D) Morton's extension.

Metatarsal pad (dome/bar)

A metatarsal dome is a pad, designed to sit centrally just proximal to the 2nd, 3rd and 4th metatarsal heads (6). The material is usually a sponge rubber but it can be moulded within the shell of a custom orthosis if required. The aim of a metatarsal dome is to influence and offload the metatarsal heads by increasing localised weight-bearing, decelerating the rate of plantarflexion of the metatarsals and widening of the intermetatarsal webspace. A dome also increases tension within the flexor tendons, thereby stretching the extensor tendons and reducing the grip reflex in patients with hammer toes. A metatarsal bar is designed to offload all the metatarsal heads and is often used when fat pad atrophy occurs.

Reverse Morton's extension

A reverse Morton's extension is a forefoot extension added plantar to the 2nd, 3rd, 4th and 5th metatarsophalangeal (MTP) joints of a foot orthosis. This extension is usually an addition to the main shell of the orthosis and its aim is to either accommodate or offload the 1st MTP joint.

Morton's extension

A Morton's extension is a continuation of an orthosis, usually in polypropylene or a composite, beyond the first MTP joint. The stiffness of the extension is determined by the severity of limitation across the joint, pain and the forces acting across the joint by the patient's body weight and foot length.

Wedging

Medial and lateral wedges can be added to the hindfoot and forefoot of any FFO. They provide either a supination or pronation force to offload pathological structures. These wedges can be added to the outside of the device (extrinsic post) or within the shell of the device during the manufacturing process (intrinsic). Intrinsic wedges are extremely hard to detect.

Ankle foot orthoses

AFOs are prescribed for patients that require both foot and ankle control for either mechanical or neuromuscular reasons. As with FFOs, their design and material choice are entirely dependent on the presentation and patients' goal. There are many different types of AFOs, both custom made and prefabricated. To a varying degree, regardless of the cost or complexity, every orthosis will improve swing phase clearance in patients with foot drop. It is what the AFO does in the stance phase that dictates the prescription and it is the skill of the orthotist to determine the most appropriate device for the patient (Figure 4.4). Information from members of the multidisciplinary team, where appropriate, is invaluable in helping to achieve the best outcome (Figure 4.4).

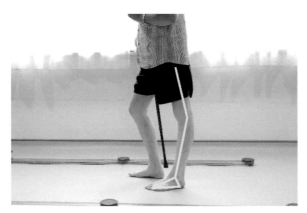
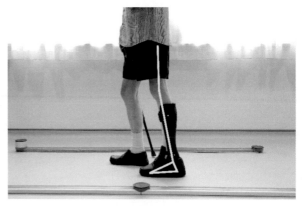

Figure 4.4 Influence of an AFO on stance phase. Demonstration of how an AFO is also designed to control stance phase, in this case, knee hyperextension in a patient who suffered a stroke.

Ground reaction ankle foot orthoses (GRAFO)

A GRAFO utilises the ground reaction force in order to apply a greater directional turning moment to resist knee flexion in those patients with foot and ankle pathology and quadriceps or triceps surae weakness. The orthosis positions the foot in slight plantarflexion, so as to limit tibial progression and further amplify the extensor moment. This type of device is often used in patients with spina bifida, or in children with cerebral palsy diplegia where a crouch pattern can be seen in those whose power to weight ratio is beginning to cause faster muscle fatigue (7).

Solid ankle foot orthoses

Solid AFOs are the strongest form of support. They restrict ankle and foot motion in all three planes so as to provide significant stability in both swing and stance phases (3). As a result of this stiffness, it is important to try and mimic a normal movement pattern where possible, and this is achieved by the tuning process (8). Heel raises, which are added underneath the AFO, help to improve the gait allowing some movement.

Hinged ankle foot orthoses

Hinged AFOs offer a varying degree of mediolateral control whilst facilitating the range of movement through the talocrural joint. There are different types of hinges that facilitate this, and their use is dependent upon the functional goal. Free moving hinges are most common. Other hinges include those with a range of movement that can be set and those with dampening springs to facilitate deceleration and return of energy at the most appropriate time of need within the gait cycle.

Posterior leaf spring ankle foot orthoses (PLS AFO)

This type of AFO is designed to offer control in swing phase with good positioning for heel strike and very minimal mediolateral control. Advances in composite materials mean that this design of AFO has improved greatly, generating energy absorption during the beginning of stance phase as the material is loaded, and energy return during the later stages of stance phase, when body weight unloads.

Supramalleolar orthosis (SMO)

The SMO is designed as a progressive step up from a heel cup. This device offers support across the ankle joint whilst still allowing a full range of movements through the ankle. This type of orthosis is used when there is deformity or weakness in the frontal plane, with normal muscle power in the sagittal plane (Figure 4.5).

Conventional ankle foot orthoses

These devices were used in the past before the recent advances in orthotic material and technology. Patients with loss of protective sensation, lower limb oedema and issues with skin integrity are still well served by this group of orthoses as they offer reduced points of skin contact and can accommodate volume changes. Conventional AFOs do not offer as much control due to poor fitting. They are also considerably heavier as they are made from steel, leather and duralumin (aluminium alloy) and more labour intensive to produce.

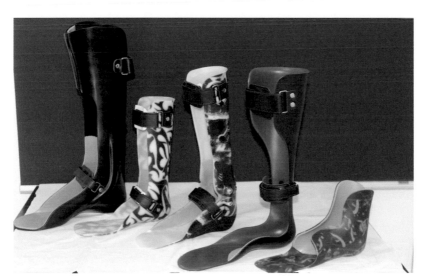

Figure 4.5 Different AFO designs. Pictured left to right: Ground reaction AFO, Solid AFO, Hinged AFO, Posterior leaf spring AFO, SMO.

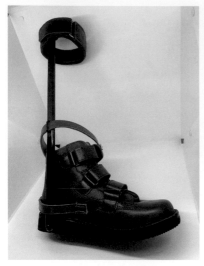 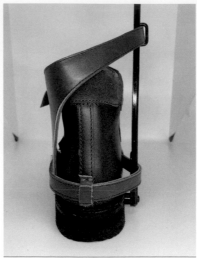 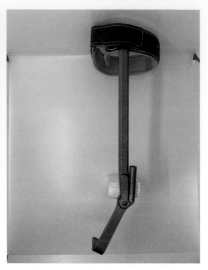

Figure 4.6 Conventional AFOs. A single stem medial below knee calliper (left) with an outside Y-strap aimed at controlling varus deformity (centre). A single stem spring assisted below knee hinged calliper (right).

The side members of a conventional AFO are inserted into the heel of the shoe via a socket. Frontal plane deformities can be controlled with the addition of a T-strap, attached to the shoe on the side of the deformity with a single stirrup on the opposing side, offering a point of anchorage to create a varus or valgus force (Figure 4.6).

Orthosis selection for different conditions (Table 4.1)

Chronic Achilles rupture

The majority of patients with untreated chronic Achilles rupture describe symptoms of instability and a lack of propulsion. Eccentric contraction of the gastrocnemius controls the rate of progression of the knee over the ankle whereas concentric contraction provides plantarflexion to facilitate propulsion. Therefore, an Achilles rupture will not only result in a loss of push off but reduced control of the tibia/fibula through stance phase. The functional goals of the orthosis are to provide stability in stance phase and an energy return and propulsive component at terminal stance.

In patients that can achieve a decent stride length, the use of a PLS AFO is indicated. The elderly patient group with reduced mobility and a higher risk of falls require an AFO that offers greater stability such as a solid AFO.

Ankle arthritis

Initial treatments such as an ankle boot, to reduce movements, should be considered and can be used in severe cases where the patient does not have the support network or the ability to manage the use of more complex orthoses. Ankle range of motion loss is common and so the sagittal plane deformity can be accommodated with a heel raise, built into an FFO in the early stages.

A solid AFO is prescribed if there is pain with all movements and the patient is not suitable for surgery. If there are significant pain levels, a patella tendon bearing AFO which can reduce axial load through the joint could be considered. These devices are more complex in nature and expensive.

Subtalar joint arthritis

The use of an FFO with a deep heel cup and a stabilising heel post to minimise movements should be considered as the first line of orthotic intervention. Should this not be enough, then the prescription of a heel cup, which is an orthosis made from polypropylene that encompasses the subtalar joint can be prescribed (Figure 4.7). These devices will require a change in footwear to accommodate the device. For patients who experience pain only with activity, an ankle brace is often a suitable recommendation.

Peroneal tendinopathy

Functional loss due to severe peroneal tendinopathy includes loss of eccentric control during midstance in resisting hindfoot inversion and, loss of concentric contraction, which aids first ray plantarflexion and helps with the windlass mechanism (9).

An FFO with a lateral heel or forefoot wedge and a cut out in the plastic shell for the first ray can reduce the load on the affected structure whilst rehabilitation

Table 4.1 Choosing the most appropriate orthosis: A quick reference table for common clinical scenarios

Presenting problem	Scenario 1	Scenario 2
Achilles rupture	Good stride length and stable gait: PLS AFO	Elderly with risk of falls: Solid AFO
Ankle arthritis	Good skin integrity with severe degeneration: Solid AFO	Poor skin integrity and reduced mobility: Stiff ankle boots
Subtalar arthritis	Symptoms due to increased activity only (mild arthritis): Ankle brace	Frequent symptoms (moderate/severe arthritis): FFO with high heel cupping
Peroneal tendinopathy	Secondary to pes cavus: FFO with lateral wedging and a reverse Morton's extension	Frequent symptoms: FFO with lateral hindfoot and forefoot wedging
Ligamentous instability	Symptoms due to increased activity only: Ankle brace	Frequent symptoms: FFO with high heel cupping
Traumatic or congenital deformities	Flexible deformity: Solid or Hinged AFO	Fixed deformity: Custom footwear with FFO
Midfoot arthritis	Occasional symptoms: Advice on the use of stiff soled shoes, e.g., walking shoes	Frequent symptoms: FFO made from stiff material
Tibialis posterior tendon dysfunction	Flexible deformity: FFO with heel cupping and medial hind foot wedging	Fixed deformity: AFO for active patients. Footwear/FFO combination for patients with fragile skin
Charcot arthropathy	Stable midfoot: FFO with offloading	Unstable midfoot: AFO/Footwear combination or CROW
Hallux rigidus	Mild to moderate: FFO	Severe: FFO with Morton's extension
Pes cavus	Flexible deformity: FFO with reverse Morton's extension	Fixed deformity: AFO
Metatarsalgia	Mild to moderate: FFO with metatarsal dome and cushioning	Severe: FFO with a rocker sole adaption
Hallux valgus	Mild to moderate: FFO	Severe: FFO with accommodative footwear

occurs. If the overload of the peroneal tendons is due to a pes cavovarus deformity, the use of a reverse Morton's extension may also be added to resist the supination forces leading to pathological overload.

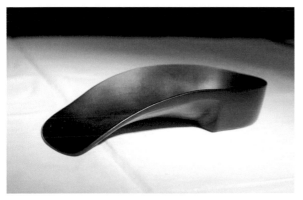

Figure 4.7 Heel cup. An effective orthosis where control of the subtalar joint is required.

Ankle ligamentous instability

Functional loss due to chronic lateral ligament rupture includes a reduction in proprioception and insufficient stability across the ankle joint.

For most patients, the use of ankle orthoses for specific activities is the most suitable orthotic intervention to run alongside effective rehabilitation. For the patient group where the instability is chronic, there are a lot of prefabricated ankle orthoses that exist. Ankle orthoses with non-elasticated straps will offer the greater level of stability (10). Care should be taken in selecting patients for this level of support as it may create muscle atrophy and dependence on the orthosis.

Traumatic or congenital deformities

The prescription is based upon whether the deformity is fixed or whether it can be controlled in a more anatomically neutral position.

If the deformity if fixed, it may be more suitable to take a custom footwear approach. The prescription of footwear also gives the option of using a conventional AFO, with a T-strap, if there is a frontal plane deformity. An equinovarus deformity will require forces to be controlled in both sagittal and frontal planes. This is best achieved with an AFO (11).

Midfoot arthritis

Excessive mechanical loading of midfoot structures is thought to contribute to symptoms associated with midfoot arthritis (12). Ensuring that this patient group is wearing appropriate footwear is a simple but important essential step. Patients should be discouraged from wearing flexible, completely flat shoes, as this can increase the bending moments across the midfoot during late mid-stance.

FFOs are prescribed with the aim of reducing the load and bending moments which are increased, especially in the presence of equinus (Figure 4.8). These devices tend to have a greater level of stiffness with the aim of reducing some movement across symptomatic joints.

Tibialis posterior tendon dysfunction

The clinical presentation is variable dependent on the stage of tibialis posterior dysfunction. Functional loss includes eccentric control of the hindfoot, and of pronation during initial contact. Also, loss of concentric

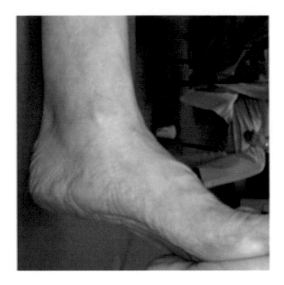

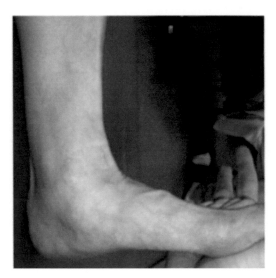

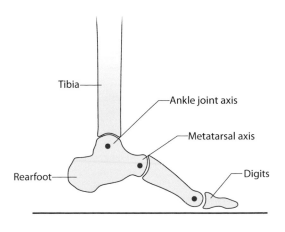

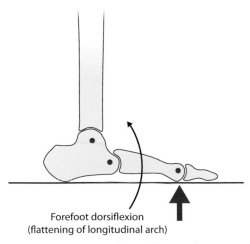

Figure 4.8 Demonstration of the impact forces and bending moments occurring across the midfoot in the presence of flexible equinus.

In the presence of an unstable midfoot, where stabilisation is not appropriate, an AFO/footwear combination or Charcot resistant orthotic walker (CROW) should be prescribed. A CROW consists of a moulded total contact insole wrapped within a clam shell polypropylene AFO with an external sole unit (Figure 4.9). This device is a highly effective method of managing the instability, but patient selection is important to ensure compliance.

Patients with diabetic ulcers in combination with plantar deformity require aggressive and effective offloading to prevent deterioration and to promote healing. In the presence of a good vascular supply and adequate diabetic control, redistributing pressure with offloading is the key to a successful outcome (Figure 4.10).

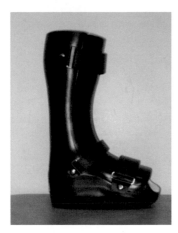

Figure 4.9 A CROW boot with both posterior and anterior shell design along with a sole unit to contain an unstable Charcot deformity.

contraction, which supinates the foot so as to achieve the rigid foot needed for push off (13).

An FFO with medial heel wedging to decelerate the uncontrolled pronation and reduce the lateral bony impingement is useful. An arch profile aims to reduce the effort required to achieve supination by the damaged structure, and use of a heel raise can also speed up the entry into, and exit from, stance phase.

In patients with spring ligament disruption, an FFO is usually not sufficient and more rigid and proximal control is required with an AFO. Should patients have swelling, poor skin quality or, a fixed deformity, then the use of custom footwear could be considered in order to increase stability and contain the deformity.

Charcot arthropathy

Early diagnosis is essential in this condition as it has a significant impact on the orthotic options and long-term management of this patient group (14). Immobilisation and off-loading should continue until there is an appropriate and successful orthotic solution in place.

Hallux rigidus

It is important to ensure that there is no tightness of soleus and gastrocnemius as this has an impact on the amount of joint dorsiflexion required for step length, e.g., reduced ankle dorsiflexion will result in early heel rise and prolonged 1st MTP joint dorsiflexion.

FFOs and footwear alterations are the commonly recommended non-surgical treatment options for hallux rigidus (15, 16). Whilst both methods have shown to be effective in reducing pain, footwear adaptions such as rocker soles are less likely to be adhered to. This is due to their impracticality, especially as some footwear types cannot be adapted and because of the wide variety of shoes that people wear (17). A Morton's extension can be considered in patients who have limited dorsiflexion due to pain.

Pes cavus

The Coleman block test is a good way to assess the likely benefit of a reverse Morton's extension, built into an orthosis (18). If the hindfoot deformity is flexible, then the use of this FFO can be considered (Figure 4.11). Other features of the prescribed FFO could include, a reduced medial arch height, a first ray cut out of the shell, metatarsal dome and lateral wedging.

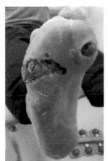 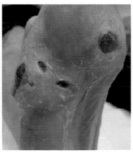 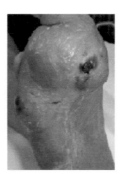 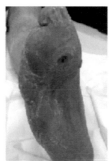 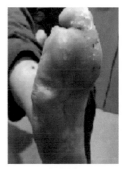

Figure 4.10 Offloading plantar ulcers in presence of deformity. Pictures depict offloading carried over an 8-week period, with 2-week interval changes, with the use of offloading felt in conjunction with a total contact cast.

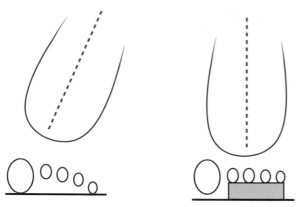

Figure 4.11 Effect of a reverse Morton's extension on hindfoot position in flexible pes cavus.

If the pes cavovarus deformity is fixed, the addition of control across the ankle, in conjunction with an FFO can be considered. This can be achieved with the use of an AFO or, custom footwear with a conventional AFO and T-strap.

Metatarsalgia

The treatment principles to manage this condition are: (a) redistribution of plantar pressure, (b) offloading of the forefoot and (c) reduction of pressure under the metatarsal heads.

First choice treatment option is to recommend the use of cushioned footwear in conjunction with stretching of the calf muscles to reduce pressure on the forefoot.

FFOs aim to achieve the above-mentioned goals and will often include additions such as metatarsal domes. The use of footwear adaptations, such as a rocker sole modification, can also be tried if surgical options are limited. This type of modification is not always accepted by patients as it limits their footwear options.

Hallux valgus

Once a hallux valgus deformity has progressed beyond a certain point, the foot loses its natural, even weight distribution between medial and lateral columns. This in turn leads to increased dorsiflexion of the first ray, and increased tension in the flexor hallucis resulting in functional hallux limitus (19). This means that the windlass mechanism is impeded and there is increased load through the medial column which further increases the abduction force upon the hallux.

An FFO is an effective method of intervention for this patient group (20). The functional goal is to ensure appropriate loading through the medial column thereby reducing the damaging forces that aim to accelerate deformity. Patients with a large medial eminence and who are not suitable for surgical intervention may first try wider footwear to relieve pressure.

Take home messages

- Functional anatomy must be understood in order to understand the biomechanical deficit and to be able to produce the most appropriate orthosis.
- An orthosis request must include the functional goals as well as the overall management plan when known.
- Orthoses do not correct but instead influence a joint or soft tissue structure by reducing the load being exerted on them.
- Patient compliance will play a large role and as a result there may a trial of more than one orthosis before a decision on surgical management is made.
- Conventional orthoses are prescribed when there is a loss of protective sensation, fragile skin or fluctuating oedema.

References

1. Zatsiorsky VM, Prilutsky BI. Biomechanics of skeletal muscles. Champaign, IL: Human Kinetics. 2012.
2. Perry J. Gait analysis normal and pathological function. Thorofare, NJ: Slack. 1992.
3. Lusardi M, Jorge M, Nielsen C. Orthotics and prosthetics in rehabilitation (3rd ed). Elsevier: 2000. pp. 219–221.
4. Collins N, Bisset L, McPoil T, Vicenzino B. Foot orthoses in lower limb overuse conditions: A systematic review and meta-analysis. Foot Ankle Int. 2007; 28:396–412.
5. Hawke F, Burns J, Radford JA, du Toit V. Custom-made foot orthoses for the treatment of foot pain. Cochrane Database Syst Rev. 2008; CD006801.
6. Koenraadt KLM, Stolwijk NM, Van den Wildenberg D, Duysens J. Effect of a metatarsal pad on the forefoot during gait. J Am Podiatr Med Assoc. 2012; 102(1):18–24.
7. Bowers R, Ross K. Development of a best practice statement on the use of ankle-foot orthoses following stroke in Scotland. Prosthet Orthot Int. 2010; 34(3):245–253.
8. Rogozinski BM, David JR, Davis RB, Jameson GG, Backhurst DW. The efficacy of the floor-reaction ankle-foot orthosis in children with cerebral palsy. J Bone Joint Surgery Am. 2009; 91(10);2440–2447.
9. Bolgla LA, Malone TR. Plantar fasciitis and the windlass mechanism: A biomechanical link to clinical practice. J Athl Train. 2004; 39(1):77–82.
10. Fatoye F, Haigh C. The cost-effectiveness of semi-rigid ankle brace to facilitate return to work following first-time acute ankle sprains. J Clin Nurs. 2016; 25(9-10):1435–1443.
11. Lin SS, Sabharwal S, Bibbo C. Orthotic and bracing principles in neuromuscular foot and ankle problems. Foot Ankle Clin. 2000; 5(2):235–264.
12. Chapman GJ, Halstead J, Redmond AC. Comparability of off the shelf foot orthoses in the redistribution of forces in midfoot osteoarthritis patients. Gait Posture. 2016; 49:235–240.
13. Durrant B, Chockalingam N, Hashmi F. Posterior tibial tendon dysfunction: A review. J Am Podiatr Med Assoc. 2011; 101(2):176–186.
14. Milne TE, Rogers JR, Kinnear EM, Martin HV, Lazzarini PA, Quinton TR, Boyle FM. Developing an evidence-based

clinical pathway for the assessment, diagnosis and management of acute Charcot neuro-arthropathy: A systematic review. J Foot Ankle Res. 2013; 6(1):30.

15. Hylton B, Maria A, Tan JM, Levinger P, Roddy E, Munteanu SE. Predictors of response to prefabricated foot orthoses or rocker-sole footwear in individuals with first metatarsophalangeal joint osteoarthritis. BMC Musculoskelet Disord. 2017; 18(1):185.

16. Menz HB, Auhl M, Tan JM, Levinger P, Roddy E, Munteanu SE. Effectiveness of foot orthoses versus rocker-sole footwear for first metatarsophalangeal joint osteoarthritis: Randomized trial. Arthritis Care Res. 2016; 68:581–589.

17. Zammit GV, Menz HB, Munteanu SE. Structural factors associated with hallux limitus/rigidus: A systematic review of case–control studies. J Orthop Sports Phys Ther. 2009; 39:733–742.

18. Burns J, Crosbie J, Ouvrier R, Hunt A. Effective orthotic therapy for the painful cavus foot: A randomized controlled trial. J Am Podiatr Med Assoc. 2006; 96(3):205–211.

19. Dananberg HJ. Functional hallux limitus and its relationship to gait efficiency. J Am Podiatr Med Assoc. 1986; 76:648–652.

20. Nakagawa R, Yamaguchi S, Kimura S, Sadamasu A, Yamamoto Y, Muramatsu Y, Sato Y, Akagi R, Sasho T, Ohtori S. Efficacy of foot orthoses as nonoperative treatment for hallux valgus: A 2-year follow-up study. J Orthop Sci. 2019; 24(3):526–531.

5

Paediatric and adolescent foot disorders

Hari Prem and Basil Budair

Introduction

It is generally accepted that children are not small adults, and this couldn't be more true when it comes to the assessment and management of paediatric foot and ankle pathologies. The paediatric foot shape changes dynamically as the child grows and deep knowledge and understanding of the natural history of foot development, anatomic variations and biomechanics is crucial to making a correct diagnosis and avoid unnecessary, stressful and potentially harmful interventions.

When assessing a paediatric foot problem, it is imperative to think of the child as a whole. Some patients will have other deformities or underlying genetic or neuromuscular disorders. Perinatal, development and family history should be part of a thorough and methodical history taking in all cases. Similarly, a head to toe clinical examination is the key to look for syndromic features, spinal deformity or dysraphism and deformities in the upper limbs, hips and knees. No assessment is complete without a full neurological and rotational profile evaluation. Addressing the parent's and child's concerns and expectations is equally as important as the interventional management.

The main remit of this book is adult foot and ankle pathology, and this chapter should supplement that by providing an overview of some high-yield paediatric foot and ankle topics.

In-toeing gait

In-toeing is a common reason for children presenting to primary care and orthopaedic clinics. It can be unilateral or bilateral and caused by excessive hip anteversion, tibial internal torsion or metatarsus adductus of the feet. In-toeing gait is a benign condition and requires no active intervention, except in rare symptomatic cases, where derotation may be indicated. Hence, only reassurance and education of the parents is needed in most cases.

Most toddlers will have an internally directed foot progression angle (FPA), which contributes to the normal clumsiness as they learn to walk. This gradually improves during growth to normal at about 8 years of age (FPA −5° to +20°) and in those who do not improve, it is very rarely a clinical problem.

At birth, normal femoral anteversion is 30–40° and it decreases to the normal adult value of about 15° by the age of 8 years in most children. Normal hip range of motion is 20–60° of internal rotation (IR) and 30–60° of external rotation (ER). IR of >70° and ER <20° represents excessive femoral anteversion.

Rotational profile (Figure 5.1) is assessed with the child prone and knees flexed to 90°. Tibial rotation is assessed by measuring the Thigh-Foot angle (TFA), an angle formed by the bisector line of the thigh and the foot bisector line (normal range −10° to +30°, mean +10° external). A TFA of >−10° denotes internal tibial torsion and a TFA of >+30° represents external tibial torsion.

Metatarsus adductus (MA) is defined as medial deviation of the forefoot with a normal hindfoot alignment. The lateral border of the foot is normally straight and the heel bisector line points towards the second web space. Convex lateral foot border, medial skin crease and a heel bisector line passing lateral to the 2nd webspace are suggestive of MA. Flexible MA is observed in >95% and they resolve spontaneously by the age of 5 years, while MA with moderate to severe rigidity might require serial casting. Surgery is rarely indicated in resistant symptomatic cases.

In-toeing gait is a benign condition that requires no treatment in the majority of cases.

Rotational profile assessment identifies the cause – Increased anteversion of the hips (prone rotation test), internal tibial torsion (Thigh Foot angle), adducted metatarsals (Heel Bisector line).

Children <8 years may trip up when running but gradually stop tripping as rotational control improves.

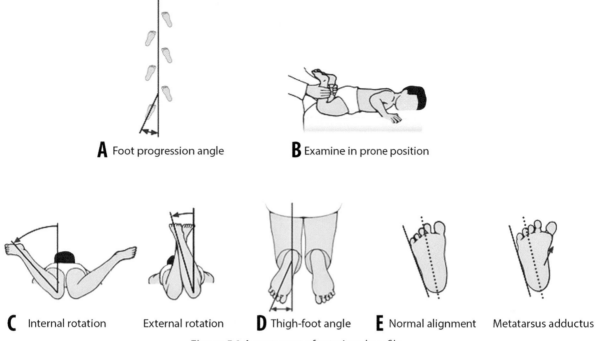

A Foot progression angle   **B** Examine in prone position

C Internal rotation   External rotation   **D** Thigh-foot angle   **E** Normal alignment   Metatarsus adductus

Figure 5.1 Assessment of rotational profile.

Clubfoot

Overview

Clubfoot, also referred to as congenital talipes equin-ovarus (CTEV), is the most common congenital foot deformity with a reported incidence of up to 27 in 1000 live births, with 50% being bilateral (1). The majority of cases are idiopathic but 20% are associated with other anomalies like arthrogryposis (Figure 5.2), neural tube defects and genetic syndromes (2). There are several theories about its causes with no confirmed aetiology. However, some genetic predispositions have been identified.

Pathoanatomy

A CTEV deformity cannot be corrected passively and is characterised by:

1. Ankle plantarflexion: the foot is in equinus position.
2. Hindfoot varus: the calcaneus is rotated inwards (inverted) with the anterior end locked under the talus and the tuberosity tilted towards the fibula in the horizontal plane. The whole talus is plantarflexed, its head and neck are rotated medially and the body is externally rotated.
3. Midfoot adduction: the navicular displaced medially on the talus and the cuboid is displaced medially at the calcaneocuboid joint.

4. Forefoot pronation: along with plantarflexion of the first metatarsal (MT), there is adduction resulting in a cavus deformity.

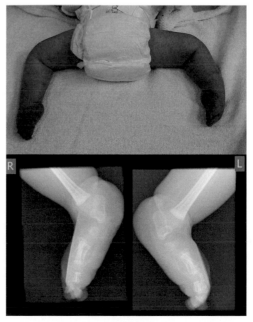

Figure 5.2 Bilateral clubfeet in a patient with arthrogryposis.

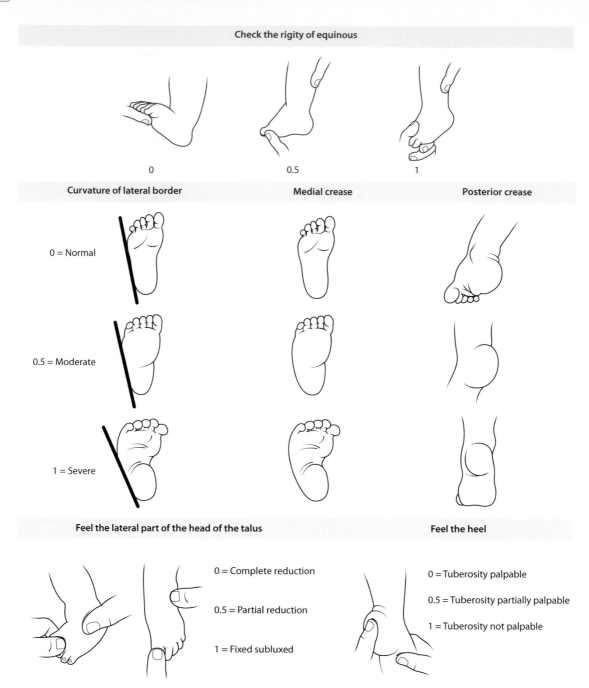

Figure 5.3 The Pirani scoring system for clubfeet.

The Pirani (Figure 5.3) and Dimeglio scores are equally useful to indicate the severity of the different components of the deformity (3–6).

Imaging

Radiographs are not routinely obtained except in atypical and resistant cases. In the dorsiflexion lateral view, the equinus position of both bones decreases the normal talocalcaneal angle and it can even approach 0°. In the anteroposterior view, the talocalcaneal angle is decreased proportional to the varus deformity. The tibiocalcaneal angle in the lateral view is useful to assess the severity of equinus in cases of relapse or residual deformity, to help choose between a revision tenotomy and open surgery, with the latter indicated for a correction of more than 10–15°.

Treatment

Non-operative treatment: Ponseti method of casting

The Ponseti method (7) of casting and treatment remains popular. His innovative concept was to avoid any manipulation of the hindfoot (where the bulk of the deformity resides) and to instead unlock and correct it by just manipulating the forefoot and the midfoot, followed by correction of the equinus with a percutaneous Achilles tenotomy.

The steps of weekly above knee casting follow the acronym 'CAVE'. **C**avus is corrected by elevating the first MT from its pronated position. **A**dduction is corrected by abducting the forefoot around the talonavicular joint by keeping a thumb on the lateral side of the head of talus while maintaining supination. **V**arus of the heel gradually corrects by itself to neutral or slight valgus, as the forefoot is maximally abducted well beyond neutral. **E**quinus is corrected by doing a percutaneous Achilles tenotomy once the heel reaches a neutral or slight valgus position. Forced dorsiflexion will cause a rocker-bottom deformity. Six to eight casts are usually needed. It is important to manipulate the foot to stretch the soft tissues *before* cast application and use the cast only to hold the correction (Figure 5.4).

The tenotomy is best done with a small ophthalmic Beaver blade to prevent neurovascular injury. It can be done under local or general anaesthesia. The post-tenotomy cast is removed after 3 weeks. A boots and bar splint (Foot Abduction Brace – FAB) is applied for 23 hours every day over 3 months and thereafter applied overnight for 4–5 years. Initial successful correction is achieved in about 90% of patients with this protocol (8).

Operative treatment

Nowadays, open surgery is preserved for relapsed and residual deformities. The term 'relapse' is used to indicate that good correction was achieved with the Ponseti method in the first attempt whereas 'residual' deformity indicates that there was only partial correction with the first attempt. The most common cause of early relapse is non-compliance with the use of the FAB. Early detection of recurrence by regular reviews, when it is mild and parental education on compliance is the key to a good outcome.

<2.5 years: Serial casting and getting back into the splint is the first step, but a revision tenotomy may be needed in recalcitrant cases. Unlike a first tenotomy, which could provide 20–30° of improvement, a second tenotomy can be expected to improve dorsiflexion by only about 10–15°. It is best to wait for at least 12 weeks before repeating the tenotomy (9).

If more correction is required, then surgical *open posterior release* is needed. The current trend is to do an *'a-la-carte'* approach and proceed in a step wise manner by initially doing a Z lengthening of the Achilles tendon and proceeding to a release of the posterior, postero-medial and posterolateral capsules of the ankle and subtalar joints as required. Release of other structures (tendons, ligaments, fascia) is done only if required. With the Ponseti type manipulations the forefoot remains flexible and an extensive medial and lateral release recommended in the pre-Ponseti era is usually needed only in those stiff clubfeet associated with other syndromes like arthrogryposis.

Most 'residual' deformities in idiopathic clubfeet are mild and still allow fitting into the splint between surgeries. Those feet associated with severe residual

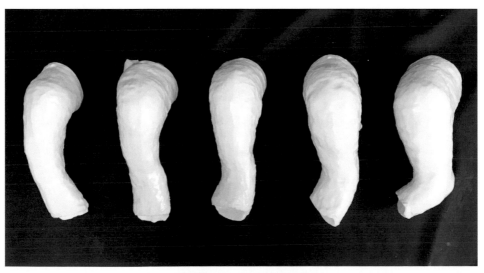

Figure 5.4 Ponseti method casting steps.

deformities cannot be splinted and are best left free until the open surgery.

>2.5 years: Even with good compliance, *Dynamic Supination (DS)* can occur due to a subtle imbalance in muscle power between the invertors and evertors. The feet can be asymptomatic but the decision to do a corrective tibialis anterior transfer should be based on the risk of DS *leading to a fixed hindfoot varus*. Serial casting to tilt the heel into valgus is the first step as a tendon transfer can only bring about correction in a supple foot and is contraindicated if the joints have stiff deformities. Adjunct muscle lengthening and joint releases should be done to correct the varus at the sub-talar joint and equinus at the ankle if needed. A total tibialis anterior transfer to the lateral cuneiform, with or without fractional lengthening at the gastrocso-leus and tibialis posterior aponeurosis, is the author's preferred option. In those who are persistently non-compliant with a splint, the tendon transfer acts as an internal brace.

>5 years: With increasing age, surgical correction is difficult and some residual deformities may persist, but the aim is to deliver a plantigrade weight-bearing foot, which fits in school shoes and trainers. The resistant cases may be 'syndromic' and one should look for associated chromosomal abnormalities, neuromuscular conditions, coalitions, absent or atrophied or adherent muscles in the anterior, medial and lateral compartments. Deformities like a flat top talus can block improvement in equinus, when it is significant, due to an anterior bone on bone block to dorsiflexion (10, 13).

Hindfoot: An extensive posterior release is the procedure of choice for equinus, with extension to the posteromedial and posterolateral corners. Anterior closing wedge osteotomy or epiphysiodesis of the distal anterior tibia is associated with recurrence but can be considered if there is a flat top talus (10). To realign the 'bean shaped' foot in the horizontal plane, a laterally based wedge of bone can either be removed as part of the calcaneocuboid joint fusion (Dillwyn-Evans procedure) or as a wedge resection osteotomy of the anterior calcaneum (Lichtblau procedure). These can be done to supplement a posteromedial release. Mild isolated heel varus can be corrected with a calcaneal tuberosity closing wedge osteotomy (Dwyer osteotomy) +/– calcaneal shift and rotation. The corrections from osteotomies improve with increase in size of the foot.

Forefoot: The adduction and cavus can be corrected with multiple closing wedge basal osteotomies of the first three MTs along with a lateral closing wedge osteotomy of the cuboid and a plantar opening wedge of the medial cuneiform (11).

The Ilizarov method can be also used to bring about gradual correction using the Ponseti principles and aided by appropriate soft tissue releases and osteotomies (12, 13).

>12 years: The Lambrinudi type of triple arthrodesis should be done after all the joint preserving options detailed earlier have been considered. The Lambrinudi procedure involves removal of large wedges of bone and it is best to wait till the foot is of adolescent size. Equinus is corrected by removing an anteriorly based wedge from the anterior subtalar joint and the varus and adduction is corrected by taking a laterally based wedge starting at the calcaneocuboid joint with the apex at the talonavicular joint. Talectomy is rarely indicated as a salvage surgery when all else fails.

Neglected Clubfoot: These are feet in older children where no treatment was provided in infancy. The Ponseti method works even up to 9 years of age with the forefoot and midfoot showing better correction than the hindfoot; however, there is a higher rate of repeated tenotomies and open posterior release (14). Corrections through a triple arthrodesis and external fixators are options (15, 16).

Deformities include – Equinus, hindfoot varus, fore-foot adduction and pronation.

Ponseti Corrective Casting Sequence – "CAVE" – Cavus, Adduction, Varus, Equinus – is very successful.

Pirani score is popular and indicates prognosis and possibility of recurrence. For extended score including toe flexor tightness and Fibula-Achilles interval reference No. 5 is recommended.

Escalating solutions for recurrence – Recasting +/– Tibialis anterior lateral tendon transfer, limited selective soft tissue 'a-la-carte' release, foot and tibial osteotomies, external fixator, fusion.

Look for clinical (bony block to dorsiflexion), radiological signs of Flat-Top Talus in recurrent cases.

Congenital vertical talus

Overview

Congenital vertical talus (CVT), also known as congenital convex pes valgus, is a foot deformity present at birth and characterised by a severe rigid "rocker-bottom" flatfoot (Figure 5.5). It is an uncommon condition of the foot with an estimated incidence of 1 in 10,000 live births and equal prevalence amongst males and females. Half of the children with the pathology have bilateral involvement (17–20). The exact aetiology remains largely unknown; however, 50% of cases are associated with neuromuscular disorders like neural tube defects, cerebral palsy and arthrogryposis, or genetic syndromes such as De Barsy syndrome, Marfan's syndrome, Prune belly syndrome, Costello syndrome and Rasmussen syndrome. Hence, a comprehensive clinical assessment

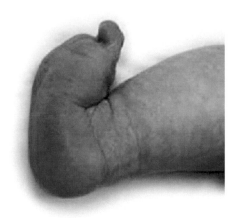

Figure 5.5 Congenital vertical talus with rocker-bottom foot shape.

looking for any syndromic features and full evaluation of the neuroaxis is mandatory for all patients presenting with CVT (17, 21–27).

The remaining 50% of cases with isolated CVT are considered idiopathic, with up to 20% of them having a strong positive family history suggesting a genetic aetiology. Though an autosomal dominant element with incomplete penetrance has been reported, no single gene defect has been found to be responsible for all idiopathic CVT (28–34).

Pathoanatomy

Anatomically, the condition results from irreducible dorsolateral dislocation of the navicular on the talus, and is associated with dorsally placed wedge-shaped navicular, flat plantarflexed talar head, shortening of the lateral column and relative lengthening of the medial column. The anterior talus, which is normally held up in position by the spring ligament, anterior calcaneum and capsular ligaments, including the anterior deltoid, is completely unsupported and in almost vertical plantarflexion. The hindfoot is in equinovalgus due to the Achilles tendon contracture. The peroneal and tibialis posterior tendons tend to dislocate anteriorly, and along with the shortened and bowstringing long extensors they exacerbate the midfoot dorsiflexion and forefoot abduction deformity. Consequently, the dorsolateral ligaments and capsules are contracted whereas those on the plantarmedial aspect of the foot are stretched. The deformity also causes morphological changes to the hindfoot and midfoot articular surfaces and could involve calcaneocuboid joint dorsal subluxation or complete dislocation (35–39).

Clinical assessment

CVT does not usually delay walking; however, if left untreated, children develop an unsteady gait with limited push off and absent heel strike, painful callosities under the dislocated talar head and difficulty finding suitable footwear. Secondary adaptive and degenerative changes develop with time leading to long-term pain and disability (40, 41).

In a new-born, it is crucial to differentiate clinically between a rigid CVT deformity and the more common flexible calcaneovalgus foot, a positional "packaging" disorder characterised by hyperdorsiflexion and eversion of the hindfoot with no joint deformity or dislocation. It appears similar to CVT but only requires reassurance of the parents with advice to perform daily stretching exercises for the dorsiflexors and evertors, which might expedite the rate of deformity correction, as almost all cases resolve completely with no active intervention (42). With CVT, the excessive forefoot dorsiflexion creates a palpable gap dorsally at the site of the dislocated talonavicular joint and a plantar medial prominence of the talar head, which does not reduce with passive plantarflexion, unlike a calcaneovalgus foot where the gap disappears as the foot alignment is restored. Other differential diagnoses to consider include posteromedial tibial bowing, paralytic calcaneus deformity, fibular hemimelia and idiopathic severe flatfoot (43–45).

Imaging

Interpretation of plain radiographs of the foot at birth could be challenging as only the calcaneum, talus and MTs are ossified. The cuboid ossifies during the first month of life and the cuneiforms and navicular ossify approximately at age 2 and 3 years, respectively. The longitudinal axis of the first MT and the talus are used instead to outline the relationship between the talus and navicular (46, 47).

On the anterior-posterior radiograph, the talocalcaneal (Kite's) angle is increased because of the equinovalgus position of the calcaneum. The talus-first MT and calcaneum-fourth MT angles are also increased indicating hindfoot eversion and forefoot abduction.

Dynamic lateral views in neutral, maximum dorsiflexion and plantarflexion are particularly useful to differentiate between CVT and other benign, more flexible, conditions (Figure 5.6). In CVT, there is very minimal change in alignment between maximum dorsiflexion and plantarflexion views. The longitudinal axis of the talus is in extreme plantarflexion and the first MT axis remains dorsally translated onto the body of the talus, indicating irreducible dorsal dislocation of the navicular. The position of the calcaneum in the maximum dorsiflexion view also indicates the degree of equinus deformity. In calcaneovalgus foot, the calcaneum is dorsiflexed, rather than in equinus, and the first MT lines up fully with the talus on plantarflexion radiographs.

Congenital oblique talus (COT) is a mild form of CVT and shares some of the pathoanatomic features but has

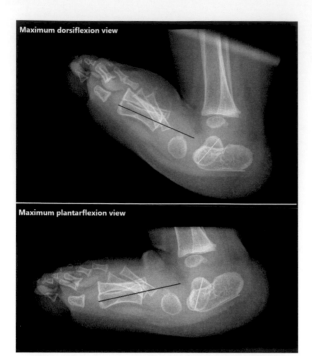

Figure 5.6 Dynamic lateral radiographs of a right foot with congenital vertical talus showing irreducible dislocation of the talonavicular joint. The first MT axis (*red line*) passes dorsal to the axis of the talus (*yellow line*) in both maximum dorsiflexion and plantarflexion views. Note the calcaneal plantarflexed position (*blue line*) which points to the severity of the hindfoot equinus deformity.

the ankle and hindfoot, avascular necrosis of the talus, wound necrosis and reported recurrence of the deformity of up to 90% (51–59).

A more recent minimally invasive approach described by Dobbs et al. has been shown to be more effective in treating CVT with good short- and mid-term outcomes in both idiopathic and those with associated neuromuscular or genetic disorders (60–69).

The "Dobbs" method consists of two stages:

1. Serial manipulation and weekly casting by the "reverse Ponseti technique" is performed to stretch contracted dorsiflexors, evertors and the dorsolateral capsular and ligamentous structures to progressively reduce the TNJ. All deformities, except equinus, are corrected simultaneously using the head of the talus as a fulcrum by manipulating the forefoot and midfoot around it into a plantarflexed and adducted position while gentle counter pressure in a dorsolateral direction is applied to the head of the talus. Manipulation of the calcaneus should be avoided. This process should continue until full reduction of the TNJ has been achieved or when correction progression ceases. In the final cast, the foot shape is in extreme equinovarus and resembles a clubfoot.

2. Minimally invasive surgery is indicated in all cases to stabilise a fully reduced TNJ with a Kirschner wire applied in a retrograde fashion either percutaneously or through a small medial incision and limited TNJ capsulotomy to ensure correct placement of the wire in young children in whom the navicular is not yet ossified and cannot be visualised under fluoroscopy, and to manually complete the reduction of the talar head in partially reduced dislocations before stabilisation. In more severe and rigid cases, an open soft tissue release of the dorsal and dorsolateral talonavicular capsule with or without tendon lengthening of the peroneus brevis, peroneus tertius and dorsiflexors, might be required in a progressive manner as needed. After the stabilisation of reduced TNJ, percutaneous tendoachilles tenotomy is performed to correct the hindfoot equinus.

a more flexible talus and tends to respond more favourably to non-surgical interventions. On maximum plantarflexion radiographs, the navicular position improves but may not reduce completely and the axis of the first MT passes slightly dorsal to the talus signifying residual subluxation of the talonavicular joint. COT should be considered as an entity along the spectrum of CVT severity and not as a separate pathology, and management should be guided by the severity and rigidity of the deformity as COT could progress to become a symptomatic flatfoot (28, 33, 42, 48–50). Those with hyperlaxity syndromes could have an oblique talus on weight-bearing lateral radiographs, which is completely reducible at the talonavicular joint and is a benign condition, which needs to be differentiated from CVT and COT.

Treatment

Traditionally, the management of CVT involved extensive surgical releases of the dorsolateral and posteromedial soft tissue structures, either as a single or two-stage procedure, to restore foot alignment. But as with conventional clubfoot treatment, this open surgical approach was associated poor long-term outcomes and high rate of complications including severe stiffness of

Postoperatively, plaster is applied with the foot in a neutral position to stretch the peroneal tendons and the ankle in slight dorsiflexion to maintain hindfoot equinus correction. The plaster and the Kirschner wire are removed at 5–6 weeks postoperatively and a bar brace is provided to be worn full time for 2 months and then at bedtime time for 2 years. The boots are set to point in a straight position, rather than external rotation in the Ponseti clubfoot method. Ankle-foot orthoses (AFOs), with moulding under the medial arch, are fitted to provide more support when the child begins to stand or walk. This minimally invasive technique helps to avoid complications of extensive surgery and is more likely to result in a relatively more flexible and less painful foot. Recurrence is still a concern, mainly with in patients with underlying comorbidities, but happens at a much lower rate.

In partially treated, neglected or resistant cases a more extensive soft tissue release, including that of the calcaneocuboid and subtalar joints, might be required, especially in children older than 2 years of age. Tenotomy of the evertors and dorsiflexors, instead of lengthening, is likely to be required in conditions like arthrogryposis and neural tube defects to achieve reduction and prevent recurrence. Naviculectomy and arthrodesis of a single of multiple joints are preserved as salvage options (42, 50).

The senior author performs medial plantar plication with advancement of the medial talonavicular capsule, spring ligament and tibialis posterior tendon in every case after stabilising the TNJ. These structures are stretched and tightening them helps buttress the talar head and provides more support against recurrence after removal of the Kirshner wire.

In our centre, in those with only 10° or less of equinus on the maximum dorsiflexion lateral radiograph, fractional lengthening of the gastrocsoleus aponeurosis is done, instead of tenotomy, to avoid overcorrection into a calcaneus deformity, a complication which in our experience becomes clinically apparent only after several years.

Congenital vertical talus is a rare rigid rocker bottom flatfoot deformity.

Differentiate it from the more common calcaneovalgus foot, which is a benign, and flexible.

Check Talo-first metatarsal line in lateral view radiographs in plantarflexion and dorsiflexion.

The "Reverse Ponseti method" involves gradual reduction of the talonavicular joint by casting.

Use the mini open method for wiring of the talonavicular joint and Achilles tenotomy or fractional gastrosoleus lengthening (Author's preferred method).

Paediatric flatfoot

Overview

The core issue with paediatric flatfeet (pes planus) has historically been the difficulty in defining what is normal and abnormal. It also raises difficult questions around the "need" for conservative or surgical treatment and the selection criteria for surgery.

Flatfoot is a very common condition with estimated incidence of 20% (1 in 5) of the general population. The foot arches develop over several years, from the age of 1–10 years old, with a wide range of normal variations. The vast majority of adults and children with flatfeet have no symptoms and their flatfeet have no impact on their daily lives, and hence need no intervention; however, flexible flatfeet with a tight tendoachilles (TA) and rigid flatfeet are likely to cause pain and some degree of disability (70, 71).

Flexible flatfeet

The alignment of the multiple bones that form the foot arch is maintained by the ligaments that connect them, with the head of the talus forming the "keystone" of the arch. The laxity/tautness of the ligaments therefore plays an important static structural role. The muscles are necessary for propulsion and balance and protect the ligaments from abnormal stresses. The "keystone" is particularly vulnerable as it rests on the edge of a bony platform, constituted by the middle and anterior facets of the calcaneum, which can be of variable width (70) and the spring ligament, which forms a "hammock" between the sustentaculum tali and the navicular. In flexible flatfeet, the subtalar joint is dorsiflexed and externally rotated, the midfoot is abducted and the forefoot is supinated relative to the hindfoot (72). This movement of the subtalar joint causes plantarflexion and medial tilt of the talus of a variable degree, resulting in the medial prominence in flatfeet.

Children, who present to a paediatric orthopaedic clinic, having seen a GP or podiatrist, are a self-selecting group who tend to have a visually obvious flatfoot on weight-bearing, causing concern for parents who are often under social pressure to seek treatment as teachers and relatives comment upon the shape of their kids' feet. However, for the surgeon the first step in the treatment of flexible flatfeet is to classify them as either "symptomatic" or "asymptomatic" feet, irrespective of the severity of heel valgus or decrease in the arch height. Only the symptomatic feet need treatment.

Role of a tight tendoachilles (TA) in a flexible flatfoot

1. *Primary TA tightness:* The joints of the foot are like links in a chain and when one is stuck the next link has to move more to compensate. A tight TA blocks dorsiflexion at the ankle. However, when this block is reached during gait, further dorsiflexion is forced by the body weight and the ground reaction forces through the subtalar joint complex, including the talonavicular joint, as part of a multiplanar movement of eversion. The movement of eversion causes the lowering of the arch, a valgus heel and plantarflexion of the talus, all combining to form a flatfoot (70).

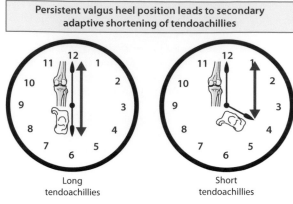

Figure 5.7 Persistent valgus heel position leads to secondary adaptive shortening of tendoachilles – the heel and tibia shown as hands on a clock with loss of height when the heel changes position.

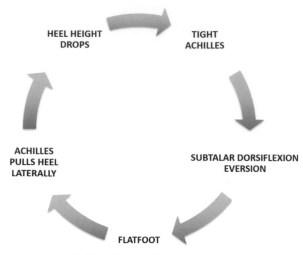

Figure 5.8 The role of Achilles tendon tightness in flatfoot.

2. *Secondary TA tightness:* Those with significantly painful flatfeet tend to avoid sports or jumping activities, which cause the heel to momentarily move to neutral or varus. As the heel remains in persistent valgus during daily activities and the TA insertion is placed lateral to the midline of the limb, its pull during gait exacerbates the heel valgus. The height of the calcaneum is also decreased and so is the distance from the origin to insertion of the gastrocsoleus muscle (Figure 5.7). This causes a further *adaptive* shortening of the TA due to the lack of stretch from sports-related activities, and lack of tension stresses on the tendon due to laxity of the tarsal joints producing subtalar dorsiflexion (70). We have noted that this mechanism causes a significant worsening of flatfeet during the growth spurts especially in adolescent boys, as the TA fails to keep pace with the growth in length of the bones and shortens even further.

It is important to understand the abnormal biomechanics caused by a tight TA as it could facilitate a cycle of progression of the deformity. The tight TA causes compensatory subtalar dorsiflexion, eversion, persistent plantarflexion of the talus, and subluxation at the talonavicular joint (Figure 5.8).

Clinical assessment

Tests for differentiating a flexible and rigid flatfoot:

1. *Toe raise 'Jack' test:* Passive dorsiflexion of the big toe will restore the arch by the windlass mechanism indicating flexibility and is the preferred test in a child under 5–6 years of age.
2. *Tiptoe standing test:* In the older child, a double or single leg tiptoe stance will tilt the heel from valgus to varus and will restore the arch indicating a flexible flatfoot. The child should be advised to do a "high" tiptoe stance, as only then will it show the effect of the tibialis posterior pulling powerfully in a straight line and causing the varus tilt of the heel. In rigid flatfeet, the heel will not tilt into varus but may tilt towards neutral as the ankle has some laxity in a fully plantarflexed position, when the narrow portion of the talar dome engages the mortise.
3. *Subtalar joint passive range of motion assessment:* The assessment is done by keeping the ankle in neutral dorsiflexion, as it locks the ankle by engaging the wide part of the anterior talar dome in the mortise and allows only subtalar motion. Flexing the knee slightly will relax the gastrocnemius and reduce the restriction caused by a tight TA. The heel is cupped in the hand and moved side to side with the forefoot resting on the examiner's forearm. In a rigid flatfoot the movements will be reduced or absent.

Note: In a small group of adolescents with severe flexible flatfeet and high BMI, the tibialis posterior, though having MRC grade 5 power, cannot work against the load of the body weight, around the curve of the subluxed talar head, to tilt the heel into varus, during a single leg tip toe stance. These patients also struggle to perform a high tiptoe stance and the heel usually tilts towards neutral but not into varus. The passive range of subtalar joint is however normal and it is still a flexible flatfoot. This is a "functional" and not a "structural" deficiency of the tibialis posterior muscle and may be due to relative weakness arising from the lack of athletic activities in this cohort.

Checking true dorsiflexion in flatfeet with a tight TA

Dorsiflexing a flexible flatfoot with a tight TA, passively or actively, could show a "false" dorsiflexion, which is partly through subtalar and talonavicular motion. Therefore, to reveal the "true" ankle dorsiflexion and to demonstrate a "hidden" equinus, the subtalar motion should be blocked. With the knee extended, the calcaneum should be passively shifted from its valgus position to neutral and held firmly with a hand to prevent subtalar motion, and passive or active motion will reveal the true ankle dorsiflexion or equinus (70). The Silfverskiöld test is useful for determining if the gastrocnemius is tight in isolation or in association with a tight soleus.

Most flatfeet with *recalcitrant* symptoms will show some degree of Achilles tightness either as equinus or at least a lack of ankle dorsiflexion beyond neutral.

Eliciting peroneal spasm

It is important to identify a rigid flatfoot with peroneal spasm, as it is of prognostic significance. The patient with peroneal spasm has a markedly out toeing gait, severe heel valgus and midfoot abduction and in severe cases the lateral border is just off the floor. Any attempt to invert the foot, and sometimes even just plantar flexing the fifth MT, will cause immediate withdrawal of the foot due to pain, as it stretches the peroneal muscles and triggers a reflex contraction/spasm.

Fixed supination in flatfeet

Passive correction of the heel valgus is likely to reveal some amount of forefoot supination in most symptomatic patients. The first MT head will be elevated relative to the lateral MTs. In the more severe cases when surgical correction of the hindfoot deformity is planned, plantarflexion of the first ray may also be needed.

Generalised hypermobility

Although it is useful to rule out hypermobility syndromes by checking the elbows, knees, fingers and spine for laxity in the joints, isolated subtalar laxity can be a finding in flatfeet.

Treatment options for flexible flatfeet

<6 years: Flatfeet are 'normal' and 'flexible' in the vast majority of infants (3). A consensus for defining by measurement what is abnormal enough to require long-term follow-up remains elusive. Fortunately, symptoms are rare and treatment is required only if they demonstrate a stiff subtalar joint with a vertical talus or oblique talus.

6–10 years: Symptoms, if present, tend to come on only with strenuous activities like long distance walking, repetitive jumping or performing sports. Insoles do not produce a permanent structural improvement in

the arch (72) and so are best prescribed for symptoms of medial overload or abnormal excessive shoe wear on the medial half of the heel. Insoles should have a medial posting (adding a wedge to increase thickness) extending from the heel to the midfoot to correct the heel valgus and support the arch. It can be off the shelf or custom made as a moulded insole.

Correcting the hindfoot valgus with the insoles, will dorsiflex the talar head by normal biomechanics, offloading it and reducing symptoms. Adding medial height to the insole in the area of the arch, without correcting the heel valgus can exacerbate the pressure and pain over the talar head, accounting for some of the complaints of insoles making the symptoms worse.

Physiotherapy for TA stretches should be done while holding the heel and foot in inversion to prevent subtalar dorsiflexion. Tibialis posterior strengthening exercises and weight loss, where applicable, should be advised.

10–14 years: For those children with symptoms recalcitrant to insoles and physiotherapy, surgical options are available mainly in the form of arthroereisis or calcaneal osteotomies with or without medial ray plantarflexion osteotomies and lengthening of the gastrocnemius/soleus.

Arthroereisis (Sinus tarsi implants)

The use of arthroereisis has yet to be accepted widely in the paediatric orthopaedic community, due to poor experiences with the early implants and the lack of criteria for case selection. The basic concept is to reduce heel valgus by blocking excessive eversion at the subtalar joint (73). Those implants, which extend into the tarsal canal, may play a role in reducing plantarflexion of the talus. Some surgeons believe that it may also improve proprioception (74) (Figure 5.9).

The use of this implant in asymptomatic flatfeet, prior to skeletal maturity as part of a guided growth process with removal after 2–3 years, remains controversial. Short-term follow-up of 2–3 years shows the correction

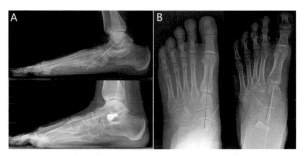

Figure 5.9 Patient with symptomatic flexible flatfoot treated with AR – weight-bearing plain radiographs showing correction of the plantar tilt of the talus on the lateral view (A) and resolution of the medial talar tilt and talonavicular subluxation on the anteroposterior view (B).

to be maintained but long-term follow-up studies are needed (73, 74).

Complications reported with this procedure include migration of the implant, lateral impingement between the implant and the bone causing pain, peroneal spasm or tightening, migration or wrong sizing requiring revision of implants, breakage of implant, early implant removal, undercorrection, over correction, bone erosion around the implant and granuloma formation with some bioabsorbable implants (72–76).

Calcaneal lengthening (CL)

The osteotomy is started laterally about 1.5 cm posterior to the calcaneocuboid joint and directed medially to end between the middle and anterior facet. CL effects a transformational correction through three joints and three planes as it moves the foot anterior to the osteotomy through the talonavicular and calcaneocuboid joints, and posterior to it at the subtalar joint. The navicular is pushed medially and slightly plantar relative to the talar head correcting the forefoot abduction and correcting the talonavicular subluxation (77). The formation of a deep arch, dorsiflexion of the talus, correction of forefoot abduction and heel valgus, and an increase in calcaneal pitch is immediate as the osteotomy site is distracted. This is achieved by correcting the deformity at the virtual CORA (centre of rotation of angulation) which is near the centre of the talar head (Figure 5.10).

Potential complications include calcaneocuboid subluxation, graft resorption, non-union, undercorrection, overcorrection, wound healing problems, nerve injury, infection and implant migration. Suh et al. (76) in their review noted that the non-union rate ranged from 3% to 4.7%, and although the calcaneocuboid subluxation rate ranged from 0.8% to 86.9%, it did not lead to local symptoms or osteoarthritis.

Posterior calcaneal displacement osteotomy

Although popular in adults it is not recommended in children as the default procedure for flexible flatfeet, as it does not alter the deformity at the CORA and only produces a compensatory shift (72). The shift does shift the pull of the TA medially and decrease the heel valgus but does not bring about decrease in forefoot abduction or improvement in the plantar tilt of the talus.

Double calcaneal osteotomy

In severe flatfeet, a second osteotomy through the calcaneal tuberosity may be necessary to correct residual valgus (78). The minimally invasive surgical technique (MIS) is useful and could reduce wound-related risks (79). The "Plantar Malleoli View Sign" is used to assess the correction after CL (74). The correction is ideal if both malleoli are seen when the hindfoot is viewed from the plantar side. If only the lateral malleolus is seen, there is overcorrection. If only the medial malleolus is seen, there is undercorrection and the calcaneum needs to be shifted further with a second osteotomy through the tuberosity. The calcaneal screws used for fixation are removed after healing of the osteotomy in immature skeleton, to allow continued growth of the calcaneal apophysis (Figure 5.11).

Arthroereisis (AR) vs calcaneal lengthening (CL)

Chong et al. (75) compared AR (7 patients, 13 feet) and CL (8 patients, 11 feet) with a 1-year follow-up, without randomization. The patients who had CL had a more severe radiological deformity. Two patients who had

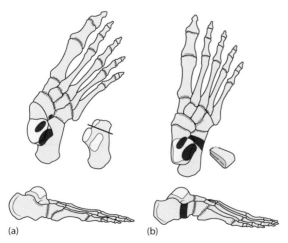

(a)　　　　　(b)

Figure 5.10 Schematic diagram showing the immediate effect of calcaneal lengthening osteotomy in correcting flatfoot deformity.

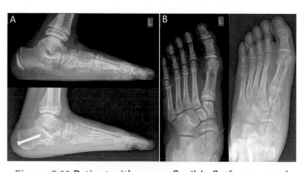

Figure 5.11 Patient with severe flexible flatfoot treated with calcaneal lengthening and posterior calcaneal shift osteotomy (double calcaneal osteotomy) – weight-bearing plain radiographs showing improvement of the talo-first MT lines alignment on the lateral view (A) and on the anteroposterior view (B).

arthroereisis required implant removal and one patient in the CL group needed removal of a staple and another had wound dehiscence. They did not find any significant difference in functional outcomes between the groups but highlighted that longer term studies were needed. They also highlight that arthroereisis is considered an experimental procedure by insurance carriers making it difficult to conduct more studies. They conclude that the less invasive nature and lower potential morbidity suggest that judicious use of arthroereisis implants is appropriate for some patients. However, this study did not have an equal distribution of the severity in the two groups, with the cases having severe forefoot abduction undergoing CL rather than AR and it does not report on the use of AR in severe cases.

Suh et al. (76), in their systematic review of AR and CL, also found that CL showed more radiographic correction, especially with forefoot abduction and also had better AOFAS outcome scores than AR. The main reasons for implant removal in AR were persistent pain and implant migration. Calcaneocuboid subluxation and non-union were the main complications in the CL group. They concluded that CL is indicated for greater than 40% uncoverage of the talonavicular joint. They felt that AR is indicated in children between 8–12 years of age with a chance of remodelling of the subtalar joint. Improvements in the talo-first MT angle and the calcaneal pitch were greater in the CL group compared to the AR group. TA lengthening or gastrocsoleus recession and lengthening of the peroneus brevis, with or without peroneus longus, were the most common additional procedures. The percentage of satisfaction ranged from 68% to 89% and from 78.5% to 96.4% in the CL and AR groups, respectively. However, the studies of CL also had non-ambulatory patients who were associated with poorer outcomes.

Author's experience with flexible flatfeet without associated neuromuscular conditions

The senior author has created a list collectively designated as "Arch at risk signs", which predict a poor prognosis with conservative treatment of flexible flatfeet. Patients with two or more of these signs are likely to fail conservative treatment and they are also a contraindication for AR (Table 5.1).

Arthroereisis: In our practice, the CL is our default procedure with arthroereisis being done only in a minority of patients. As part of the case selection for arthroereisis, De Pellegrin et al. (74) identified two anatomical types of flexible paediatric flatfeet in their cohort of 732 treated with a "calcaneo-stop" type of screw arthroereisis:

1. Pes planovalgus
2. Pes calcaneus valgus (marked flexible valgus of the hindfoot)

Table 5.1   Flatfoot 'Arch at Risk' signs
1. Callosity under the talonavicular joint
2. Femoral retroversion or tibial external torsion or both
3. Genu valgum
4. Severe forefoot abduction (>30% uncovering of the talonavicular joint in the anteroposterior plain film view)
5. Lateral pain (impingement in the sinus tarsi)
6. Inability to do a high tiptoe stance tilting the heel into varus
7. High BMI
8. Equinus greater than 10°

While the first category reflects the common type of flatfoot with a collapsed medial arch, forefoot abduction and hindfoot valgus, the second category reflects an atypical flatfoot where the arch is maintained or only slightly lowered even on a weight-bearing lateral view radiographs but visually demonstrates an obvious excessive heel tilt into valgus, due to marked laxity at the subtalar joint (Figure 5.12). It is possible that the talar heads in these feet have a wider support from the sustentaculum tali and anterior facet preventing it from collapsing (70), while the subtalar joint has ligamentous laxity. These patients do not have excessive forefoot abduction and are ideally suited for AR, as the focus of correction is to reduce the subtalar joint eversion and valgus of the heel.

The senior author uses a titanium implant (80), which has a conical lateral end for seating in the sinus tarsi and has a cylinder extending into the tarsal canal. Our review (81) of the results of the first of 31 patients with painful flatfeet (56 feet) who underwent AR, with a mean follow-up of 51.3 months and age range of 9–17 years, showed that 12 had no pain with any activity, 4 had occasional pain with no restriction of any activity and 11 had pain with sports but not with other activities and 4 failed to improve. The average talar-second MT angle was 35° for those who had postoperative peroneal spasm and 26° for the remaining group, indicating that severe forefoot abduction was a contraindication. Additional procedures included excision of the accessory navicular bone in 8 patients and 1 patient each had a medial cuneiform osteotomy and a gastrocsoleus fractional lengthening. The importance of calf muscle stretching exercises on a daily basis was stressed. In spite of persistence of some limitations in function, 81% were satisfied with the procedure, due to the relative improvement.

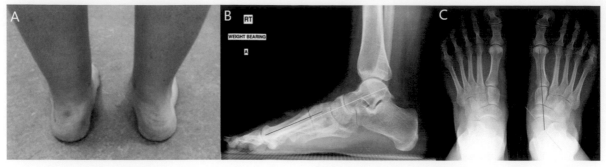

Figure 5.12 Pes calcaneus valgus with isolated subtalar laxity (De Pellegrin type 2) – (A) a weight-bearing clinical photograph showing flatfoot with heel valgus on the right side. Weight-bearing plain radiograph showing no excessive plantar tilt of the talus with well-maintained arch on the lateral view (B), but subluxation of the talus in the anteroposterior view (C).

This study reflects our first attempt at evaluating AR and resulted in the development of the *Arch at risk signs* to help the case selection for AR and CL. There is a steep learning curve in terms of case selection. The ideal patient for AR is an active but symptomatic child who has no *Arch at risk signs* and has Pes calcaneus valgus (subtalar hyperlaxity with increased heel valgus but minimal forefoot abduction). We do not perform surgeries on asymptomatic flatfeet.

Careful case selection and counselling the parents and patients about the limitations of AR is important to achieve a high-satisfaction rate. They should be made aware that if AR succeeds the more complex CL surgery can be avoided and if it fails, the AR implant can be removed and correction by CL can be considered. However, the psychological ill effects on children of multiple interventions should be considered (82, 83).

Calcaneal lengthening: We use the technique described by Mosca (84) (Figure 5.12). We harvest iliac crest graft and fix the calcaneocuboid joint and graft with a K wire. A trapezoid shaped graft which opens the medial cortex rather than a wedge graft is more effective as the procedure is not an "open-wedge" but a "distraction-wedge" osteotomy (84). Although lateral plates incorporating wedges are available for distraction, they provide only an open-wedge type correction. Large and small Hintermann distractors are useful tools to distract the calcaneum and cunciform, respectively, and they provide a clear view for inserting the graft.

The full extent of the equinus is only revealed when the heel is corrected from excessive valgus to neutral. The increase in the calcaneal pitch further tightens the TA. As CL is selected for the more severe deformities, gastrocsoleus fractional lengthening (GSFL) is needed in almost all the cases. An ankle without true dorsiflexion after CL will again force dorsiflexion and eversion through the subtalar joint, causing a recurrence of a flatfoot.

Although there is an immediate transfer of weight-bearing forces from the medial to the lateral side of the foot after CL, the normal loading of the first MT head is not usually restored, as most severe deformities have a hidden supination deformity, which is revealed after correction of the hindfoot valgus. This is borne out by the pressure studies (85), which show a lateral transfer but not loading of the first MT head, in spite of cadaver studies (77) showing some correction of the supination by the plantar translation of the navicular during CL. Palpation of the transverse MT arch after a CL, with the ankle in neutral dorsiflexion, will demonstrate the first MT elevation relative to the second MT, in cases with a residual supination deformity. In our experience, a dorsal open wedge osteotomy of the medial cuneiform (MCO) is needed in most cases to restore loading of the first MT head and this plantarflexion of the first ray further improves the arch. No fixation is needed as the wedge-shaped graft has a tight fit.

Peroneal spastic flatfoot and the accessory anterolateral talar facet

The majority of patients with peroneal spasm and a rigid type of flatfoot have a tarsal coalition; however, a minority has no coalition. All patients with peroneal spasm tend to have lateral sinus tarsi pain and tenderness from impingement between the lateral process of the talus and the calcaneum. It can occur without a tarsal coalition if there is an *Accessory Anterolateral Talar Facet* (AATF) and the heel valgus is severe (86) (Figure 5.13). A high BMI is also a risk factor for lateral impingement (87).

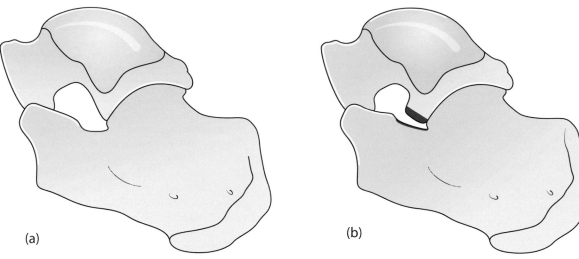

(a)

(b)

Figure 5.13 Accessory anterolateral talar facet (AATF) – schematic diagram of the ankle lateral view showing (a) a normal talus without AATF and (b) an abnormal talus with AATF.

This facet is easily missed on radiographs and is best seen on CT or MRI scans. An MRI scan will also show a typical area of soft tissue and bone oedema at the site of impingement in the sinus tarsi (Figure 5.14). An

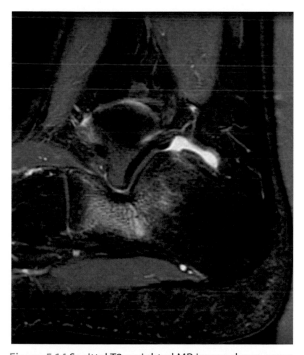

Figure 5.14 Sagittal T2-weighted MR image shows accessory anterolateral talar facet with soft tissue and bone oedema of the talus and calcaneum suggestive of lateral impingement.

injection with steroid and a local anaesthetic drug into the sinus tarsi is a useful diagnostic test, as it temporarily reduces the pain and peroneal spasm.

The lateral pain at the sinus tarsi should be differentiated from the more common anterolateral ankle pain along the stressed Anterior Talofibular Ligament. Resection of this facet is important, when correcting flatfeet with peroneal spasm. Although isolated excision has been reported (88) It has not been effective in our experience, without concurrent joint sparing procedures for flatfoot correction (87).

Majority asymptomatic, symptomatic feet associated with tight Achilles. Examine Achilles tightness locking the subtalar joint. Use insoles with medial posting from heel to midfoot and physiotherapy.

Look for 'Arch at Risk Signs' as poor prognostic indicators for conservative management.

Single leg tip-toe test useful for differentiating mobile and rigid flatfoot with coalition and/or peroneal spasm.

Sinus Tarsi Implant requires more long-term studies. Currently limited use by author for Pes Calcaneus Valgus and not for Pes Planovalgus.

Calcaneal lengthening with bone graft, lengthening of gastro-soleus aponeurosis +/− medial cuneiform open wedge osteotomy currently the mainstay of author's surgical management.

Tarsal coalition

Overview

Tarsal coalition is an abnormal connection between two or more tarsal bones. The majority are congenital resulting from mesenchymal segmentation failure during fetal development of the tarsal bones. An autosomal dominant inheritance pattern with a high penetrance has been suggested (89–94). The bridging may be fibrous (syndesmosis), cartilaginous (synchondrosis), or osseous (synostosis). It is generally estimated to affect 1–2% of the population; however, recent radiological and cadaveric studies described an incidence of up to 13%. Coalitions are bilateral in approximately 50% of cases with no sex predilection. The talocalcaneal coalition (TCC), primarily at the middle facet, and the calcaneonavicular coalition (CNC), between the anterior process of the calcaneus and the navicular, equally account for more than 90% of all cases. It can occur infrequently in any other 2 adjacent bones of the foot (95–100).

Tarsal coalition is classically an isolated pathology, but also known to occur in association with other congenital disorders including carpal coalition, fibular hemimelia, symphalangism, phocomelia, clubfoot, arthrogryposis, Apert syndrome, and Nievergelt–Pearlman syndrome. Rarely, tarsal coalitions can be acquired secondary to trauma, degenerative joint diseases like inflammatory arthritis, neoplasia, infection or be iatrogenic (93, 101–105).

Presentation and clinical assessment

Although tarsal coalition is present at birth, the condition is generally asymptomatic in early years but could become gradually symptomatic in late childhood and adolescence as the coalition ossifies and restricts subtalar motion. Due to the natural ossification progression of the tarsal bones, CNC tends to present at a younger age, 8–12 years old, than TCCs, 12–16 years old (96, 106–109). If bilateral, it is not unusual for one side only to be symptomatic.

Patients mainly complain of vague and diffuse mechanical pain that exacerbates during activity and improves with rest and can be triggered by a minor trauma. The child may be reluctant to partake in physical activities and becomes more sedentary (110).

They can also present with any of the following symptoms:

- *Repetitive ankle sprains and anterolateral ankle ligament pain:* It tends to follow walking or running on uneven ground when the ankle ligaments are stretched and sprained in the process of trying to compensate for the decreased subtalar movements, especially in TCCs. CNCs generally cause less deformity and rigidity as they do not bridge cross the subtalar joint.

- *Pain at the site of the coalition:* This is thought to occur only in cartilaginous type coalitions (osteochondrosis) secondary to microfractures. Often, the pain is localised dorsolateral aspect of the foot and over sinus tarsi in CNC, and under the medial malleolus in TCC.

- *Intense pain over lateral subtalar joint:* TCC is the most common cause of peroneal spastic flatfoot, a syndrome characterised by hindfoot rigid valgus, forefoot abduction, and apparent involuntary painful spasms of the peroneal tendons with foot inversion. These reflex spasms are a result of adaptive peroneal shortening in response to heel valgus. This presentation is often associated with an *accessory facet on the lateral process of talus* and talocalcaneal impingement. Peroneal spastic flatfoot is not pathognomonic for tarsal coalition and may be seen in other forms of rigid flatfoot deformity. Also, patients with tarsal coalition can also present with a normal foot alignment and infrequently with a rigid cavovarus deformity (86, 105, 111–114).

- *Pain over the medial talonavicular joint and spring ligament:* This is due to medial overloading caused by a plantarflexed talus in rigid flatfoot.

Clinically, patients should be thoroughly assessed for foot alignment, gait pattern, points of tenderness, calf muscles tightness and hindfoot joints range of motion. Pes planovalgus and hindfoot stiffness are generally detected. With subtalar coalition, the hindfoot valgus does not correct and the arch does not reconstitute during standing heel-rise test or with the Jack toe-raising manoeuvre (115–117). With longstanding subtalar rigidity, the Chopart's (calcaneocuboid and talonavicular) joints can develop compensatory hypermobility, which can be potentially confused with true subtalar motion.

Imaging

Initial assessment with weight-bearing plain radiography of anteroposterior, lateral and 45° internal oblique views are recommended.

Calcaneonavicular osseous coalitions are best visualised on 45° internal oblique radiographs (Figure 5.15).

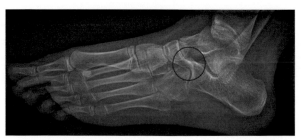

Figure 5.15 Oblique radiograph showing calcaneonavicular coalition and the "Anteater nose sign".

For cartilaginous and fibrous CNCs, the plain radiographs are likely to show irregularity and sclerosis of the bone edges, subchondral cysts, and narrowing of the gap between the calcaneus and the navicular. The "Anteater nose sign", caused by an elongated anterior process of the calcaneus and the "reverse anteater sign", caused by elongated lateral navicular, are two fairly reliable described indicators of CNC (118–120).

TCCs are more difficult to visualise on standard radiographs given the hindfoot anatomy complexity and the overlapping of multiple bony structures. The "C sign", seen on lateral radiographs, is a continuous C-shaped line formed by the confluence of the medial subchondral outline of the talar dome and the posteroinferior aspect of the sustentaculum tali of the calcaneus due to their bony bridging, and is an important radiographic sign of TCC; however, it can also be present in other pathologies mainly severe pes planus deformity. Other radiographic features include narrowing of the subtalar posterior facet joint, overgrowth and rounding of the lateral process of the talus, absent middle facet sign, and a "ball and socket" adaptive ankle changes in early onset and syndromic subtalar rigid coalitions. The dorsal "talar beak sign" can be present in both types of tarsal coalition and is caused by traction of the capsule secondary to altered subtalar mechanics and should not be misjudged as arthritic changes (92, 101, 102, 121–127) (Figure 5.16).

Cross-sectional imaging should always be utilised whenever a tarsal coalition diagnosis is suspected, even when plain radiographs do not show any obvious abnormal findings. Computed tomography (CT) with two- and three-dimensional reconstructions is vital for surgical planning and provides valuable information regarding the precise location, size and extent of the pathology, severity of hindfoot malalignment,

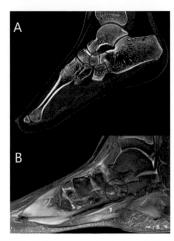

Figure 5.17 (A) Calcaneonavicular coalition on a sagittal slice CT image, (B) cartilaginous coalition diagnosis confirmed on T2-weighted MRI scan.

signs of joint degenerative changes and to rule out any concomitant coalitions. Magnetic resonance imaging (MRI) is more helpful for evaluating non-osseous coalitions, allows assessment of bone marrow oedema and concomitant soft tissue pathology with the additional benefit of avoiding radiation exposure (109, 128–134) (Figure 5.17). In cases with an atypical clinical picture of tarsal coalition, single photon emission computed tomography–CT (SPECT-CT) can help identify the true source of pain to distinguish a symptomatic coalition from an incidental finding.

Management

The main aim of treatment is to provide pain relief. Asymptomatic coalitions should not be treated as there is no evidence in the literature that they lead to future disability and neither does resection of incidental coalitions improve functional outcomes (92, 115, 122, 135, 136).

Conservative measures should be first attempted in all painful tarsal coalitions as the first line of treatment. These measures include activity modification, nonsteroidal anti-inflammatory drugs (NSAIDs), corticosteroid injections, cushioning flat bottom orthoses and physiotherapy for calf stretching and rehabilitation of ankle sprains (96, 137). Short-term immobilisation for 3–6 weeks in a boot or a below-knee walking cast with hindfoot maintained neutral alignment can be offered, with an estimated 30% of patients remaining symptom-free after cast removal for at least 6 weeks. TCCs tend to respond better to conservative treatment than CNCs (108–115).

Surgery is typically reserved for recalcitrant or recurrent cases after exhaustion of all appropriate conservative options. It is vital to counsel patients, and their

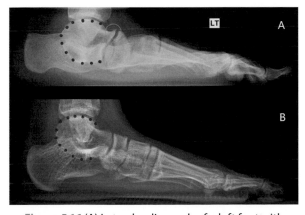

Figure 5.16 (A) Lateral radiograph of a left foot with talocalcaneal coalition with severe pes planus and demonstrating the "C sign" (*red dots*) and dorsal "talar beak sign" (*blue circle*). (B) Talocalcaneal coalition in a foot with relatively normal alignment.

parents, that the goal of surgery is not to restore normal anatomy, as the articulations have never been entirely "normal"; however, any surgical intervention should aim to improve pain and mobility.

There is a lot of controversy in the literature about the ideal surgical management of symptomatic tarsal coalitions. Decision-making is based on multiple factors like age, site and size of the coalition, number of coalitions in the ipsilateral foot, foot alignment and the presence of degenerative joint changes. In general, the options include resection of the coalition with or without interposition in the gap, single or multiple joint arthrodesis, deformity corrective osteotomy or a combination of any of these interventions. Resection at a younger age and that of fibrocartilaginous coalitions could yield better results.

Surgical management of CNC

Isolated CNC with no signs of arthritic changes are best treated with resection of the bridging bar, with good outcomes reported in up to 90% of cases regardless of interposition graft use (115, 138–146). At least a 1 cm thick bone block resection is recommended to avoid recurrence. The lateral border of the talar neck medially and the medial border of the cuboid laterally can be used as landmarks for the resection. Preoperative planning with cross sectional imaging is crucial to ensure adequate resection and avoid iatrogenic chondral injury (147–149). Multiple studies have recommended the use of interposition graft to minimise the risk of recurrence and prolong pain relief. Options for interposition include extensor digitorum brevis (EDB) muscle, at, bone wax, fibrin glue and silicone sheets. Although the use of EDB has shown inferior results compared to fat graft, there is no conclusive evidence to support the use of one type of graft over another, with good results reported even with no graft interposition as with procedures performed arthroscopically (135, 150–159). Arthritic changes are rarely present in the talonavicular and calcaneocuboid joints and considered a contraindication to bar resection. Selective or triple arthrodesis is advocated in these cases.

Surgical management of TCC

This is still a subject of considerable debate, especially with regards to decision-making between resection and arthrodesis.

Wilde et al. (160) suggested that resection should be offered only if three parameters, measured on coronal CT, are met (Figure 5.18):

1. The ratio of the *surface area* of the coalition of the middle facet to the surface area of the posterior facet is not more than 50%.

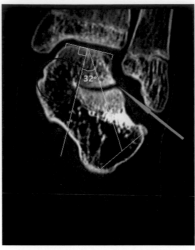

Figure 5.18 Coronal CT scan slice showing severe hindfoot valgus, narrowing of the subtalar joint space (*blue arrow*) compared to the ankle joint and extensive TCC area of 69% measured as a ratio of the middle facet (*red circle*) coalition surface area to the posterior facet surface area; hence, it cannot be assessed on a single CT slice.

2. Less than 16° of heel valgus measured as 90° minus the angle formed between a line extending from the midpoint of the trochlear surface of the talus to the centre of the plantar surface of the calcaneum.

3. Normal posterior talocalcaneal joint space with no narrowing, degenerative changes or evidence of impingement of the lateral talar process on the calcaneum.

Although these measures are widely adopted, more recent studies found quite favourable outcomes in patients with relative area of coalition greater than 50%, and more severe hindfoot valgus but with little or no evidence of subtalar arthrosis (150, 161, 162). Both, open resection of the TCC through a medial approach and arthroscopic techniques, are well established; however, the latter provides much better visualisation of the posterior facet for assessment and to ensure full resection of the coalition, with lower morbidity albeit with longer learning curve (163, 164).

Simple resection of TCC, with or without graft interposition, provides satisfactory symptomatic relief, functional improvement and low recurrence rates in the majority of cases (114, 117, 145, 160, 165–170).

Coalitions and severe flatfoot: In patients with associated severe pes planovalgus especially with pain under the talonavicular joint, coalition resection alone could lead to further worsening of the deformity due to the loss of the medial tether on the tension side of the deformity. In addition the lateral soft tissue contractures and ongoing deforming forces, mainly calf muscles and peroneal tendons, will pull the heel into more valgus. Combining resection with flatfoot reconstruction in a single-stage operation has shown significant improvement in radiological parameters and long-term clinical outcomes (84, 171–174).

Reconstruction surgery is undertaken using an Evan's type CL osteotomy and/or medialising calcaneal osteotomy, a medial cuneiform opening wedge plantarflexion osteotomy, lengthening of gastrocnemius or Achilles tendon and peroneal tendons if clinically indicated. The use of subtalar joint arthroereisis concomitantly with coalition resection has also been reported with acceptable results (79, 137, 175, 176).

Flatfoot reconstruction without coalition resection has also been suggested for patients with extensive coalitions and severe flatfoot deformity even when evidence of posterior facet degenerative changes is present on imaging, as the pain is thought to be related to the deformity itself rather than the coalition (42, 84, 106, 113, 147, 173, 174, 177–180).

Arthrodesis is reserved as a salvage procedure for failed primary resections, multiple coalitions or associated degenerative disease and correction of the hindfoot valgus should be attained. In skeletally immature children, extra-articular arthrodesis, like the Grice procedure or any of its modifications, is preferred to avoid potential growth disturbances of the hindfoot. Triple arthrodesis should be exploited as a last resort, especially in young patients, given the well-documented long-term poor outcomes (113, 181–187).

Tarsal coalition results from failure of mesenchymal segmentation.

Asymptomatic in early years but could become symptomatic in late childhood and adolescence as the coalition ossifies and restricts subtalar motion.

Identifying source/site of pain– Lateral ankle ligaments, Coalition site, Talonavicular joint (Flatfoot).

Imaging – CT / MRI – Identify abnormal Accessory Anterolateral Talar facet causing impingment.

Initially treat conservatively. If symptoms persist, consider surgical intervention - coalition excision, with or without correction of pes planovalgus. Arthrodesis is advocated as a salvage procedure.

Paediatric ankle fractures

Overview

Paediatric ankle fractures are relatively common, accounting for 5% of all fractures (188–192) and about 2% of presentations to paediatric accident and emergency departments (193). In regard to growth plate injuries, the distal tibia is the third most common physeal injury site, after the hand digits and distal radius (194–198). However, it carries a much higher risk of complications and long-term sequela like growth arrest and 3-dimensional deformity. Most of these fractures are from low-energy twisting mechanisms, i.e., rotation about a planted foot, incurred during sports requiring sudden changes in direction like football. Other causes include higher energy mechanisms like crush injuries and fall from heights or as part of polytrauma. Children with a high body mass index (BMI) have been found to be at a higher risk of athletic ankle fractures and sprains (199–202).

The presence of an epiphyseal growth plate is the crucial difference between paediatric and adult injuries. Due to the strong ligaments and tendons in childhood relative to the weaker physis, as it has high turnover of cells, injuries tend to cause physeal fractures instead of sprains as seen in adulthood. However, recent studies looking at distal fibula injuries showed that ligamentous injuries may be more common than previously reported (203, 204).

The distal tibial secondary ossification centre appears at around 6 months of age, whereas the distal fibular ossification centre appears at 1–3 years of age. The distal tibia and fibula contribute 4–6 mm of longitudinal growth per year. This accounts for 40% and 17% of the overall tibial growth and lower extremity growth, respectively. Hence, physeal injury at a young age can lead to significant angular deformity and limb length discrepancy. High-energy fractures, like motor vehicle injuries, and initial displacement are the main predictive factors associated with growth disturbance, and surgical fixation does not seem to reduce the incidence of growth arrest in these injuries (205, 206).

Classification

Salter and Harris (SH) classified physeal fractures anatomically to 5 types. Their classification is still the most widely used system to describe physeal injuries, as it is easy to apply, reproducible and has good interobserver and intraobserver reliability (207–211). The risk of premature physeal closure increases as the severity of growth plate fractures increases with the SH grade. Mercer Rang added a 6th type to this classification to describe a crush or avulsion injury to the zone of Ranvier (Table 5.2).

The Dias-Tachdjian classification is a modification of the adult Lauge-Hansen model in conjunction with SH classification. It categorises paediatric ankle fractures based on the mechanism of injury by describing the foot position at the time of trauma and the direction of the force (29). This system could be potentially useful to facilitate fracture reduction by reversing the applied force. However, it is less popular due to its complexity and poor interobserver reliability (212, 213) (Table 5.3).

Table 5.2 Salter-Harris (SH) classification

Type	Incidence (%)	Description	
SH-I	5–15	Fracture runs along the width of the physis. It is a pure physeal injury with no bony involvement. Only visible on plain films if the growth plate is widened or the epiphyseal and metaphyseal components are malaligned	
SH-II	30–45	Fracture involves at least part of the physis width and exits through the metaphysis, which create a wedge-shaped Thurston-Holland fragment	
SH-III	25	Fracture involves at least part of the physis width and exits through the epiphysis, often involving the articular surface	
SH-IV	<25	Fracture extends vertically across the physis, involving the epiphysis and metaphysis	
SH-V	1	Crush injury to the physis caused by axial compression. These are often diagnosed retrospectively as they cause premature growth arrest	
SH-VI	Rare	Injury to the perichondral ring from open injury or during surgery (iatrogenic). May cause an osseous bridge between the metaphysis and epiphysis and growth deformity	

Table 5.3 Dias-Tachdjian classification

Mechanism	Description		Management and prognosis	
Supination-Inversion (SI)	Grade 1	Traction by the lateral ligaments will produce a SH type I or II injury or lateral ligamentous sprain/rupture	Can be treated conservatively Good prognosis	
	Grade 2	Grade 1 + SH type III or IV of the medial malleolus. Rarely, a medial displacement of the entire tibial epiphysis will occur with a SH type I or II	Requires anatomical reduction of the medial malleolus (closed or open) due to the risk of growth arrest which could lead to a varus deformity of the ankle joint	
Supination-External Rotation (SER)	Grade 1	Distal tibia SH type II fracture with posterior displacement of the distal fragment and posteromedial displacement of the Thurston-Holland	Requires anatomical reduction of the distal tibial metaphysis (closed or open) +/− trans-metaphyseal screw fixation <35% risk of distal tibial growth arrest	
	Grade 2	Grade 1 + spiral fracture of the fibula metaphysis starting medially and running superior and posterior		
Pronation/Eversion-External Rotation (PER)	SH type II fracture of the distal tibia with posterolateral Thurston-Holland fragment and a short oblique fibular fracture		Requires anatomical reduction of the distal tibial metaphysis (closed or open) +/− trans-metaphyseal screw fixation >50% risk of distal tibial growth arrest	
Supination-Plantarflexion (SPF)	SH type II fracture of the distal tibia (rarely SH type I) with posterior Thurston-Holland metaphyseal fragment. No fibular fracture but could be associated with syndesmotic injury		Requires anatomical reduction of the distal tibial metaphysis (closed or open) +/− trans-metaphyseal screw fixation Good prognosis	

Transitional fractures

Distal tibial physeal closure occurs over a transitional period of 18 months. This process typically starts at 13 years of age in girls and 15 years in boys and follows a unique and predictable eccentric pattern. It begins centrally and extends anteromedially then posteromedially, with the anterolateral portion (Chaput tubercle) fusing last. This slow and gradual ossification of the physis presents distinct mechanical and biological environment, which leads to unique fracture patterns in adolescents referred to as transitional fractures. During the earlier phases of closure patients often present with triplane fractures. These injuries are usually caused by an external rotation mechanism. Complications related to physeal arrest are rare with transitional fractures, because patients are already near skeletal maturity; however, poorly reduced fractures could lead to post-traumatic arthritis.

Triplane fractures are multiplanar injuries extending through the epiphysis in a sagittal direction, then axial (horizontal) though the physis, and coronal in the distal tibia metaphysis. They appear as SH type III injury on the AP radiographs and SH type II on the lateral view (Figure 5.19). They have been classified into 2-, 3-, and 4-part fractures (198, 214, 215).

Tillaux fractures occur in the later phases where only the lateral aspect of the physis is open. Juvenile Tillaux fractures are SH type III injuries due to the avulsion of the unfused anterolateral distal tibial epiphysis by the strong anterior-inferior tibiofibular ligament (Figure 5.20).

Imaging

Plain x-ray radiography is the imaging standard to evaluate paediatric ankle injuries. Anteroposterior, lateral, and mortise views of the ankle should be obtained. The mortise radiograph is particularly helpful in identifying subtle intra-articular fracture patterns, such as a triplane or Tillaux fracture. Physeal widening is an important sign to look for as it could be suggestive of SH type 1 injury. Weight-bearing views to assess for syndesmotic injury and full-length tibia radiograph to rule out Maisonneuve-type high fibula fracture should be considered if any clinical suspicion. Good knowledge of normal anatomical variants, such as Os Subtibiale and Os Subfibulare, is key to avoid false-positive diagnoses.

CT imaging is recommended for accurate assessment of fracture patterns and should be obtained routinely for all intra-articular and multiplanar ankle injuries. CT scanning is crucial to evaluate articular congruity before and after attempted closed reduction if there is any doubt on plain radiographs. It also helps with preoperative planning and improve accurate interfragmentary screw placement. A standard ankle CT is

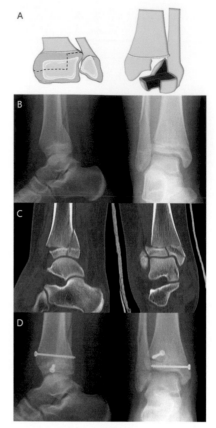

Figure 5.19 (A) Triplane fracture diagram showing a SH-III fracture line on the sagittal plane extending into the joint, a transverse line through the physis and a SH-II fracture line on the coronal plane through the posterior metaphysis. Plain radiographs (B) and CT images (C) of a triplane fracture. (D) Postoperative radiographs showing the fixation with compression screws.

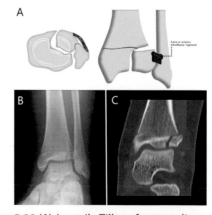

Figure 5.20 (A) Juvenile Tillaux fracture diagram. The anteroinferior tibiofibular ligament (AITFL) avulses a fragment of the anterolateral tibial epiphysis corresponding to the portion of the remaining unfused physis. Plain radiographs (B) and CT images (C) of a Tillaux fracture.

estimated to have a radiation dose lower than a conventional chest radiograph (216).

MRI scanning has a limited role but may be useful to diagnose occult fractures and osteochondral injuries or to rule out infections and or tumours. However, they should be reviewed with special care to avoid confusing paediatric normal marrow signal with potential pathology (217).

Management

The main aim of treatment in paediatric ankle fractures is to preserve physeal anatomy and restore joint alignment and articular congruency to achieve a fully mobile and pain-free joint and minimise long-term complication of deformity, leg length discrepancy and post-traumatic arthritis.

As a general rule, nondisplaced and stable paediatric ankle fractures can be managed conservatively with cast immobilisation and protected weight-bearing for three to 6 weeks. If there is any concern about rotational stability, long leg cast with the knee flexed is advisable.

Tibial fractures

Distal tibia fractures with displacement of more than 2 mm or unacceptable malalignment (any varus, >10° of valgus/recurvatum/procurvatum) should undergo closed reduction. No more than two attempts should be performed to prevent further iatrogenic physeal injury. If satisfactory reduction achieved, fractures are treated in a cast and should be closely monitored with weekly radiographs for the first 2–3 weeks for any signs of redisplacement. Widening of the physis in excess of 3 mm after a closed reduction attempt is suggestive of soft tissue interposition, mainly periosteum, at the physis and open reduction with or without skeletal fixation is warranted.

Post reduction CT scan is recommended for intraarticular fractures (i.e., SH type III and IV, triplane and Tillaux fractures). Articular step-off of >2 mm or widening of >3 mm is an indication for surgical treatment using open or percutaneous techniques. It is imperative to avoid extensive dissection and periosteal stripping at the physis, as this may cause further injury to the growth plate.

Screw removal may be offered after fracture healing, but delayed removal of partially threaded screws may be difficult. Bioabsorbable screw fixation can be used safely in some fractures to obviate the need for hardware removal, but the very high cost of these implants is a major drawback (218, 219).

Fibula fractures

Isolated fibular fractures are often low risk minimally or non-displaced SH type I or II fractures and can be treated with immobilisation in a below-knee cast and protected weight-bearing. MRI studies of children with suspected SH type 1 injuries of the distal fibula identified a much higher incidence of high-grade ligament sprains and very few SH type 1 fractures, challenging the widely adopted concept that skeletally immature children do not get sprains. These sprains can be managed with a removable splint (203, 220–222).

Displaced distal fibula fractures frequently accompany distal tibia fractures and may require closed or open reduction if displaced (>2 mm) with 2 or more years of growth remaining, or if blocking the reduction of the tibial fracture. Smooth wires, instead of screws, should be used if fixation across the physis is needed.

McFarland fractures

These are SH type III or IV fracture of the medial malleolus. This distinct category of injuries can result in growth disturbances and angular deformity in up to 50% of patients. Surgical treatment for these injuries should be considered if initial displacement is more than 1 mm on CT scan and no preoperative attempt at closed reduction should be performed (223–226).

Monitoring: Biannual radiographic monitoring of children who have more than 2 years of growth remaining and have sustained a physeal ankle fractures is recommended until definitive evidence of the resumption of growth in the form of symmetric Park-Harris (PH) growth arrest lines are noted or they achieve natural skeletal maturity. Tenting or angulation of the PH growth lines into the fracture site is suspicious for a growth arrest or a bony bridge formation (196, 227).

Physeal ankle injuries could lead to growth arrest and significant angular deformity and should be monitored for at least one year.

Transitional fractures (Triplane and Tillaux) occur near skeletal maturity and, if inadequately reduced, could lead to post-traumatic arthritis.

CT scanning is very beneficial for preoperative planning of intra-articular fracture reduction.

Undisplaced ankle fractures can be predictively managed conservatively in a plaster, while displaced fractures require anatomical reduction (closed or open) +/– screw fixation.

Take home messages

- Children less than 8 years may trip up when running but gradually stop tripping as the rotational control improves.
- Ponseti corrective casting Sequence – "CAVE" – Cavus, Adduction, Varus, Equinus – is very successful for treatment of clubfoot.

- Congenital vertical talus should be differentiated from the more common calcaneovalgus foot, which is a benign, and flexible.
- 'Arch at Risk Signs' are poor prognostic indicators for conservative management of paediatric flatfoot.
- Physeal ankle injuries could lead to growth arrest and significant angular deformity and should be monitored for at least 1 year.

References

1. Stoll C, Alembick Y, Dott B, Roth MP. Associated anomalies in cases with congenital clubfoot. *Am J Med Genet A*. 2020;182(9):2027–2036.
2. Sharon-Weiner M, Sukenik-Halevy R, Tepper R, Fishman A, Biron-Shental T, Markovitch O. Diagnostic accuracy, work-up, and outcomes of pregnancies with clubfoot detected by prenatal sonography. *Prenat Diagn*. 2017;37(8): 754–763.
3. Pirani S, Outerbridge H, Moran M, Sawatsky BJ. *A Method of Evaluating the Virgin Clubfoot with Substantial Interobserver Reliability*. Vol. 71. Miami, FL: POSNA; 1995.
4. Diméglio A, Bensahel H, Souchet P, Mazeau P, Bonnet F. Classification of clubfoot. *J Pediatr Orthop B*. 1995;4(2): 129–136.
5. Flynn JM, Donohoe M, Mackenzie WG. An independent assessment of two clubfoot-classification systems. *J Pediatr Orthop*. 1998;18(3):323–327.
6. Cosma D, Vasilescu DE. A clinical evaluation of the Pirani and Dimeglio idiopathic clubfoot classifications. *J Foot Ankle Surg*. 2015;54(4):582–585.
7. Ponseti IV. *Congenital Clubfoot: Fundamentals of Treatment*. Oxford: Oxford University Press; 1996.
8. Laaveg SJ, Ponseti IV. Long-term results of treatment of congenital club foot. *J Bone Joint Surg Am*. 1980;62(1):23–31.
9. Mangat KS, Kanwar R, Johnson K, Korah G, Prem H. Ultrasonographic phases in gap healing following Ponseti-type Achilles tenotomy. *J Bone Joint Surg Am*. 2010;92(6):1462–1467.
10. Malik SS, Knight R, Ahmed U, Prem H. Role of a tendon transfer as a dynamic checkrein reducing recurrence of equinus following distal tibial dorsiflexion osteotomy. *J Pediatr Orthop B*. 2018;27(5):419–424.
11. Mubarak SJ, Van Valin SE. Osteotomies of the foot for cavus deformities in children. *J Pediatr Orthop*. 2009;29(3): 294–299.
12. Eidelman M, Kotlarsky P, Herzenberg JE. Treatment of relapsed, residual and neglected clubfoot: Adjunctive surgery. *J Child Orthop*. 2019;13(3):293–303.
13. Prem H, Zenios M, Farrell R, Day JB. Soft tissue Ilizarov correction of congenital talipes equinovarus–5 to 10 years postsurgery. *J Pediatr Orthop*. 2007;27(2):220–224.
14. Lourenço AF, Morcuende JA. Correction of neglected idiopathic club foot by the Ponseti method. *J Bone Joint Surg Br*. 2007;89(3):378–381.
15. Penny JN. The neglected clubfoot. *Tech Orthop*. 2005;20(2):153–166.
16. Kelly DM. *Campbell's Operative Orthopaedics*. 12th Ed. Philadelphia: Elsevier; 2013. pp. 994–1012.
17. Lamy L, Weissman L. Congenital convex pes valgus. *J Bone Joint Surg*. 1939;21:79–91.
18. Jacobsen ST, Crawford AH. Congenital vertical talus. *J Pediatr Orthop*. 1983;3(3):306–310.
19. Dodge LD, Ashley RK, Gilbert RJ. Treatment of the congenital vertical talus: A retrospective review of 36 feet with long-term follow-up. *Foot Ankle*. 1987;7(6):326–332.
20. Outland T, Sherk HH: Congenital vertical talus. *Clin Orthop Relat Res*. 1960;16(16):214–218.
21. Sharrard WJ, Grosfield I. The management of deformity and paralysis of the foot in myelomeningocele. *J Bone Joint Surg Br*. 1968;50(3):456–465.
22. Townes PL, Dehart GK Jr, Hecht F, Manning JA. Trisomy 13-15 in a male infant. *J Pediatr*. 1962;60:528–532.
23. Uchida IA, Lewis AJ, Bowman JM, Wang HC. A case of double trisomy: Trisomy No. 18 and triplo-X. *J Pediatr*. 1962;60:498–502.
24. Stanton RP, Rao N, Scott CI Jr. Orthopaedic manifestations in de Barsy syndrome. *J Pediatr Orthop*. 1994;14(1):60–62.
25. Green NE, Lowery ER, Thomas R. Orthopaedic aspects of prune belly syndrome. *J Pediatr Orthop*. 1993;13(4):496–501.
26. Yassir WK, Grottkau BE, Goldberg MJ. Costello syndrome: Orthopaedic manifestations and functional health. *J Pediatr Orthop*. 2003;23(1):94–98.
27. Julia S, Pedespan JM, Boudard P, et al. Association of external auditory canal atresia, vertical talus, and hypertelorism: Confirmation of Rasmussen syndrome. *Am J Med Genet*. 2002;110(2):179–181.
28. Ogata K, Schoenecker PL, Sheridan J. Congenital vertical talus and its familial occurrence: An analysis of 36 patients. *Clin Orthop Relat Res*. 1979;(139):128–132.
29. Stern HJ, Clark RD, Stroberg AJ, Shohat M. Autosomal dominant transmission of isolated congenital vertical talus. *Clin Genet*. 1989;36(6):427–430.
30. Dobbs MB, Schoenecker PL, Gordon JE. Autosomal dominant transmission of isolated congenital vertical talus. *Iowa Orthop J*. 2002;22:25–27.
31. Dobbs MB, Gurnett CA, Pierce B, et al. HOXD10 M319K mutation in a family with isolated congenital vertical talus. *J Orthop Res*. 2006;24(3):448–453.
32. Gurnett CA, Keppel C, Bick J, Bowcock AM, Dobbs MB. Absence of HOXD10 mutations in idiopathic clubfoot and sporadic vertical talus. *Clin Orthop Relat Res*. 2007;462: 27–31.
33. Hamanishi C. Congenital vertical talus: Classification with 69 cases and new measurement system. *J Pediatr Orthop*. 1984;4:318–326.
34. Thomas JT, Kilpatrick MW, Lin K, Erlacher L, Lembessis P, Costa T, Tsipouras P, Luyten FP. Disruption of human limb morphogenesis by a dominant negative mutation in CDMP1. *Nat Genet*. 1997;17(1):58–64.
35. Drennan JC, Sharrard WJ. The pathological anatomy of convex pes valgus. *J Bone Joint Surg Br*. 1971;53(3):455–461.
36. Patterson WR, Fitz DA, Smith WS. The pathologic anatomy of congenital convex pes valgus. Post mortem study of a newborn infant with bilateral involvement. *J Bone Joint Surg Am*. 1968;50(3):458–466.
37. Seimon LP. Surgical correction of congenital vertical talus under the age of 2 years. *J Pediatr Orthop*. 1987;7(4):405–411.
38. Specht EE. Congenital paralytic vertical talus. An anatomical study. *J Bone Joint Surg Am*. 1975;57(6):842–847.

39. Alaee F, Boehm S, Dobbs MB. A new approach to the treatment of congenital vertical talus. *J Child Orthop.* 2007;1(3):165–174.

40. Lloyd-Roberts GC, Spence AJ. Congenital vertical talus. *J Bone Joint Surg Br.* 1958;40-B(1):33–41.

41. McKie J, Radomisli T. Congenital vertical talus: A review. *Clin Podiatr Med Surg.* 2010;27(1):145–156.

42. Mosca VS. *Principles and Management of Pediatric Foot and Ankle Deformities and Malformations.* Philadelphia: Wolters Kluwer/Lippincott Williams & Wilkins; 2014.

43. Sankar WN, Weiss J, Skaggs DL. Orthopaedic conditions in the newborn. *J Am Acad Orthop Surg.* 2009;17(2):112–122.

44. Sullivan JA. Pediatric flatfoot: Evaluation and management. *J Am Acad Orthop Surg.* 1999;7(1):44–53.

45. Harrold AJ. Congenital vertical talus in infancy. *J Bone Joint Surg Br.* 1967;49(4):634–643.

46. Oestreich AE. Radiology. In: Drennan JC (ed). *The Child's Foot and Ankle.* New York, NY: Raven Press; 1992, pp. 37–70.

47. Katz MA, Davidson RS, Chan PS, Sullivan RJ. Plain radiographic evaluation of the pediatric foot and its deformities. *University of Pennsylvania Orthopaedic Journal (UPOJ).* 1997;10:30–39.

48. Gould N, Moreland M, Alvarez R, Trevino S, Fenwick J. Development of the child's arch. *Foot Ankle.* 1989;9(5): 241–245.

49. Kumar SJ, Cowell HR, Ramsey PL. Vertical and oblique talus. *Instr Course Lect.* 1982;31:235–251.

50. Miller M, Dobbs MB. Congenital vertical talus: Etiology and management. *J Am Acad Orthop Surg.* 2015;23(10):604–611.

51. Bosker BH, Goosen JH, Castelein RM, Mostert AK. Congenital convex pes valgus (congenital vertical talus). The condition and its treatment: A review of the literature. *Acta Orthop Belg.* 2007;73(3):366–372.

52. Zorer G, Bagatur AE, Dogan A. Single stage surgical correction of congenital vertical talus by complete subtalar release and peritalar reduction by using the Cincinnati incision. *J Pediatr Orthop B.* 2002;11(1):60–67.

53. Kodros SA, Dias LS. Single-stage surgical correction of congenital vertical talus. *J Pediatr Orthop.* 1999;19(1):42–48.

54. Mazzocca AD, Thomson JD, Deluca PA, Romness MJ. Comparison of the posterior approach versus the dorsal approach in the treatment of congenital vertical talus. *J Pediatr Orthop.* 2001;21:212–217.

55. Saini R, Gill SS, Dhillon MS, Goyal T, Wardak E, Prasad P. Results of dorsal approach in surgical correction of congenital vertical talus: An Indian experience. *J Pediatr Orthop B.* 2009;18(2):63–68.

56. Napiontek M. Congenital vertical talus: A retrospective and critical review of 32 feet operated on by peritalar reduction. *J Pediatr Orthop B.* 1995;4(2):179–187.

57. Hootnick DR, Dutch WM Jr, Crider RJ Jr. Ischemic necrosis leading to amputation following surgical correction of congenital vertical talus. *Am J Orthop (Belle Mead NJ).* 2005;34(1):35–37.

58. DeRosa GP, Ahlfeld SK. Congenital vertical talus: The Riley experience. *Foot Ankle.* 1984;5(3):118–124.

59. Fitton JM, Nevelös AB. The treatment of congenital vertical talus. *J Bone Joint Surg Br.* 1979;61-B(4):481–483.

60. Dobbs MB, Purcell DB, Nunley R, Morcuende JA. Early results of a new method of treatment for idiopathic congenital vertical talus. *J Bone Joint Surg Am.* 2006;88(6):1192–1200.

61. Dobbs MB, Purcell DB, Nunley R, Morcuende JA. Early results of a new method of treatment for idiopathic congenital vertical talus. Surgical technique. *J Bone Joint Surg Am.* 2007;89(Suppl 2 Pt.1):111–121.

62. Chalayon O, Adams A, Dobbs MB. Minimally invasive approach for the treatment of non-isolated congenital vertical talus. *J Bone Joint Surg Am.* 2012;94(11):e73.

63. Wright J, Coggings D, Maizen C, Ramachandran M. Reverse Ponseti-type treatment for children with congenital vertical talus: Comparison between idiopathic and teratological patients. *Bone Joint J.* 2014;96-B(2):274–278.

64. Jowett CR, Morcuende JA, Ramachandran M. Management of congenital talipes equinovarus using the Ponseti method: A systematic review. *J Bone Joint Surg Br.* 2011;93(9): 1160–1164.

65. Bhaskar A. Congenital vertical talus: Treatment by reverse Ponseti technique. *Indian J Orthop.* 2008;42(3):347–350.

66. David MG. Simultaneous correction of congenital vertical talus and talipes equinovarus using the Ponseti method. *J Foot Ankle Surg.* 2011;50(4):494–497.

67. Aydın A, Atmaca H, Müezzinoğlu ÜS. Bilateral congenital vertical talus with severe lower extremity external rotational deformity: Treated by reverse Ponseti technique. *Foot (Edinb).* 2012;22(3):252–254.

68. Hader A, Huntley JS. Congenital vertical talus in Cri du Chat syndrome: A case report. *BMC Res Notes.* 2013;6:270.

69. Eberhardt O, Fernandez FF, Wirth T. The talar axis-first metatarsal base angle in CVT treatment: A comparison of idiopathic and non-idiopathic cases treated with the Dobbs method. *J Child Orthop.* 2012;6(6):491–496.

70. Harris R, Beath T. Hypermobile flatfoot with short tendo Achilles. *J Bone Joint Surg Am.* 1948;30(1):116–150.

71. Staheli LT, Chew DE, Corbett M. The longitudinal arch. A survey of eight hundred and eighty two feet in normal children and adults. *J Bone Joint Surg Am.* 1987;69(3): 426–428.

72. Mosca VS. Flexible flatfoot in children and adolescents. *J Child Orthop.* 2010;4(2):107–121.

73. Needleman RL. Current topic review: Subtalar arthroereisis for the correction of flexible flatfoot. *Foot Ankle Int.* 2005;26(4):336–346.

74. De Pellegrin M, Moharamzadeh D, Strobl WM, Biedermann R, Tschauner C, Wirth T. Subtalar extra-articular screw arthroereisis (SESA) for the treatment of flexible flatfoot in children. *J Child Orthop.* 2014;8(6):479–487.

75. Chong DY, Macwilliams BA, Hennessey TA, Teske N, Stevens PM. Prospective comparison of subtalar arthroereisis with lateral column lengthening for painful flatfeet. *J Pediatr Orthop B.* 2015;24(4):345–353.

76. Suh DH, Park JH, Lee SH, et al. Lateral column lengthening versus subtalar arthroereisis for paediatric flatfeet: A systematic review. *Int Orthop.* 2019;43(5):1179–1192.

77. Dumontier TA, Falicov A, Mosca V, Sangeorzan B. Calcaneal lengthening: Investigation of deformity correction in a cadaver flatfoot model. *Foot Ankle Int.* 2005;26(2):166–170.

78. Xu Y, Cao YX, Li XC, Zhu Y, Xu XY. Double calcaneal osteotomy for severe adolescent flexible flatfoot reconstruction. *J Orthop Surg Res.* 2017;12(1):153.

79. Mourkus H, Prem H. Double calcaneal osteotomy with minimally invasive surgery for the treatment of severe flexible flatfeet. *Int Orthop.* 2018;42(9):2123–2129.

80. Bali N, Theivendran K, Prem H. Computed tomography review of tarsal canal anatomy with reference to the fitting of sinus tarsi implants in the tarsal canal. *J Foot Ankle Surg.* 2013;52(6):714–716.

81. Bali N, MacLean S, Prem H. British Society for Children's Orthopaedic Surgery Meeting. Leicester, UK: 2013. Arthroereisis for symptomatic paediatric flatfeet – early results.

82. Hu AC, Bertrand AA, Dang BN, Chan CH, Lee JC. The effect of multiple surgeries on psychosocial outcomes in pediatric patients: A scoping review. *Ann Plast Surg.* 2020;85(5): 574–583.

83. Driano AN, Staheli L, Staheli LT. Psychosocial development and corrective shoewear use in childhood. *J Pediatr Orthop.* 1998;18(3):346–349.

84. Mosca VS. Calcaneal lengthening for valgus deformity of the hindfoot. Results in children who had severe, symptomatic flatfoot and skewfoot. *J Bone Joint Surg Am.* 1995;77(4):500–512.

85. Davitt JS, MacWilliams BA, Armstrong PF. Plantar pressure and radiographic changes after distal calcaneal lengthening in children and adolescents. *J Pediatr Orthop.* 2001;21(1):70–75.

86. Martus JE, Femino JE, Caird MS, Hughes RE, Browne RH, Farley FA. Accessory anterolateral facet of the pediatric talus. An anatomic study. *J Bone Joint Surg Am.* 2008;90(11): 2452–2459.

87. Martus JE, Femino JE, Caird MS, Kuhns LR, Craig CL, Farley FA. Accessory anterolateral talar facet as an etiology of painful talocalcaneal impingement in the rigid flatfoot: A new diagnosis. *Iowa Orthop J.* 2008;28:1–8.

88. Niki H, Aoki H, Hirano T, Akiyama Y, Fujiya H. Peroneal spastic flatfoot in adolescents with accessory talar facet impingement: A preliminary report. *J Pediatr Orthop B.* 2015;24(4):354–361.

89. Gardner E, Gray DJ, O'Rahilly R. The prenatal development of the skeleton and joints of the human foot. *J Bone Joint Surg Am.* 1959;41-A(5):847–876.

90. Harris BJ. Anomalous structures in the developing human foot. *Anat Rec.* 1955;121:399.

91. Harris RI. Rigid valgus foot due to talocalcaneal bridge. *J Bone Joint Surg Am.* 1955;37-A(1):169–183.

92. Harris RI, Beath T. Etiology of peroneal spastic flat foot. *J Bone Joint Surg Br.* 1948;30B(4):624–634.

93. Leonard MA. The inheritance of tarsal coalition and its relationship to spastic flat foot. *J Bone Joint Surg Br.* 1974;56B(3):520–526.

94. Graham JM Jr, Braddock SR, Mortier GR, Lachman R, Van Dop C, Jabs EW. Syndrome of coronal craniosynostosis with brachydactyly and carpal/tarsal coalition due to Pro250Arg mutation in FGFR3 gene. *Am J Med Genet.* 1998;77(4): 322–329.

95. Lysack JT, Fenton PV. Variations in calcaneonavicular morphology demonstrated with radiography. *Radiology.* 2004;230(2):493–497.

96. Nalaboff KM, Schweitzer ME. MRI of tarsal coalition: Frequency, distribution, and innovative signs. *Bull NYU Hosp Jt Dis.* 2008;66(1):14–21.

97. Wray JB, Herndon CN. Hereditary transmission of congenital coalition of the calcaneus to the navicular. *J Bone Joint Surg Am.* 1963;45(2):365.

98. Rühli FJ, Solomon LB, Henneberg M. High prevalence of tarsal coalitions and tarsal joint variants in a recent cadaver sample and its possible significance. *Clin Anat.* 2003;16(5):411–415.

99. Solomon LB, Rühli FJ, Taylor J, Ferris L, Pope R, Henneberg M. A dissection and computer tomograph study of tarsal coalitions in 100 cadaver feet. *J Orthop Res.* 2003;21(2): 352–358.

100. Stormont DM, Peterson HA. The relative incidence of tarsal coalition. *Clin Orthop Relat Res.* 1983;(181):28–36.

101. Grogan DP, Holt GR, Ogden JA. Talocalcaneal coalition in patients who have fibular hemimelia or proximal femoral focal deficiency. A comparison of the radiographic and pathological findings. *J Bone Joint Surg Am.* 1994;76: 1363–1370.

102. Spero CR, Simon GS, Tornetta P 3rd. Clubfeet and tarsal coalition. *J Pediatr Orthop.* 1994;14(3):372–376.

103. Mah J, Kasser J, Upton J. The foot in Apert syndrome. *Clin Plast Surg.* 1991;18:391–397.

104. Zaw H, Calder JD. Tarsal coalitions. *Foot Ankle Clin.* 2010;15(2):349–364.

105. Mosier KM, Asher M. Tarsal coalitions and peroneal spastic flat foot. A review. *J Bone Joint Surg Am.* 1984;66(7):976–984.

106. Vincent KA. Tarsal coalition and painful flatfoot. *J Am Acad Orthop Surg.* 1998;6(5):274281.

107. Warren MJ, Jeffree MA, Wilson DJ, MacLarnon JC. Computed tomography in suspected tarsal coalition. Examination of 26 cases. *Acta Orthop Scand.* 1990;61(6):554–557.

108. Jayakumar S, Cowell HR. Rigid flatfoot. *Clin Orthop Relat Res.* 1977;(122):77–84.

109. Newman JS, Newberg AH. Congenital tarsal coalition: Multimodality evaluation with emphasis on CT and MR imaging. *Radiographics.* 2000;20(2):321–532.

110. Linklater J, Hayter CL, Vu D, Tse K. Anatomy of the subtalar joint and imaging of talo-calcaneal coalition. *Skeletal Radiol.* 2009;38(5):437–449.

111. Stuecker RD, Bennett JT. Tarsal coalition presenting as a pes cavo-varus deformity: Report of three cases and review of the literature. *Foot Ankle.* 1993;14(9):540–544.

112. Thorpe SW, Wukich DK. Tarsal coalitions in the adult population: Does treatment differ from the adolescent? *Foot Ankle Clin.* 2012;17(2):195–204.

113. Zhou B, Tang K, Hardy M. Talocalcaneal coalition combined with flatfoot in children: Diagnosis and treatment: A review. *J Orthop Surg Res.* 2014;9:129.

114. Gantsoudes GD, Roocroft JH, Mubarak SJ. Treatment of talocalcaneal coalitions. *J Pediatr Orthop.* 2012;32:301–307.

115. Mosca VS. Flexible flatfoot and tarsal coalition. *Orthopaedic Knowledge Update: Pediatrics.* Rosemont, IL: American Academy of Orthopaedic Surgeons; 1996, pp. 211–221.

116. Jack EA. Naviculo-cuneiform fusion in the treatment of flat foot. *J Bone Joint Surg Br.* 1953;35B:75 82.

117. Mosca VS. Subtalar coalition in pediatrics. *Foot Ankle Clin.* 2015;20(2):265–281.

118. Conway JJ, Cowell HR. Tarsal coalition: Clinical significance and roentgenographic demonstration. *Radiology.* 1969;92:799–811.

119. Oestreich AE, Mize WA, Crawford AH, Morgan RC Jr. The "anteater nose": A direct sign of calcaneonavicular coalition on the lateral radiograph. *J Pediatr Orthop.* 1987;7(6): 709–711.

120. Ridley LJ, Han J, Ridley WE, Xiang H. Anteater nose and reverse anteater signs: Calcaneo-navicular coalition. *J Med Imaging Radiat Oncol.* 2018;62(Suppl 1):118–119.

121. Resnick D. Talar ridges, osteophytes and beaks: A radiologic commentary. *Radiology.* 1984;151:329–332.

122. Taniguchi A, Tanaka Y, Kadono K, Takakura Y, Kurumatani N. C sign for diagnosis of talocalcaneal coalition. *Radiology.* 2003;228(2):501–505.

123. Liu PT, Roberts CC, Chivers FS, et al. "Absent middle facet": A sign on unenhanced radiography of subtalar joint coalition. *AJR Am J Roentgenol.* 2003;181(6):1565–1572.

124. Lateur LM, Van Hoe LR, Van Ghillewe KV, Gryspeerdt SS, Baert AL, Dereymaeker GE. Subtalar coalition: Diagnosis with the C sign on lateral radiographs of the ankle. *Radiology.* 1994;193:847–851.

125. Sakellariou AS, Sallomi D, Janzen DL, Munk PL, Claridge RJ, Kiri VA. Talocalcaneal coalition: Diagnosis with the C-sign on lateral radiographs of the ankle. *J Bone Joint Surg Br.* 2000;82:574–578.

126. Crim J. Imaging of tarsal coalition. *Radiol Clin North Am.* 2008;46(6):1017–1026.

127. Brown RR, Rosenberg ZS, Thornhill BA. The C sign: More specific for flatfoot deformity than subtalar coalition. *Skeletal Radiol.* 2001;30:84–87.

128. Clarke DM. Multiple tarsal coalitions in the same foot. *J Pediatr Orthop.* 1997;17:777–780.

129. Herzenberg JE, Goldner JL, Martinez S, Silverman PM. Computerized tomography of talocalcaneal tarsal coalition. A clinical and anatomic study. *Foot Ankle.* 1986;6(6): 273–288.

130. Cooperman DR, Janke BE, Gilmore A, Latimer BM, Brinker MR, Thompson GH. A three-dimensional study of calcaneonavicular tarsal coalitions. *J Pediatr Orthop.* 2001;21(5): 648–651.

131. Upasani VV, Chambers RC, Mubarak SJ. Analysis of calcaneonavicular coalitions using multi-planar three-dimensional computed tomography. *J Child Orthop.* 2008;2(4): 301–307.

132. Kernbach KJ. Tarsal coalitions: Etiology, diagnosis, imaging, and stigmata. *Clin Podiatr Med Surg.* 2010;27:105–117.

133. Guignand D, Journeau P, Mainard-Simard L, Popkov D, Haumont T, Lascombes P. Child calcaneonavicular coalitions: MRI diagnostic value in a 19-case series. *Orthop Traumatol Surg Res.* 2011;97(1):67–72.

134. Deutsch AL, Resnick D, Campbell G. Computed tomography and bone scintigraphy in the evaluation of tarsal coalition. *Radiology.* 1982;144(1):137–140.

135. Cowell HR. Tarsal coalition – review and update. *Instr Course Lect.* 1982;31:264–271.

136. Drennan JC. Tarsal coalitions. *Instr Course Lect.* 1996;45: 323–329.

137. Gougoulias N, O'Flaherty M, Sakellariou A. Taking out the tarsal coalition was easy: But now the foot is even flatter. What now? *Foot Ankle Clin.* 2014;19(3):555–568.

138. Bauer T, Golano P, Hardy P. Endoscopic resection of a calcaneonavicular coalition. *Knee Surg Sports Traumatol Arthrosc.* 2010;18(5):669–672.

139. Knorr J, Accadbled F, Abid A, Darodes P, Torres A, Cahuzac JP, Sales de Gauzy J. Arthroscopic treatment of calcaneonavicular coalition in children. *Orthop Traumatol Surg Res.* 2011;97(5):565–568.

140. Molano-Bernardino C, Golanó P, Garcia MA, López-Vidriero E. Experimental model in cadavera of arthroscopic resection of calcaneonavicular coalition and its first in-vivo application: preliminary communication. *J Pediatr Orthop B.* 2009;18(6):347–353.

141. Singh AK, Parsons SW. Arthroscopic resection of calcaneonavicular coalition/malunion via a modified sinus tarsi approach: An early case series. *Foot Ankle Surg.* 2012;18(4):266–269.

142. O'Neill DB, Micheli LJ. Tarsal coalition. A follow up of adolescent athletes. *Am J Sports Med.* 1989;17(4):544–549.

143. Skwara A, Zounta V, Tibesku CO, Fuchs-Winkelmann S, Rosenbaum D. Plantar contact stress and gait analysis after resection of tarsal coalition. *Acta Orthop Belg.* 2009;75(5):654–660.

144. Saxena A, Erickson S. Tarsal coalitions. Activity levels with and without surgery. *J Am Podiatr Med Assoc.* 2003;93(4): 259–263.

145. Khoshbin A, Bouchard M, Wasserstein D, Leroux T, Law PW, Kreder HJ, Daniels TR, Wright JG. Reoperations after tarsal coalition resection: A population-based study. *J Foot Ankle Surg.* 2015;54(3):306–310.

146. Fuson S, Barrett M. Resectional arthroplasty: Treatment for calcaneonavicular coalition. *J Foot Ankle Surg.* 1998;37(1): 11–15.

147. Klammer G, Espinosa N, Iselin LD. Coalitions of the tarsal bones. *Foot Ankle Clin.* 2018;23(3):435–449.

148. Swensen SJ, Otsuka NY. Tarsal coalitions–calcaneonavicular coalitions. *Foot Ankle Clin.* 2015;20(4):669–679.

149. Espinosa N, Dudda M, Andersen J, Bernardi M, Kasser JR. Prediction of spatial orientation and morphology of calcaneonavicular coalitions. *Foot Ankle Int.* 2008;29(2): 205–212.

150. McCormack T, Olney B, Asher M. Talocalcaneal coalition resection: A 10-year follow-up. *J Pediatr Orthop.* 1997;17: 13–15.

151. Mubarak SJ, Patel PN, Upasani VV, Moor MA, Wenger DR. Calcaneonavicular coalition: Treatment by excision and fat graft. *J Pediatr Orthop.* 2009;29(5):418–426.

152. Weatherall JM, Price AE. Fibrin glue as interposition graft for tarsal coalition. *Am J Orthop (Belle Mead NJ).* 2013;42(1): 26–29.

153. Masquijo J, Allende V, Torres-Gomez A, Dobbs MB. Fat graft and bone wax interposition provides better functional outcomes and lower reossification rates than extensor digitorum brevis after calcaneonavicular coalition resection. *J Pediatr Orthop.* 2017;37(7):e427–e431.

154. Gonzalez P, Kumar SJ. Calcaneonavicular coalition treated by resection and interposition of the extensor digitorum brevis muscle. *J Bone Joint Surg Am.* 1990;72:71–77.

155. Moyes ST, Crawford EJ, Aichroth PM. The interposition of extensor digitorum brevis in the resection of calcaneonavicular bars. *J Pediatr Orthop.* 1994;14:387–388.

156. Chambers RB, Cook TM, Cowell HR. Surgical reconstruction for calcaneonavicular coalition. Evaluation of function and gait. *J Bone Joint Surg Am.* 1982;64(6):829–836.

157. Bosch P, Musgrave DS, Lee JY, Cummins J, Shuler F, Ghivizzani SC, Evans C, Robbins PD, Huard J. Osteoprogenitor cells within skeletal muscle. *J Orthop Res.* 2000;18(6):933–944.

158. Okada M, Saito H. Resection interposition arthroplasty of calcaneonavicular coalition using a lateral

supramalleolar adipofascial flap: Case report. *J Pediatr Orthop B*. 2013;22(3):252–254.

159. Sperl M, Saraph V, Zwick EB, Kraus T, Spendel S, Linhart WE. Preliminary report: Resection and interposition of a deepithelialized skin flap graft in tarsal coalition in children. *J Pediatr Orthop B*. 2010;19(2):171–176.

160. Wilde PH, Torode IP, Dickens DR, Cole WG. Resection for symptomatic talocalcaneal coalition. *J Bone Joint Surg Br*. 1994;76(5):797–801.

161. Luhmann SJ, Schoenecker PL. Symptomatic talocalcaneal coalition resection: Indications and results. *J Pediatr Orthop*. 1998;18(6):748–754.

162. Khoshbin A, Law PW, Caspi L, Wright JG. Long-term functional outcomes of resected tarsal coalitions. *Foot Ankle Int*. 2013;34(10):1370–1375.

163. Bonasia DE, Phisitkul P, Amendola A. Endoscopic coalition resection. *Foot Ankle Clin*. 2015;20(1):81–91.

164. Bonasia DE, Phisitkul P, Saltzman CL, Barg A, Amendola A. Arthroscopic resection of talocalcaneal coalitions. *Arthroscopy*. 2011;27(3):430–435.

165. Mahan ST, Spencer SA, Vezeridis PS, Kasser JR. Patient-reported outcomes of tarsal coalitions treated with surgical excision. *J Pediatr Orthop*. 2015;35(6):583–588.

166. Scranton PE Jr. Treatment of symptomatic talocalcaneal coalition. *J Bone Joint Surg Am*. 1987;69(4):533–539.

167. Swiontkowski MF, Scranton PE, Hansen S. Tarsal coalitions: Long-term results of surgical treatment. *J Pediatr Orthop*. 1983;3(3):287–292.

168. Takakura Y, Sugimoto K, Tanaka Y, Tamai S. Symptomatic talocalcaneal coalition. Its clinical significance and treatment. *Clin Orthop Relat Res*. 1991;(269):249–256.

169. Kumar SJ, Guille JT, Lee MS, Couto JC. Osseous and non-osseous coalition of the middle facet of the talocalcaneal joint. *J Bone Joint Surg Am*. 1992;74(4):529–535.

170. Olney BW, Asher MA. Excision of symptomatic coalition of the middle facet of the talocalcaneal joint. *J Bone Joint Surg Am*. 1987;69(4):539–544.

171. Kernbach KJ, Blitz NM, Rush SM. Bilateral single-stage middle facet talocalcaneal coalition resection combined with flatfoot reconstruction: A report of 3 cases and review of the literature. Investigations involving middle facet coalitions–part 1. *J Foot Ankle Surg*. 2008;47(3):180–190.

172. Kothari A, Masquijo J. Surgical treatment of tarsal coalitions in children and adolescents. *EFORT Open Rev*. 2020;5(2):80–89.

173. Mosca VS, Bevan WP. Talocalcaneal tarsal coalitions and the calcaneal lengthening osteotomy: The role of deformity correction. *J Bone Joint Surg Am*. 2012;94(17):1584–1594.

174. Javier Masquijo J, Vazquez I, Allende V, Lanfranchi L, Torres-Gomez A, Dobbs MB. Surgical reconstruction for talocalcaneal coalitions with severe hindfoot valgus deformity. *J Pediatr Orthop*. 2017;37(4):293–297.

175. Giannini S, Ceccarelli F, Vannini F, Baldi E. Operative treatment of flatfoot with talocalcaneal coalition. *Clin Orthop Relat Res*. 2003;(411):178–187.

176. Koutsogiannis E. Treatment of mobile flat foot by displacement osteotomy of the calcaneus. *J Bone Joint Surg Br*. 1971;53(1):96–100.

177. Dwyer FC. President's address. Causes, significance and treatment of stiffness of the subtaloid joint. *Proc R Soc Med*. 1976;69(2):97–102.

178. Cain TJ, Hyman S. Peroneal spastic flat foot. Its treatment by osteotomy of the os calcis. *J Bone Joint Surg Br*. 1978;60-B(4):527–529.

179. Evans D. Calcaneo-valgus deformity. *J Bone Joint Surg Br*. 1975;57(3):270–278.

180. Mosca VS. Calcaneal lengthening osteotomy for valgus deformity of the hindfoot. *Master Techniques in Orthopaedic Surgery: Pediatrics*. Philadelphia: Lippincott Williams & Wilkins; 2008, pp. 263–276.

181. Grice DS. An extra-articular arthrodesis of the subastragalar joint for correction of paralytic flat feet in children. *J Bone Joint Surg Am*. 1952;34 A(4):927–940.

182. Høiness PR, Kirkhus E. Grice arthrodesis in the treatment of valgus feet in children with myelomeningocele: A 12.8-year follow-up study. *J Child Orthop*. 2009;3(4):283–290.

183. Drew AJ. The late results of arthrodesis of the foot. *J Bone Joint Surg Br*. 1951;33-B(4):496–502.

184. Adelaar RS, Dannelly EA, Meunier PA, Stelling FH, Goldner JL, Colvard DF. A long term study of triple arthrodesis in children. *Orthop Clin North Am*. 1976;7(4):895–908.

185. Southwell RB, Sherman FC. Triple arthrodesis: A long-term study with force plate analysis. *Foot Ankle*. 1981;2(1):15–24.

186. Angus PD, Cowell HR. Triple arthrodesis. A critical long-term review. *J Bone Joint Surg Br*. 1986;68(2):260–265.

187. Saltzman CL, Fehrle MJ, Cooper RR, Spencer EC, Ponseti IV. Triple arthrodesis: Twenty-five and forty-four-year average follow-up of the same patients. *J Bone Joint Surg Am*. 1999;81(10):1391–1402.

188. Barmada A, Gaynor T, Mubarak SJ. Premature physeal closure following distal tibia physeal fractures: A new radiographic predictor. *J Pediatr Orthop*. 2003;23(6):733–739.

189. Mann DC, Rajmaira S. Distribution of physeal and nonphyseal fractures in 2,650 long-bone fractures in children aged 0-16 years. *J Pediatr Orthop*. 1990;10(6):713–716.

190. Mizuta T, Benson WM, Foster BK, Paterson DC, Morris LL. Statistical analysis of the incidence of physeal injuries. *J Pediatr Orthop*. 1987;7(5):518–523.

191. Worlock P, Stower M. Fracture patterns in Nottingham children. *J Pediatr Orthop*. 1986;6(6):656–660.

192. Landin LA, Danielsson LG. Children's ankle fractures. Classification and epidemiology. *Acta Orthop Scand*. 1983;54(4):634–640.

193. Boutis K, Von Keyserlingk C, Willan A, Narayana UG, Brison R, Grootendorst P, Plint AC, Parker M, Goeree R. Cost consequence analysis of implementing the low risk ankle rule in emergency departments. *Ann Emerg Med*. 2015;66(5):455–463.e4.

194. Peterson CA, Peterson HA. Analysis of the incidence of injuries to the epiphyseal growth plate. *J Trauma*. 1972;12(4):275–281.

195. Peterson HA, Madhok R, Benson JT, Ilstrup DM, Melton LJ 3rd. Physeal fractures: Part 1. Epidemiology in Olmsted County, Minnesota, 1979–1988. *J Pediatr Orthop*. 1994;14(4):423–430.

196. Hynes D, O'Brien T. Growth disturbance lines after injury of the distal tibial physis. Their significance in prognosis. *J Bone Joint Surg Br*. 1988;70:231–233.

197. W H O, Craig C, Banks HH. Epiphyseal injuries. *Pediatr Clin North Am*. 1974;21(2):407–422.

198. Rapariz JM, Ocete G, González-Herranz P, López-Mondejar JA, Domenech J, Burgos J, Amaya S. Distal tibial

triplane fractures: Long-term follow-up. *J Pediatr Orthop.* 1996;16(1):113–118.

199. Ebbeling CB, Pawlak DB, Ludwig DS. Childhood obesity: Public-health crisis, common sense cure. *Lancet.* 2002;360(9331):473–482.

200. McHugh MP. Oversized young athletes: A weighty concern. *Br J Sports Med.* 2010;44(1):45–49.

201. Tyler TF, McHugh MP, Mirabella MR, Mullaney MJ, Nicholas SJ. Risk factors for noncontact ankle sprains in high school football players: The role of previous ankle sprains and body mass index. *Am J Sports Med.* 2006;34(3):471–475.

202. Zonfrillo MR, Seiden JA, House EM, Shapiro ED, Dubrow R, Baker MD, Spiro DM. The association of overweight and ankle injuries in children. *Ambul Pediatr.* 2008;8(1):66–69.

203. Boutis K, Narayanan UG, Dong FF, Mackenzie H, Yan H, Chew D, Babyn P. Magnetic resonance imaging of clinically suspected Salter-Harris I fracture of the distal fibula. *Injury.* 2010;41(8):852–856.

204. Mallick A, Prem H. Physeal injuries in children. *Surgery (Oxford).* 2017;35(1):10–17.

205. Leary JT, Handling M, Talerico M, Yong L, Bowe JA. Physeal fractures of the distal tibia: Predictive factors of premature physeal closure and growth arrest. *J Pediatr Orthop.* 2009;29(4):356–361.

206. Russo F, Moor MA, Mubarak SJ, Pennock AT. Salter-Harris II fractures of the distal tibia: Does surgical management reduce the risk of premature physeal closure? *J Pediatr Orthop.* 2013;33(5):524–529.

207. Salter RB. Injuries of the ankle in children. *Orthop Clin North Am.* 1974;5(1):147–152.

208. Salter RB. Injuries of the epiphyseal plate. *Instr Course Lect.* 1992;41:351–359.

209. Cepela DJ, Tartaglione JP, Dooley TP, Patel PN. Classifications in brief: Salter-Harris classification of pediatric physeal fractures. *Clin Orthop Relat Res.* 2016;474(11):2531–2537.

210. Podeszwa DA, Mubarak SJ. Physeal fractures of the distal tibia and fibula (Salter-Harris Type I, II, III, and IV fractures). *J Pediatr Orthop.* 2012;32(Suppl 1):S62 S68.

211. Salter RB, Harris WR. Injuries involving the epiphyseal plate. *J Bone Joint Surg Am.* 1963;45(3):587–622.

212. Dias LS, Tachdjian MO. Physeal injuries of the ankle in children: Classification. *Clin Orthop Relat Res.* 1978;(136):230–233.

213. Eduardo B, Fernando M, Bibiana DR. A comparison of two classification systems for pediatric ankle fractures. *J Clin Exp Orthop.* 2016;2(3):22.

214. Kärrholm J. The triplane fracture: Four years of follow-up of 21 cases and review of the literature. *J Pediatr Orthop B.* 1997;6(2):91–102.

215. Cooperman DR, Spiegel PG, Laros GS. Tibial fractures involving the ankle in children: The so-called triplane epiphyseal fracture. *J Bone Joint Surg Am.* 1978;60(8):1040–1046.

216. Biswas D, Bible JE, Bohan M, Simpson AK, Whang PG, Grauer JN. Radiation exposure from musculoskeletal computerized tomographic scans. *J Bone Joint Surg Am.* 2009;91(8):1882–1889.

217. Shabshin N, Schweitzer ME, Morrison WB, Carrino JA, Keller MS, Grissom LE. High-signal T2 changes of the bone marrow of the foot and ankle in children: Red marrow or traumatic changes? *Pediatr Radiol.* 2006;36(7):670–676.

218. Podeszwa DA, Wilson PL, Holland AR, Copley LA. Comparison of bioabsorbable versus metallic implant fixation for physeal and epiphyseal fractures of the distal tibia. *J Pediatr Orthop.* 2008;28(8):859–863.

219. Böstman OM. Metallic or absorbable fracture fixation devices. A cost minimization analysis. *Clin Orthop Relat Res.* 1996;(329):233–239.

220. Launay F, Barrau K, Petit P, Jouve JL, Auquier P, Bollini G. Traumatismes de la cheville sans fracture chez l'enfant. Etude prospective par résonance magnétique de 116 patients [Ankle injuries without fracture in children. Prospective study with magnetic resonance in 116 patients]. *Rev Chir Orthop Reparatrice Appar Mot.* 2008;94(5):427–433.

221. Lohman M, Kivisaari A, Kallio P, Puntila J, Vehmas T, Kivisaari L. Acute paediatric ankle trauma: MRI versus plain radiography. *Skeletal Radiol.* 2001;30(9):504–511.

222. Stuart J, Boyd R, Derbyshire S, Wilson B, Phillips B. Magnetic resonance assessment of inversion ankle injuries in children. *Injury.* 1998;29(1):29–30.

223. McFarland B. Traumatic arrest of epiphysial growth at the lower end of the tibia. *Br J Surg.* 1931;19(73):78–82.

224. Cass JR, Peterson HA. Salter-Harris Type-IV injuries of the distal tibial epiphyseal growth plate, with emphasis on those involving the medial malleolus. *J Bone Joint Surg Am.* 1983;65(8):1059–1070.

225. Seel EH, Noble S, Clarke NM, Uglow MG. Outcome of distal tibial physeal injuries. *J Pediatr Orthop B.* 2011;20(4):242–248.

226. Spiegel PG, Cooperman DR, Laros GS. Epiphyseal fractures of the distal ends of the tibia and fibula. A retrospective study of two hundred and thirty-seven cases in children. *J Bone Joint Surg Am.* 1978;60(8):1046–1050.

227. Mencio GA, Swiontkowski MF. *Green's Skeletal Trauma in Children.* 5th Ed. Philadelphia: Elsevier/Saunders; 2014.

Rajesh Kakwani

Introduction

Amongst the forefoot pathologies seen in outpatient clinics, most relate to the first ray either directly or indirectly. The majority of forefoot conditions can be treated conservatively with footwear modifications. Surgery generally attempts to restore the mechanics of the foot and transfer the weight-bearing function back to the first ray. Heel weight-bearing in a protective shoe is commonly allowed for the first 6 weeks. It can take up to 6 months for the swelling and discomfort to improve following forefoot surgery.

Hallux valgus

Introduction

Hallux valgus is one of the most common pathologies encountered in the outpatient clinic. First ray surgery was one of the indexed surgical procedures on the orthopaedic curriculum. There are hundreds of operations described for the treatment of hallux valgus, which itself demonstrates that no single operation addresses the varied spectrum of hallux valgus presentation.

Aetiology

Up to two-thirds of patients with hallux valgus have a family history of similar affection. Narrow shoes and high heeled shoes have also been associated with a higher incidence of hallux valgus. The common associations being pes planus and hypermobility syndrome (1).

Pathogenesis

Stephens attributes weakening of the medial capsular structures of the great toe metatarsophalangeal joint which allows the proximal phalanx to move into valgus and the 1st metatarsal move into varus (2). This causes prominence of the 1st metatarsal head medially. The constant rubbing of the metatarsal head against footwear can lead to the development of a bursa over the medial aspect of the metatarsal head. Eventually, the line of action of the extensor hallucis longus and the flexor hallucis longus moves lateral to the 1st metatarsophalangeal joint which renders them to become deforming forces along with the adductor hallucis, hence worsening the deformity. The ridge on the plantar aspect of the metatarsal head between the medial and lateral sesamoid eventually gets eroded and the metatarsal head subluxes medially beyond the sesamoids. The factor to note is that the sesamoids remain in the same position and it is the metatarsal head which subluxes medially. The resulted imbalance of forces at the metatarsophalangeal joint causes pronation of the big toe and also dorsiflexes the first ray and thus renders the first ray dysfunctional. This leads to overloading of the lesser rays and transfer metatarsalgia, as well as, deformities of the 2nd toe in the form of a hammer or a claw toe.

Clinical examination

Clinical presentation

The common presenting symptoms, in addition to pain, are cosmetic deformity in almost two-thirds of cases or transfer metatarsalgia in about 40%.

The pain can be localised to the metatarsal head prominence medially. It is worse whilst wearing tight footwear and is eased when the shoes are removed. Patients struggle in finding appropriate footwear to accommodate their deformity. Occasionally, patients complain of a neuropathic type of pain in the distribution of the dorsomedial cutaneous nerve of the great toe, due to the pressure symptoms. The patients can also present with lesser toe deformities and crowding of the lesser rays (Figure 6.1).

Examination

Standing position

The deformities are exaggerated when weight-bearing. There would be an obvious hallux valgus deformity with prominence of the medial aspect of the metatarsal head, i.e., the bunion (Figure 6.1). The common association would be a planovalgus foot, lesser toe deformities

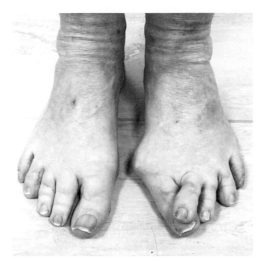

Figure 6.1 Severe hallux valgus with pronation of great toe and crossover second toe.

especially claw or hammer toes +/– lateral deviation of lesser toes.

Single leg heel raise is performed to assess hindfoot flexibility as well as the integrity of the tibialis posterior tendon.

Gait is examined for restoration of medial arch during toe-off position.

Sitting position

The correctability of the deformity is assessed by compressing the metatarsals together. The sole of the foot is inspected for any callosities especially under the lesser toe metatarsal heads or over the medial border of the big toe. Interdigital spaces are examined for interdigital neuromas as well as for any corns or callosities between the lesser toes. The range of movements of the great toe metatarsophalangeal joint has to be documented in the deformed position and in the corrected position, if possible.

Pain and crepitus within the range of movement of the great toe metatarsophalangeal joint, when the deformity is corrected, suggests intra-articular pathology. A positive grind test suggests arthritis affecting the great toe metatarsophalangeal joint. The 1st tarsometatarsal joint needs to be assessed for any instability by doing a Lachman test type of ballottement between the medial cuneiform and the 1st metatarsal base.

Movements of more than 9 mm suggest hypermobility. If this is found, it should be supplemented with a Beighton score. If the deformity is correctable passively, one can note the improvement of the power of the flexor hallucis longus in the corrected position, when compared to the same power in the deformed position. The lesser toe deformities need to be assessed for their flexibility. Silfverskiöld test is performed to rule out

any gastrocnemius tightness. Complete neurovascular examination would be performed at this stage. It is important to document the sensation assessment in the dorsomedial cutaneous nerve of the first ray, especially in cases where a curvilinear incision was used during previous first ray surgery.

Footwear and insoles are examined for any wear due to the prominence of the 1st metatarsal head.

Investigations

Weight-bearing anteroposterior and lateral radiographs of the foot performed to assess the degree of deformity and assist management decision. The congruency of the 1st metatarsophalangeal joint is noted. The following angles are calculated and recorded (Figure 6.2) and the severity is assessed to help guide the most appropriate management (Table 6.1).

1. **Hallux valgus angle:** angle between the long axis of the 1st metatarsal and the proximal phalanx
2. **Intermetatarsal angle:** angle between the 1st and 2nd metatarsal
3. **Distal metatarsal articular angle:** the angle between the distal articular surface and the perpendicular line to the long axis of 1st metatarsal

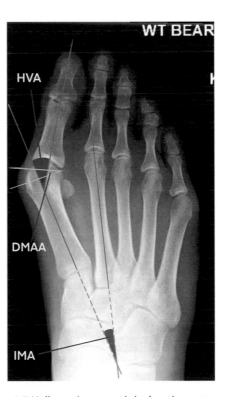

Figure 6.2 Hallux valgus – weight-bearing anteroposterior radiographs demonstrating the various angles. (Abbreviations: DMAA, distal metatarsal articular angle; HVA, hallux valgus angle; IMA, intermetatarsal angle.)

Table 6.1 Table illustrating the severity of hallux valgus (1)

	Hallux valgus angle	Intermetatarsal angle	Author's preferred surgical option
Normal	Up to 15°	Up to 9°	
Mild	15°–19°	9°–13°	Distal metatarsal osteotomy
Moderate	20°–40°	14°–20°	Metatarsal shaft osteotomy
Severe	More than 40°	More than 20°	Lapidus/Proximal osteotomy

Source: Robinson AHN (1).

Management

Conservative management

The mainstay of conservative management would be patient education, reassurance, activity modification and accommodative footwear with wide toe box shoes and gastrocnemius stretching exercises (if Silfverskiöld test positive). Foot orthoses, in the form of spacers between the big toe and lesser toe or straps to adduct the big toe proximal phalanx, can be utilised for symptomatic relief.

Operative management

The main indication for operative management is failure of control of pain despite conservative measures. Correction of the hallux valgus, for cosmetic reasons only, is not recommended. Be ready to say 'NO' if unrealistic improvements are expected after surgical correction. It is important to match patient's and surgeon's expectations and surgery is considered only as part of a shared decision-making process.

The *mainstay of deformity correction surgery* is to restore the mechanics of the big toe:

1. Restoring the 1st metatarsal head over the sesamoids,
2. Reducing the intermetatarsal angle back to normal,
3. A congruous 1st metatarsophalangeal joint and
4. Correction of rotational deformity, e.g., pronation.

The type of operation generally depends on the severity of the hallux valgus. Hundreds of osteotomies have been described for correction of hallux valgus.

The 1st metatarsal osteotomy involves translation of the distal fragment laterally to reposition the metatarsal head over the sesamoids. In order to create space for the metatarsal head to move laterally, the soft tissue release needed would include a metatarsal sesamoid suspensory (Figure 6.3) +/- the adductor hallucis tendon.

The blood supply to the 1st metatarsal head is derived from the 1st dorsal and 1st plantar metatarsal artery on the lateral side and medially from the superficial branch of the medial plantar artery. These generally form a leash of vessels which enter the 1st metatarsal head just proximal to its inferior articular surface (Figure 6.4). It is important to be careful so that the essential vascular supply on the plantar aspect of the 1st metatarsal neck is not compromised.

Damage to blood supply of the 1st metatarsal head can lead to avascular necrosis of the 1st metatarsal head. Therefore, it is important when performing a distal metatarsal osteotomy to ensure that the dorsal and plantar cuts of the Chevron extend proximal to the capsular attachments of the 1st metatarsal head. Also, that the cuts do not extend beyond the lateral cortex of the 1st metatarsal.

Distal Chevron osteotomy

This is a v-shaped osteotomy of the 1st metatarsal with the apex distal (Figure 6.4). Lateral displacement of the 1st metatarsal head fragment is performed to restore the 1st metatarsal head over the sesamoids.

The main complication of the Chevron osteotomy is avascular necrosis of the 1st metatarsal head which is seen in up to 20% of cases in certain studies especially if simultaneous lateral release is performed.

Diaphyseal Scarf osteotomy

Scarf osteotomy (Figure 6.4) involves a z-shaped diaphyseal osteotomy of the 1st metatarsal. A slight plantar slope is recommended, to allow plantar translation of the 1st metatarsal head as the distal fragment is displaced laterally. This allows restoration of the loading of the first ray. The osteotomy is held rigidly with two compression screws.

The main complication is guttering of the two osteotomy fragments leading to dorsal displacement of the 1st metatarsal head fragment and increasing the risk of transfer metatarsalgia.

Basal osteotomies

Medial opening wedge osteotomies of the 1st metatarsal base with bone grafting have been associated with a high risk of non-union.

Lateral closing wedge osteotomies of the base of first ray increases the risks of transfer metatarsalgia due to shortening of the metatarsal.

Crescentic/dome osteotomies of the 1st metatarsal base are technically more difficult and can lead to minimal shortening of the first ray. They have demonstrated excellent results in various studies (3).

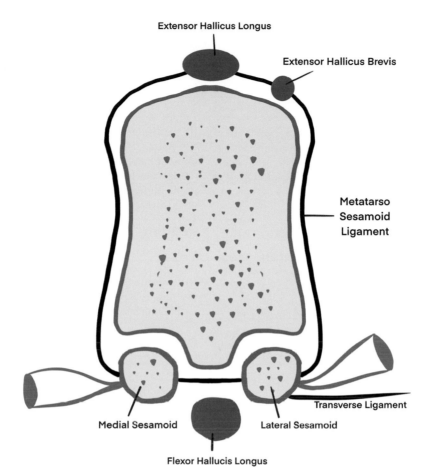

Extensor Hallicus Longus

Extensor Hallicus Brevis

Metatarso
Sesamoid
Ligament

Transverse Ligament

Medial Sesamoid   Lateral Sesamoid

Flexor Hallucis Longus

Figure 6.3 Axial anatomy of the 1st metatarsal head at the level of the sesamoids.

Akin osteotomy

A medial closing wedge osteotomy of the proximal phalanx of the first ray is recommended in certain cases to restore alignment, especially ones with hallux valgus interphalangeus and excessive pronation of the big toe.

First tarsometatarsal fusion (Lapidus procedure)

Lapidus fusion is indicated in patients with instability of the 1st tarsometatarsal joint/severe hallux valgus. It is not recommended in adolescents with open growth

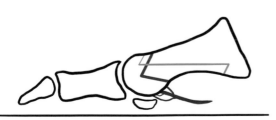

Figure 6.4 Blood supply of the 1st metatarsal. Also showing the Chevron osteotomy (purple) and Scarf osteotomy (green/teal).

plates at the base of the 1st metatarsal or in concomitant presence of 1st metatarsophalangeal arthritis. The aim would be to restore the intermetatarsal angle and avoid dorsiflexion of the first ray.

First metatarsophalangeal joint fusion

Fusion is indicated when there is significant osteoarthritis of the 1st metatarsal joint and in rheumatoid patients with severe deformities (especially in older patients). There is a 10% risk of non-union.

Hallux rigidus

Introduction

Arthritis of the great toe metatarsophalangeal joint is associated with pain, reduced range of movement and osteophyte formation. It is the most common site for arthritis affecting the foot (3). Primary osteoarthritis is the most prevalent aetiology of arthritis of the 1st metatarsophalangeal joint. Other causes include metabolic (gout), inflammatory (psoriatic arthropathy and rheumatoid arthritis), infection and post-traumatic.

Clinical examination

Clinical presentation

Most cases have bilateral affection and a positive family history. The pain in hallux rigidus is generally due to the arthritis. Other causes of pain being pressure on the dorsomedial cutaneous nerve of the first ray or the osteophytes rubbing against footwear. The incidence of night pain is uncommon. Activities such as running, going up and down the stairs and wearing high heels are associated with worsening of pain. The alteration of gait may cause pain across the outer border of the foot.

Examination

Standing

It is a frequent finding to have large tender osteophytes on the dorsal and medial aspect of the great toe metatarsophalangeal joint. The skin overlying the osteophyte may be thinned, stretched and erythematous, with or without an overlying bursa. Patients tend to walk on the outer border of the foot. Single leg heel raise reveals the patient rolling over to the outer side of the foot, due to reduce dorsiflexion at the great toe metatarsophalangeal joint.

Sitting

Inspection of the sole of the foot may reveal callosities under the lesser toe metatarsal heads. The dorsal osteophytes over the great toe metatarsophalangeal joint could be tender on palpation. There is likelihood of reduced motion of the joint with pain and crepitus. Tinel's sign of the dorsomedial cutaneous nerve of the big toe may reproduce some of the nerve-related symptoms. It is important to examine the joint above (tarsometatarsal) and joint below (interphalangeal) for tenderness and range of movement as it would have implications in your final management, if these joints are arthritic.

Imaging

Weight-bearing radiographs of the foot: anteroposterior and lateral views reveal joint space narrowing, subchondral sclerosis and osteophytes especially on the dorsal aspect (over the proximal phalanx as well as the metatarsal head). Harcup and Johnson classification of hallux rigidus (Figures 6.5–6.7) is based on radiographic changes of the great toe metatarsophalangeal joint.

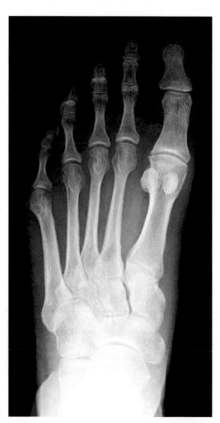

Figure 6.5 Grade 1 Hallux rigidus with mild/moderate osteophytes and preservation of joint space.

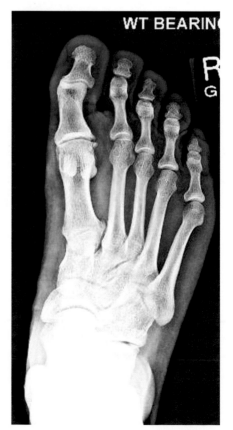

Figure 6.6 Grade 2 Hallux rigidus with moderate osteophytes and joint space narrowing.

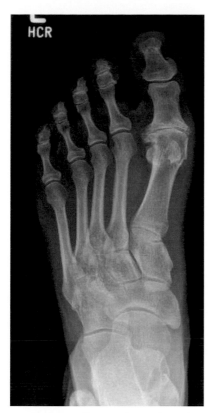

Figure 6.7 Grade 3 Hallux rigidus with marked osteophyte formation and severe reduction in joint space.

Management

Conservative management

Most patients with great toe metatarsophalangeal arthritis can be treated with conservative methods including activity modification, anti-inflammatories and modification of footwear. Activities that cause dorsiflexion of the great toe metatarsophalangeal joint (and associated pain) should be avoided. A stiff soled shoe with a forefoot rocker under the metatarsophalangeal joints may be recommended as it allows the patient to avoid dorsiflexing the great toe metatarsophalangeal joint during the push-off phase.

Injection therapy

Steroid injections into the great toe metatarsophalangeal joint show a significant improvement in pain both when resting and walking, but are only effective for up to 3 months.

Surgical management

Cheilectomy

Cheilectomy involves shaving of the dorsal osteophytes from the metatarsal head and the proximal phalanx along with the dorsal portion of the articular surface (Figure 6.8). A high incidence of revision surgery is noted in patients with advanced arthritis treated with cheilectomy. The patient should therefore be appropriately counselled. It is important to retain the collateral ligaments to avoid angular deformities. Minimally invasive and arthroscopic cheilectomy have shown excellent results in the short term with a faster recovery time.

Moberg osteotomy

Dorsal closing wedge osteotomy of the base of the proximal phalanx helps shift the arc of motion of the great toe metatarsophalangeal joint allowing more dorsiflexion. The biggest drawback of this method is the difficulty when converting to arthrodesis, especially when using pre-contoured metatarsophalangeal joint plating systems.

Keller's excision arthroplasty

Involves decompression of the metatarsophalangeal joint where resection of the base of the proximal phalanx allows maintenance of range of movement in the great toe metatarsophalangeal joint. However, it is associated with complications such as transfer metatarsalgia, cock-up deformity and weakness of push-off

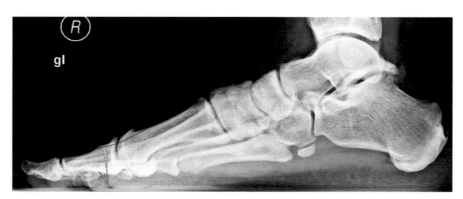

Figure 6.8 Hallux rigidus lateral radiograph demonstrating the extent of cheilectomy and Moberg osteotomy.

strength. This is best reserved for older patients with less functional demand.

Metatarsophalangeal joint arthroplasty

Various forms of arthroplasty have been attempted including a silastic hinge implants, metallic implants, hemiarthroplasty, polyvinyl alcohol hydrogel hemiarthroplasty. These stand a high risk of osteolysis and implant failure. Revision to fusion generally needs a bone block arthrodesis to maintain the length of the first ray. Additionally, the bone bridge fusion has associated risks of delayed union or non-union.

First metatarsophalangeal joint arthrodesis

Fusion remains the gold standard treatment for advanced arthritis of the great toe metatarsophalangeal joint. Various techniques and fixation methods have been described for fusion of the big toe. The preparation of the joint surfaces can be done with osteotomes, nibblers and conical reamers. The position of the fusion would be dictated by the patient's demands and occupation. Ideally, it should allow good ground clearance as well as easy use of footwear.

In general, neutral rotation, 5–10° of valgus and 10° of dorsiflexion with reference to the floor (25° to the long axis of 1st metatarsal) is recommended. The pad of the big toe should be able to touch the ground with interphalangeal joint flexion. Intraoperatively, the author recommends the use of a flat plate under the foot, to mimic weight-bearing status, and hence ensure optimal fusion position. Shortening of the length of the first ray can be associated with an increased risk of transfer metatarsalgia. Various methods of fixation have been described including cortical screws, partial threaded cancellous screws with or without dorsal plates. Brodsky showed improvement in gait following great toe MTP fusion with increased ankle range of movement, especially plantarflexion. Patients were able to bear weight on the big toe with increased force at toe-off. More than two-thirds of patients were able to return to golf, tennis and hiking (4).

Morton's neuroma

Introduction

Morton described a case series in 1876 comprising of patients with pain in the toes especially in the 3rd and 4th toes, some of which were relieved by excision of the metatarsal head. Since then the interdigital neuroma has been commonly known as a Morton's neuroma. It is not a true neuroma but thickening of the digital nerve due to perineural fibrosis, demyelination and neural oedema. Predominantly, it affects the third web space. This is likely due to the fact that the third interdigital nerve is formed by the confluence of branches from the medial and lateral plantar nerves (hence, slightly less mobile).

Clinical presentation

The most common presentations are pain and paraesthesia in the region of the affected digital nerve, particularly a burning type of pain. Patients most often describe a feeling of having a pebble in their shoe, which is worsened with enclosed tight footwear. Night pain and rest pain can occur in about one-fourth of cases. Mulder's click is performed by squeezing the metatarsal heads together in a dorsiflexed foot to produce an audible click associated with pain. Dorsal to plantar pressure in the affected webspace can also reproduce the symptoms (5). Greis' digital nerve stretch test involves hyperextension of the toes to reproduce the symptoms of Morton's neuroma (6).

Imaging

Ultrasound scan and MRI scan are extremely sensitive for a diagnosis of Morton's neuroma, with an ultrasound scan providing the additional opportunity for ultrasound-guided injection therapy. MRI is the gold standard for diagnostic accuracy (Figure 6.9) (5).

Management

Conservative management

A metatarsal dome is used to offload the metatarsal heads from the weight-bearing pressure and improve symptoms.

Injection therapy

Steroid injections around the Morton's neuroma are the mainstay of treatment in most cases. Mahadevan did not find any statistical difference in the outcomes following steroid injections for Morton's neuroma with or without an ultrasound scan in a randomised controlled trial (7).

Other modalities of treatment include ethanol/alcohol injections or radiofrequency ablation. In patients with recurrent symptoms, surgery is more difficult, due to the fibrosis causes by such treatments.

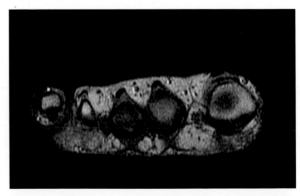

Figure 6.9 Morton's neuroma on T1 axial sections of MRI scan.

Surgical excision

Both dorsal and plantar approaches have been described for excision of a Morton's neuroma. The author's preferred approach is a dorsal approach, which allows immediate weight-bearing following the operation. A plantar approach can be associated with a tender plantar scar and wound complications. It is important to excise the nerve proximally up to the plantar branches to reduce the risk of recurrent neuromas.

Complications

Recurrence/persistence of symptoms following surgical excision is generally due to one of the following: incorrect diagnosis, incomplete resection, recurrence of the neuroma in the stump of the nerve, complex regional pain syndrome, further neuromas in the intermetatarsal spaces and metatarsalgia.

Metatarsalgia

Introduction

Pain under the lesser toe metatarsal head (plantar aspect) is referred to as metatarsalgia. This is generally due to a locally concentrated force in the forefoot during gait. It can be classified into the following categories: primary, secondary and iatrogenic.

Primary metatarsalgia

Abnormalities in the patient's anatomy can lead to overload of the affected metatarsal. This may be due to a disproportionately long or a plantarflexed metatarsal relative to the remaining metatarsal heads. The 2nd metatarsal is generally the most affected in such cases. Pain is mainly experienced during the impact of force whilst walking, i.e., the third rocker. The patient may develop callosities/intractable plantar keratosis under the metatarsal heads. This can be localised to a single metatarsal or multiple metatarsals. Other contributory factors may be enlarged metatarsal head or its condyles. Tightness of the gastrocnemius complex can be an additional contributory factor of primary metatarsalgia.

Secondary metatarsalgia

The causes of secondary metatarsalgia may include inflammatory arthropathy; instability of the metatarsophalangeal joint; Morton's neuroma; tarsal tunnel syndrome and Freiberg's infraction. Previous fractures can cause plantarflexed malunion of metatarsals leading to metatarsalgia. Inflammatory arthropathy can lead to dorsal subluxation/dislocation of the metatarsophalangeal joint with a plunger effect of the proximal phalanx on the metatarsal head. The atrophy or distal migration of the plantar fat pad can also cause excessive overload of the metatarsal head.

Iatrogenic metatarsalgia

Iatrogenic shortening or malalignment of metatarsal osteotomies can lead to offloading of the involved ray and transfer metatarsalgia affecting the other rays. For example, dorsiflexion of the first ray after 1st metatarsal osteotomy can offload the first ray and lead to pain under the lesser metatarsal heads due to excessive overload. The elevation of the ray can cause metatarsalgia during the third rocker phase, whereas shortening can cause second rocker metatarsalgia (8).

Clinical examination

Callosities are often seen under the affected metatarsal heads. The Silfverskiöld test would be performed to assess for gastrosoleus tightness. Examination of the metatarsophalangeal joints and interphalangeal spaces is conducted to rule out subluxation/dislocation of the metatarsophalangeal joints and Morton's neuroma, respectively. Palpation of the plantar aspect of the metatarsal head is performed to assess for any prominence of the plantar condyles.

Imaging

Weight-bearing anteroposterior, lateral and oblique radiographs of the feet. A CT scan (especially weight-bearing CT), SPECT scan, MRI scan and pedobarography would all be helpful in localising the pressure areas.

Management

Conservative management

Modifications of footwear, insoles/selective padding to offload the pressure areas. These include metatarsal domes and moulded total contact type insoles. Stretching exercises in patients with gastrosoleus tightness and shaving of callosities is recommended.

Surgical management

The aim is to restore the metatarsal parabola to allow more symmetric weight distribution along the metatarsal heads. This could involve plantar condylectomy, distal metatarsal osteotomy, which could be minimally invasive (Figure 6.10) or diaphyseal metatarsal

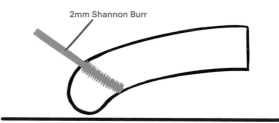

Figure 6.10 Minimally invasive lesser toe metatarsal osteotomy.

osteotomies and metatarsal head excision in certain cases.

Lesser toe metatarsophalangeal joint instability could be treated with flexor to extensor transfer.

Freiberg's disease

Introduction

Avascular necrosis of the 2nd metatarsal head is the fourth most common osteochondrosis in the body (9). It predominantly affects the 2nd metatarsal head (68%), although the lesser toe metatarsal heads can be affected as well. Freiberg's disease generally affects teenage females with a ratio of 5:1 female to male (10).

Etiopathology

Various factors such as trauma, impaired vascular supply and systemic disorders (systemic lupus erythematosus, hypercoagulability, etc.) have been included as risk factors. The 2nd metatarsal is generally the longest of the metatarsals and the keystone configuration of the 2nd tarsometatarsal joint makes it the least mobile. Hence, potentially increasing the stresses on the 2nd metatarsal head (11). High heeled shoes with repetitive dorsiflexion and dorsal impingement of the metatarsophalangeal joint may be a contributing factor.

The blood supply to the 2nd metatarsal is derived from the deep medial plantar artery and the dorsal metatarsal artery (12). Any alteration in the blood supply can generate a watershed area in the 2nd metatarsal head, thus rendering it prone to avascular necrosis.

Clinical presentation

The most common presenting symptom is pain in the 2nd metatarsal head region, mechanical in nature, with increased pain on weight-bearing and walking. The patient may have occasional history of night pain. There would be tenderness and swelling in the 2nd metatarsophalangeal joint region with possible osteophytes on the dorsal aspect of the 2nd metatarsal head. Crepitus may be palpable on movements of the 2nd metatarsophalangeal joint. Lachman test would detect metatarsophalangeal joint instability.

Classification

Smillie categorised Freiberg's disease in to five stages (13):

1. Fissure develops in the ischaemic epiphysis (Visible on MRI).
2. Central resorption of bone within the metatarsal head causing subchondral bone to subside (Visible on plain radiographs).
3. Continued resorption allows the subchondral bone to sink further centrally into the head creating peripheral irregularities of the intact joint surface (Plantar articular surface still intact).
4. Fractures of the peripheral projections and plantar isthmus of the articular cartilage (collapse of entire metatarsal head).
5. Flattening and deformity of the metatarsal head with arthrosis.

Imaging

Standard weight-bearing anteroposterior, lateral and oblique radiographs of the foot would help clarify the relative length of the 2nd metatarsal and help classify the stage of the disease. The oblique lateral radiographs generally demonstrate the lesion on the dorsum of the metatarsal head and also help identify any loose bodies.

An MRI scan allows early detection and classification of the osteonecrosis.

Treatment

Conservative management

This would entail activity modification, analgesics, insole modification to help offload the 2nd metatarsophalangeal joint. A stiff soled shoe with a forefoot rocker and a metatarsal dome is generally recommended.

Surgical management

Failure of conservative management with persistent symptoms may necessitate surgical intervention. The selection amongst the following options will depend on the individual patient needs.

Joint debridement of the 2nd metatarsophalangeal joint with excision of the synovial hypertrophy, removal of loose bodies, any unstable cartilage flaps and osteophytes may help improve symptoms.

Drilling of the sclerotic subchondral bone with or without cancellous bone graft into the defect of the metatarsal head has produces a good result in a few retrospective case series.

Osteochondral grafting as well as a dorsal closing wedge osteotomy of the affected metatarsal head have also shown good result (13).

Osteotomies of the affected metatarsal can be of two types:

1. Shortening of the metatarsal by about 4 mm can offload the ray but can lead to an unpleasant short toe (14).
2. Dorsiflexion closing wedge osteotomy with excision of the damaged articular portion and allowing the intact plantar surface to articulate with the phalanx has shown good results (10).

Excision interposition arthroplasty using the flexor and extensor tendons as well as the joint capsule have been shown to be good pain-relieving operations although the range of movement of the joint seldom improves (15, 16).

Replacement arthroplasty using simple hinged interposition spacers have good results in around 60% of feet. These are associated with problems of inappropriate fit, poor material strength, loosening and foreign body reaction (17).

Bunionette

Introduction

The term bunionette refers to the painful prominence of the lateral aspect of the 5th metatarsal head. It is commonly called the 'Tailor's bunion' because of the habit of sitting cross legged, and, consequently, the rubbing of the lateral border of the foot against the ground.

Classification

The classification of the bunionette is according to the following characteristics:

1. Enlarged 5th metatarsal head
2. Congenital bowing of the 5th metatarsal with normal 4/5 intermetatarsal angle
3. Widened 4/5 intermetatarsal angle (commonest) (Figure 6.11)

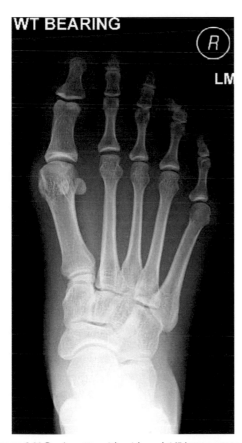

Figure 6.11 Bunionette with widened 4/5 intermetatarsal angle.

Clinical findings

Most often presents bilaterally in females, adolescents and young adults. The pain is in the lateral border of the foot, especially with enclosed footwear. Bunionettes are commonly associated with hallux valgus/rigidus, hammer toes, pes planus and valgus heel (18). Callosities over the lateral and plantar aspect of 5th metatarsal head are frequently present.

Imaging

Weight-bearing radiographs of the foot, anteroposterior/lateral and oblique, are recommended to guide management. The angles calculated are: the 5th metatarsophalangeal angle (average 10.2°) and the 4/5 intermetatarsal angle (average 10.8°). The normal width of the 5th metatarsal head is between 11–14 mm.

Management

Conservative management

Conservative management may include: activity modification, footwear modification (wide toe box shoes), padding around the callosities, shaving of the callosity.

Surgical management

Type 1: Distal metatarsal osteotomy: Chevron/oblique/minimally invasive (Figure 6.10)
Type 2/3: Reverse Ludloff/Scarf osteotomy
    Proximal osteotomy of the 5th metatarsal should be avoided due to the precarious blood supply of the metaphyscal/diaphyseal region of the 5th metatarsal.

Lesser toe deformities

The deformities of the lesser toes can account for significant morbidity. According to Swedish registry data, one-fourth of all forefoot surgeries include lesser toe deformity correction (19). The common causes of lesser toe deformities are trauma, ill-fitting shoes, hallux valgus, inflammatory arthritis, diabetes mellitus and neurological dysfunction (20).

Deformities can be either in the sagittal plane (claw/hammer/mallet toe) or in the axial plane (crossover toe) (Table 6.2). The deformities are initially flexible, but over time, the capsule, collateral ligaments and tendons tighten to render the deformity to become fixed. Nonoperative management measures include toe sleeves, padding over the PIP joint and under the MTP joint. Steroid injections can be used for MTP joint capsulitis.

Crossover toe

Medial deviation of the lesser toes is more common than lateral deviation. This is commonly associated

Table 6.2 Table illustrating the common sagittal plane lesser toe deformities (21, 22)

| | MTP joint | PIP joint | DIP joint | Operative management | |
				Flexible	Fixed
Hammer	Neutral	Flexion	Neutral/ hyperextension	Flexor to extensor transfer	Excision arthroplasty/ fusion
Claw	Hyperextension	Flexion	Flexion	Flexor to extensor transfer	Fusion
Mallet	Neutral	Neutral	Flexion	Flexor tenotomy	Fusion

with hallux valgus. The second toe is most commonly affected (Figure 6.1).

Mallet toe

Generally associated with contracture of the long flexor tendon which is commonly attributed to tight shoes.

Hammer toe

Commonly associated with hallux valgus and inflammatory arthritis. The plantar plate attenuation can lead to metatarsophalangeal joint instability.

Claw toe

Generally neurological in origin. The intrinsic muscles being weak, there is loss of the stabilising force over the MTP joint. The unopposed action of the extensors leads to hyperextension at the MTP joint and the long flexors cause flexion at the interphalangeal joints.

Take home messages

- The aim of surgical correction of hallux valgus is to restore metatarsal head over the sesamoids.
- Cheilectomy +/– Moberg osteotomy is indicated for mild to moderate hallux rigidus whereas severe arthritis is treated with first MTP joint fusion.
- Morton's neuroma is not a true neuroma but is due to thickening of the interdigital nerve due to perineural fibrosis, demyelination, and neural oedema.
- Freiberg's disease mostly affects the 2nd metatarsal. MRI is helpful in early detection. Treatment involves off-loading the second ray with conservative or operative means.
- The majority of patients with bunionette can be treated conservatively. Osteotomy with lateral condylectomy may be needed when conservative management fails to control symptoms.

Acknowledgement

Author would like to thank Mehak Kakwani (Medical Student, Leeds University) for all the fantastic illustrations in this chapter, as well as for collecting all the evidence, and proofreading the manuscript.

References

1. Robinson AHN, Limbers JP. Modern concepts in the treatment of hallux valgus. J Bone Joint Surg Br. 2005; 87-B(8):1038–1045.
2. Stephens M. Pathogenesis of hallux valgus. Foot Ankle Surg. 1994; 1(1):7–10.
3. Anderson M, Bryant S, Baumhauer J, Current concepts review: Hallux rigidus. Foot & Ankle Orthopaedics. 2018; 3(2):1–11.
4. Brodsky J, Passmore R, Pollo F, Shabat S. Functional outcome of arthrodesis of the first metatarsophalangeal joint using parallel screw fixation. Foot Ankle Int. 2005; 26(2):140–146.
5. Mahadevan D, Venkatesan M, Bhatt R, Bhatia M. Diagnostic accuracy of clinical tests for Morton's neuroma compared with ultrasonography. J Foot Ankle Surg. 2015; 54(4):549–553.
6. Cloke D, Greiss M. The digital nerve stretch test: A sensitive indicator of Morton's neuroma and neuritis. J Foot Ankle Surg. 2006; 12(4):201–203.
7. Mahadevan D, Attwal M, Bhatt R, Bhatia M. Corticosteroid injection for Morton's neuroma with or without ultrasound guidance. Bone Joint J. 2016; 98-B(4):498–503.
8. Espinosa N, Maceira E, Myerson M. Current concept review: Metatarsalgia. Foot Ankle Int. 2008; 29(8):871–879.
9. Omer GE. Primary articular osteochondroses. Clin Orthop. 1981; 158:33.
10. Morandi A, Prina A, Verdoni F. Treatment of Kohler's second syndrome by continuous skeletal traction. Ital J Orthop Traumatol. 1990; 16(3):363–368.
11. Carmont MR, Rees RJ, Blundell CM. Current concepts review: Freiberg's disease. Foot Ankle Int. 2009; 30(2):167–176.
12. Petersen WJ, Lankes JM, Paulsen F, Hassenpflug J. The arterial supply of the lesser metatarsal heads: A vascular injection study in human cadavers. Foot Ankle Int. 2002; 23(6):491–495.
13. Smillie IS. Treatment of Freiberg's infraction. Proc R Soc Med. 1967; 60(1):29–31.
14. Smith TDW, Stanley D, Rowley DI. Treatment of Freiberg's disease: A new operative technique. J Bone Joint Surg Br. 1991; 73(1):129–130.
15. Thompson FM, Hamilton WG. Problems of the second metatarsophalangeal joint. Orthopedics. 1987; 10(1):83–89.
16. Lui TH. Arthroscopic interpositional arthroplasty for Freiberg's disease. Knee Surg Sports Traumatol Arthrosc. 2007; 15: 555–559. http://dx.doi.org/10.1007/s00167-006-0189-4

17. Beito SB, Lavery LA. Freiberg's disease and dislocation of the second metatarsophalangeal joint: Aetiology and treatment. Clin Pod Med Surg. 1990; 7(4):619–631.

18. Coughlin MJ. Treatment of bunionette deformity with longitudinal diaphyseal osteotomy with distal soft tissue repair. Foot Ankle. 1991; 11:195–203.

19. Cooper MT, Granadillo VA, Coughlin MJ. The bunionette deformity—evaluation and management. Ann Joint. 2020; 5(7):1–7. http://dx.doi.org/10.21037/aoj.2019.10.03

20. Saro C, Bengtsson AS, Lindgren U, et al. Surgical treatment of hallux valgus and forefoot deformities in Sweden: A population-based study. Foot Ankle Int. 2008; 29:298–304.

21. Malhotra K, Davda K, Singh D. The pathology and management of lesser toe deformities. EFORT Open Rev. 2016; 1:409–419.

22. Coughlin M. Common causes of pain in the forefoot in adults. J Bone Joint Surg [Br]. 2000; 82-B:781–790.

7 The rheumatoid foot

Patricia Allen and Jasdeep Giddie

Introduction

Rheumatoid arthritis (RA) is a chronic systemic auto-immune disease characterised by synovitis and peri-articular bone loss. It affects the diarthrodial joints with a predilection for the small joints of the hands and feet and often has a symmetric presentation. Females are more commonly affected than males (4F: 1M), with the onset of presentation between 35 and 45 years (1).

Approximately 20% of patients initially present with foot and ankle symptoms (2), with the forefoot more commonly affected earlier in the course of the disease process (3).

The goals of treatment are control of pain and preservation of movement (4). A multidisciplinary approach is key, and should include rheumatologists, orthotists, surgeons, physical and occupational therapists.

This chapter aims to provide a guide on how to assess a patient with RA, including commonly encountered anti-arthritic medications, conservative measures and surgical options available.

Diagnostic criteria

In 2010, there was a revision of the RA classification criteria, which now includes polyarthropathy, serology testing, acute phase reactants and duration of symptoms (greater than 6 weeks). Symmetry of joint involvement, duration of morning stiffness and the presence of rheumatoid nodules are no longer considered (5).

Clinical evaluation

With 20% of first time presentations to a foot and ankle clinician, a detailed history should elicit the duration of symptoms, nature of pain and associated aggravating and relieving factors. Often, multiple joints will simultaneously be involved. A change in activity levels and a basic functional assessment such as putting on a pair of shoes or tying laces should be noted. Stiffness in patients with RA is often present on waking up and is unremitting and prolonged. A brief systemic history is relevant so as to exclude any of the extra-articular manifestations of RA, which are presented in Table 7.1.

The clinical examination should begin with an assessment for scars, foot posture, lower limb alignment and gait. Any cutaneous signs such as rheumatoid nodules should be looked for. Individual joints should be palpated to identify the probable source of pain and pulses checked for. Individual tendons and their power should be elicited. Any deformities should be assessed so as to determine whether they are fixed or flexible.

Laboratory investigations that should be performed in patients with suspected RA include erythrocyte sedimentation rate (ESR), C-reactive protein (CRP), rheumatoid factor and anti-cyclic citrullinated peptide antibodies (CCP).

Radiographic evaluation should include weight-bearing views of the foot and ankle. Subtle features present early in the disease process can be missed; these include soft tissue swelling, diffuse juxta-articular osteoporosis and periarticular erosions. Late changes include joint space narrowing, subluxation and dislocation. An additional imaging modality such as magnetic resonance imaging (MRI) is beneficial early in the disease process as it identifies inflammatory changes, joint erosions and chondrolysis. Computerised tomography (CT) scans are a useful adjunct when planning surgery both to define joint involvement and for planning deformity correction (Figure 7.1).

Pathophysiology

The aetiology of the disease remains unknown. However, environmental and genetic causes are thought to play a role. It is also hypothesised that viral infections may directly or indirectly trigger an inflammatory reaction, by activation of the human leucocyte antigen, HLA-II locus, resulting in a T-lymphocyte cell mediated immune response. The T cells incite and upregulate endothelial adhesion molecules and leucocyte migration into the proliferative synovial tissue, stimulating chondrocytes and fibroblasts to release degradative enzymes (6). There is subsequent destruction of the

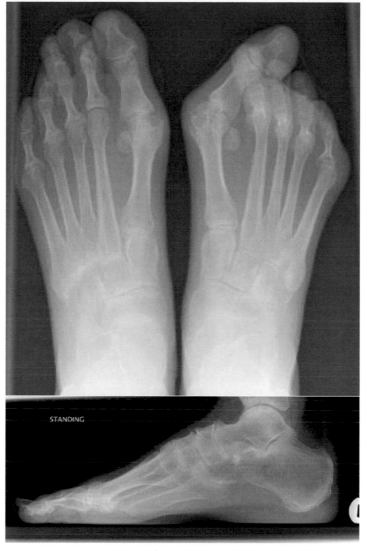

Figure 7.1 Periarticular erosions around the 1st metatarsophalangeal joint with midfoot involvement on the left and bilateral hindfoot involvement.

Table 7.1 Extra-articular manifestations of rheumatoid arthritis and associated syndromes
1. Pericarditis
2. Pulmonary disease
3. Rheumatoid vasculitis
4. Ophthalmic inflammatory disease
Associated syndromes include:
Felty's syndrome – Combined leucopaenia and splenomegaly
Still's disease – Acute onset RA with splenomegaly, fever and a rash

articular cartilage and surrounding soft tissues, leading to severe deformities (Figure 7.2).

Medical management

Medical treatment has evolved over the past 30 years, from providing symptomatic relief, to the implementation of therapeutic regimens that slow/arrest the disease process and structural joint damage which, in turn, has led to a decrease in the numbers requiring surgery.

The treatment approach starts with non-steroidal anti-inflammatory drugs (NSAIDs), corticosteroids and disease modifying anti-rheumatic drugs (DMARDs). Some patients will be managed well with monotherapy, whereas others may require combination regimens.

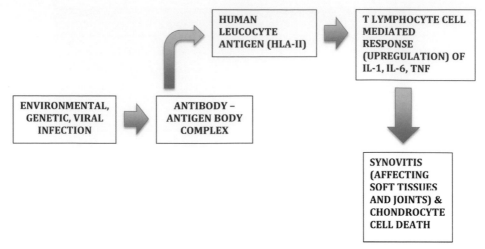

Figure 7.2 Pathophysiology of rheumatoid arthritis.

The different groups of DMARDs are demonstrated in Figure 7.3.

Perioperative management of DMARDs is fundamental to ensure surgical risks are kept to a minimum and disease remission is maintained. The decision to stop and re-start biologics should be done in conjunction with a rheumatologist. Temporary discontinuation of drug therapy remains a controversial topic, with divided opinions regarding the use of anti-tumour necrosis factor alpha inhibitors. Table 7.2 summarises the different classes of pharmacological therapies, their mechanisms of action and current guidance in the United Kingdom on management during the perioperative period.

Physical therapy

With an increasing number of lower extremity joints involved, gait assessment, training and provision of walking aids maybe necessary to maintain ambulatory independence. In addition, physical therapy helps maintain motion through the use of stretching, passive and active movements.

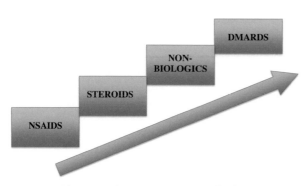

Figure 7.3 Stepwise treatment for RA.

Orthotics

Prescription footwear is an important adjunct therapy in RA patients because they have lost the fatty protective plantar tissue, have hypersensitive and inflamed skin and unstable joints. The orthotics function to: redistribute weight-bearing forces, decrease vertical and shear pressure and also horizontal movement within the foot (7).

Injections

A combination of local anaesthetic and steroid injections can be used to control localised symptoms. The anti-inflammatory and analgesic actions allow an improvement in function. Patients should be counselled regarding the variable response to injections, which may range from complete resolution of symptoms, to minimal effect and a reduced efficacy with continued use.

In the ankle and hindfoot, fluoroscopic guided injections have been shown to be superior to blind injections for diagnostic purposes and temporary relief of synovitis or arthritis (8). They can prove helpful in defining which joints are symptomatic so that surgery can be limited to just those joints, thus preserving movement wherever possible.

Surgical management

Indications for surgical management include failure to prevent deformity progression and to maintain ambulatory capacity with nonoperative measures.

Perioperative workup

Blood work analysis should be performed on all perioperative patients who are receiving DMARDs, so as to exclude bone marrow suppression and hepatotoxicity.

Table 7.2 Pharmacology of anti-arthritic medication

Drug	Mechanism of action	Perioperative period	Re-start
	Non-biological DMARDs		
Methotrexate	A folate analogue which inhibits purine and pyrimidine synthesis, reduction of antigen-dependent T cell proliferation and promotion of adenosine release with adenosine-mediated suppression of inflammation	Continue	
Leflunomide	An inhibitor of pyrimidine synthesis by inhibiting the mitochondrial enzyme dihydroorotate dehydrogenase	Stop 1–2 days prior major procedures	Re-start once wounds have healed
Hydroxychloroquine	Interference with 'antigen processing' in macrophages and other antigen presenting cells, as a result diminish formation of peptide MHC class II proteins required to stimulate CD4 – T cells	Continue	
Sulfasalazine	Mechanism of action – uncertain	Continue	
	Biological DMARDs **TNF-α antagonists**		
Etanercept (Enbrel)	Etanercept inhibits the activity of TNF-α by competitively binding to this proinflammatory cytokine and preventing interactions with its cell surface receptors	Stop for 2 weeks prior surgical procedures	Re-start 10–14 days after
Infliximab (Remicade)	Human mouse chimeric alpha monoclonal antibody, binding to TNF-α, forming stable non-disassociating immune complexes preventing binding of TNF to its receptors	Stop for 2 weeks prior surgical procedures	Re-start 10–14 days after
Adalimumab (Humira)	Human anti-TNF-α monoclonal antibody – blocking interaction of TNF with the p55 and p75 cell surface TNF receptors	Stop for 2 weeks prior surgical procedures	Re-start 10–14 days after
	Interleukin 1 (IL-1) antagonists		
Anakinra (Kineret)	Blocks IL-1 receptor 1, antagonising the effects of both IL-1 α and IL-1 β	Stop 1–2 days prior surgical procedures	Re-start 10 days after
Rituximab (Rituxan)	Monoclonal antibody to CD20 antigen (inhibits B cells).	Stop 4–7 months prior major surgery	
Abatacept (Orencia)	Prevention of T cell activation by blocking interaction of CD28 on T cells by binding to the costimulatory molecules CD80 and CD86 on antigen presenting cells	Stop 1–2 days prior surgical procedures	Re-start 10 days after
	Non-steroidal anti-inflammatories		
NSAIDs	Inhibition of cyclo-oxygenase enzymes (COX-1 and COX-2), preventing synthesis of prostaglandins	Continue	
	Corticosteroids		
Glucocorticoid	Binds to the glucocorticoid receptor within the cell cytoplasm forming the glucocorticoid/glucocorticoid receptor complex, which then binds to specific DNA binding sites resulting in the blocking of the transcription of inflammatory genes	Continue	

Other general considerations include adrenal insufficiency with long-term use of corticosteroid therapy, which will require intravenous hydrocortisone perioperatively. Flexion–extension cervical spine radiographs should be obtained to assess for any atlantoaxial instability.

Forefoot

Pathophysiology of metatarsophalangeal joint (MTPJ) deformity

Forefoot pathology is characterised by inflammation of the synovium, which results in proliferation and distension of the MTPJ capsule. Untreated, the distension progresses, leading to a loss of integrity of the stabilising structures (collateral ligaments and the plantar plate) (9, 10).

The small 1st MTPJ contact area and shallow articular profile of the proximal phalanx provides little inherent stability, most of which is provided by the capsuloligamentous and tendinous structures surrounding the joint (11). The loss of capsular integrity of the hallux causes the medial stabilising structures to become deficient resulting in a hallux valgus deformity or, less commonly, a dorsal or varus deformity.

Ongoing destruction of articular cartilage creates further instability and a worsening deformity. This compromises the weight-bearing function of the first ray leading to transfer of forces to the lesser rays (10).

The increasing load, together with capsular and ligamentous destruction of the lesser ray MTPJs, results in dorsal subluxation of the proximal phalanges. The MTPJ is subject to further deformity through external forces created by ambulation, constrictive footwear and an imbalance of the flexor and extensor tendons (3). The once primary plantar flexors of the MTPJ, the interossei and lumbricals, which act through the insertion onto the plantar aspect of the proximal phalanx, move dorsally with the dorsal subluxation of the proximal phalanx, relegating the interossei to weak, effectively functionless extensors (12). The metatarsal head is forced plantar-ward and the plantar fat pad is pulled distally, exposing the now prominent metatarsal heads, leading to keratotic lesions, which may ulcerate (3, 9).

Flexor-extensor tendon imbalance worsens the deformity. With chronic dorsiflexion at the MTPJ, the extensor tendons become inefficient, and the now unopposed flexors cause a flexion deformity at the proximal interphalangeal joint (PIPJ). These contractures can become fixed deformities leading to callosities forming over the dorsal aspect of the PIPJs (10).

The aim of surgical correction of the forefoot should be a well-aligned, stable foot that is able to bear weight. In order to achieve this, arthrodesis of the first ray, in combination with correction of hammer toes and shortening or resection of the metatarsal heads, is an accepted treatment (7).

Surgical treatment of the first MTPJ

MTPJ arthrodesis

MTPJ arthrodesis is considered the treatment of choice when treating both a hallux valgus and rigidus. Coughlin et al. recommended stable realignment of the first ray with an arthrodesis that allows for permanent correction. This provides stability to the medial column, minimising the stresses to the lesser MTP joints and thereby protecting them (13).

MTPJ preparation can be performed using a number of different techniques including cup and cone reamers, proposed by Coughlin, which create domed shaped fusion surfaces (13), hand preparation to create domed surfaces or, horizontal cuts, which create flat bony surfaces. Either technique of joint preparation will work as long as all cartilage is removed, down to the subchondral bone surface and that the cancellous bone is exposed fully, or in part (with multiple perforations of the subchondral bone plate), and that good bony apposition and compression are achieved.

Various methods of internal fixation have been described including Kirschner wire (k-wire) stabilisation, Steinman pin, staples, cortical screws, standard and contoured locking plates and a combination of plates and screws. The risk of non-union following 1st MTPJ arthrodesis is higher in cases done for degenerative disease with an associated hallux valgus deformity. Thus, whichever fixation is used, it is imperative to achieve a stable construct. A biomechanical study by Politi et al. showed a combination of a dorsal plate and compression screw with power conical reaming of the surfaces provided the most stable construct (14).

Whichever method of stabilisation is used, postoperative alignment is key. To assess alignment intraoperatively, simulated weight-bearing is performed to determine the optimal position of fusion. The rotation should be neutral. The degree of valgus and dorsiflexion varies between patients. As a general rule the pulp of the great toe should just be touching the ground (or a flat surface when tested in theatre on simulated weight-bearing).

Resection arthroplasty

Resection arthroplasty of the 1st MTPJ is now infrequently performed. Despite initial symptom relief, patients often go on to develop recurrent deformities, have poor push off and pain.

Joint preservation

With the success of DMARDs, joint preserving procedures are likely to be utilised more, with good long-term results (10). Indications include patients with a hallux valgus deformity with relatively well preserved joint cartilage. A number of procedures can be performed including Scarf and Akin osteotomies, or a Lapidus procedure if there is 1st TMTJ instability. If joint preservation techniques are to be used, patients must be counselled properly and warned of the higher risk of recurrent deformity. This has been reported in a number of studies and is likely due to capsular and ligamentous incompetence (15, 16). In younger patients, however, preservation of movement, even if it can only be achieved for a number of years before the deformity recurs, is still worthwhile as long as the patients understand that conversion to fusion is likely at some point in the future.

1st MTPJ arthroplasty

A wide variety of materials have been used for replacement arthroplasty in hallux rigidus including metal, ceramic and silastic. The aim is to maintain flexibility whilst providing stability for the joint. Despite some studies showing good results (16), the number of complications, particularly implant failure as a result of wear with microparticle release, initiating synovitis and bony osteolysis, is high (17). Other reported complications include dorsiflexion ('cock up') deformity of the toe, stiffness and transfer metatarsalgia. Given the complications and challenges of revision surgery we do not advocate the use of silicone implants as a prosthetic replacement for the MTPJ in RA patients. There are few studies of other 1st MTPJ replacements in rheumatoid patients.

Lesser rays

Synovectomy

Synovectomy of the lesser MTPJs may be indicated for painful symptomatic joints early in the disease process. Debridement of the hypertrophic synovial tissue reduces MTPJ distension, decreasing soft tissue deformation and arresting the degenerative process.

Surgical reconstruction

Lesser toe deformities are commonly associated with 1st MTPJ pathology and both are usually addressed at the same sitting.

The procedure chosen will depend on the extent of involvement of the joints. If the joints are irreducibly dislocated, the deformity can only be corrected by resection of bone. This can be achieved by resecting the metatarsal head, the base of the proximal phalanx, resecting the base of the proximal phalanx with extensor tendon interposition (Stainsby's technique) or, shortening osteotomies of the metatarsals. The latter is only indicated in those cases where the MTPJs are well preserved: once the joints are degenerate then part of the joint itself will need to be excised both to correct the

deformity and control symptoms. Whatever technique is chosen, all lesser rays must be treated with the same procedure to ensure reconstitution of the metatarsal parabola in a smooth arc, as this provides even distribution of forefoot weight and prevents recurrence of pain and deformity (11).

Over the years, several different approaches have been advocated for metatarsal head or proximal phalangeal resection, utilising both dorsal and plantar incisions. Metatarsal head excision is performed either via a plantar incision, commonly excising an ellipse of plantar skin in an attempt to bring the plantar fat pad back proximally so that it lies under the metatarsal necks or, via dorsal longitudinal incisions in the 2nd and 4th web spaces. Proximal phalangeal resection can only be achieved through dorsal incisions. Stainsby described a technique utilising four separate Chevron-shaped incisions, apex medial, over the individual rays, so as to allow exposure for resection of the proximal three quarters of the proximal phalanx and harvest of the individual extensor tendons for interposition arthroplasty. The plantar plates (and thus plantar fat pad) are repositioned under the metatarsal heads, and the toes are then stabilised with a k-wire into the metatarsal shaft (12). Meticulous attention to the soft tissues is required to avoid wound complications. The metatarsal heads are part of the weight-bearing system of the foot and retaining them helps restore a more normal weight-bearing function of the foot as well as re-establishing the transverse tie-bar system.

Based on Coughlin's landmark study, resection of lesser MTPJs has been considered the standard of care in a forefoot reconstruction (13). The amount resected should allow for deformity correction, provide an even distribution of forefoot load, permit wound closure and, as previously mentioned, allow for reduction of the plantar fat pad. With resection of the metatarsal heads or proximal phalanges, in association with 1st MTPJ fusion, good long-term results can be achieved both with control of symptoms and correction of deformity.

With increasing and earlier use of modern drug therapy, patients may now present with an earlier deformity without destruction of the lesser MTPJ surfaces. In these cases, reconstruction of the lesser rays can be achieved with release of the joints alone (+/– correction of the PIP/DIP joints) or, by shortening osteotomies of the lesser metatarsals. These can be performed either open (with a Weil osteotomy) or, with percutaneous distal metatarsal osteotomies. The advantage, as with the first ray, is preservation of the joints themselves and thus more normal function of the forefoot. Again, the patient must be adequately counselled about the risk of disease progression and thus the need to convert to a more traditional forefoot reconstruction in the future. Joint preservation also tends to stiffen the lesser

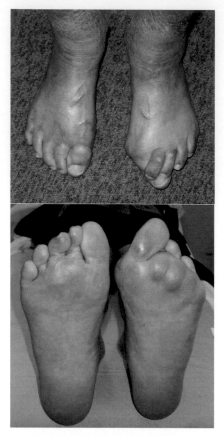

Figure 7.4 Showing typical forefoot deformities of rheumatoid arthritis with plantar callosities on the left foot and resolution of both deformity and callosities on the right foot following 1st MTPJ arthrodesis and Stainsby procedures to 2nd–5th toes.

MTPJs, which the patient must also be made aware of (Figures 7.4 and 7.5).

Lesser toes

Proximal and distal interphalangeal joint deformities are addressed following MTPJ correction if necessary. Flexible deformities can be managed with Z-lengthening of the extensor tendon, whereas fixed deformities are managed with an arthrodesis, excision arthroplasty or osteoclasis with or without k-wire stabilisation. Following excision arthroplasty of the lesser MTPJs, we recommend k-wire insertion into the metatarsal shafts for a minimum of 6 weeks.

Midfoot

Pathophysiology of midfoot disease

Although there is a high radiological incidence of midfoot disease, this does not appear to correlate clinically with symptoms and, consequently, there is little reported on the surgical outcomes of midfoot surgery in the rheumatoid patient (18).

The talonavicular (TN) and naviculocuneiform joints are most often affected causing a midfoot collapse (pes planus) (7). With the collapse of the midfoot, a valgus deformity of the hindfoot ensues. As the disease and deformity progress, the talar head is displaced medially and plantar-ward, causing the medial structures supporting the talar head (spring ligament and joint capsule) to fail, accentuating the collapse. In addition, tibialis posterior dysfunction due to synovitis is likely to contribute to the development of the planovalgus foot (Figure 7.6).

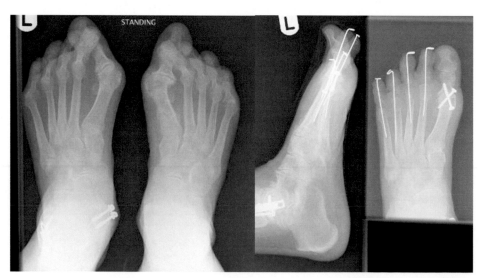

Figure 7.5 The same patient as Figure 7.4. Standing x-rays prior to surgery on either foot. Immediate postoperative x-rays following left 1st MTPJ arthrodesis and Stainsby procedure to 2nd–5th toes.

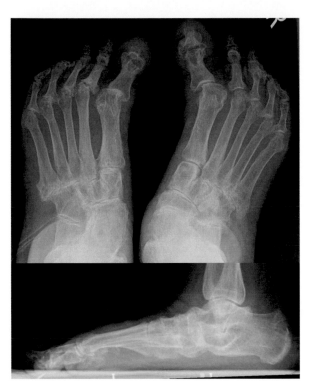

Figure 7.6 Severe planovalgus feet secondary to multiple joint involvement in patient with rheumatoid arthritis.

Hindfoot

Pathophysiology of hindfoot disease

Hindfoot involvement is a more common feature amongst patients with chronic disease (10). The subtalar, TN and calcaneocuboid (CC) are all synovial joints and can therefore be affected resulting in joint destruction, subluxation and dislocation. Instability of the subtalar joint occurs due to loss of integrity of its capsular and ligamentous structures. The subtalar instability then drives the deformity within the hindfoot, causing a planovalgus deformity. Progressive displacement of the talus can cause ankle instability due to deltoid ligament stretching and consequent incompetence and, eventually, arthritis. With the valgus deformity of the hindfoot, the gastrocnemius and soleus muscles can become contracted. These deformities are not only painful but also alter the mechanical axis of the limb and affect the ability to walk.

A careful examination is key to identifying which of the hindfoot joints are affected and should include an assessment for tightness of the gastrocnemius (Silfverskiöld test). It is imperative to assess the integrity of both the medial and lateral ligaments of the ankle as any residual deformity, in the presence of more proximal ligamentous involvement, will inevitably lead to progressive ankle deformity once the hindfoot is fused.

Function of the peroneal and tibialis posterior tendons must likewise be assessed. Radiological imaging and selective joint injections may help provide a conclusive diagnosis and determine which joints are symptomatic.

Surgical options include soft tissue releases and a corrective arthrodesis, a combination of an arthrodesis and osteotomy or, specific to the ankle joint, arthroplasty. Gastrocnemius release or Achilles lengthening can be performed if deemed necessary.

Triple arthrodesis

A fixed valgus deformity of the hindfoot with the forefoot in abduction and supination requires a triple arthrodesis. Union rates of between 92% and 98% are reported (19–21). There tends to be a higher rate of union at the subtalar joint compared to the TN and CC joints. Risks include malunion, which has been attributed to inadequate deformity correction, and the development of ankle arthritis (21). Immobilisation for a minimum of 12 weeks is required after triple fusion. This can be challenging in patients with multiple joint involvement, particularly upper limb involvement and thus an early weight-bearing protocol is preferred, allowing patients to partially weight-bear from 2 weeks postoperatively.

Talonavicular joint arthrodesis

Indications for a TN joint arthrodesis include isolated joint destruction and tibialis posterior dysfunction with a flexible/correctable hindfoot. Arthrodesis of TN joint enhances stabilisation of the hindfoot by restricting the subtalar joint to 8% of its native motion (22). This indirect stabilisation of the subtalar joint means that formal fusion of the subtalar joint is potentially avoided.

Union rates vary between 63% and 97% (23, 24) and this may be due to the challenges of accessing and exposing the joint and the forces through the fusion because of the effect on the surrounding joints. Meticulous joint preparation is key, and stabilisation thereafter, can be achieved with a combination of screws and/or staples or, indeed, plate fixation.

The ankle

The prevalence of ankle arthritis in patients who have documented RA is reported to be between 9% and 70% (25). The treatment for end stage tibiotalar arthritis in RA patients remains contentious, and it is still a matter of debate whether an ankle should be fused or replaced. In this section we shall explore both treatment options in detail.

Ankle synovectomy

Ankle joint synovectomy has a limited role in treatment and is not routinely performed. Indications include synovitis without the presence of arthritis. Although this provides initial symptomatic relief, it does not halt progression of the disease or the development of ankle arthritis.

Arthrodesis versus arthroplasty

Ankle arthrodesis has been the gold standard surgical treatment for many years. The ability of the hindfoot to compensate for the loss of movement following tibiotalar arthrodesis may be limited in rheumatoid patients due to stiffness of the remaining hindfoot joints. This, in turn, will increase stresses on adjacent joints as well as increase the amount of forefoot overload. The long period of immobilisation following an arthrodesis, requiring the use of ambulatory aids, can be a challenge for patients with upper extremity involvement, although this can be minimised with an early weight-bearing protocol.

Advocates for ankle arthroplasty argue that there is quicker recovery and that through preservation of motion there is decreased stress on adjacent joints. Whether this makes a difference to the development of hindfoot arthritis in the long term, remains to be proven. Disadvantages include intraoperative malleolar fracture, ongoing pain and loosening of implant components.

Comparison of arthrodesis and arthroplasty is difficult as the two operations have different end goals and outcome measures, and this is often ignored when comparing the two surgical treatments. Gait analysis following an ankle arthroplasty shows patients have a more symmetrical gait, whereas there is a faster gait with a longer step in the arthrodesed group (26).

Ankle arthrodesis

Following an ankle arthrodesis, union rates have been reported between 60% and 95% (25, 27, 28). Recent results have demonstrated better union rates due to improved instrumentation and surgical experience. The average time to union is between 10 and 12 weeks (28).

The position of arthrodesis is critical. The ideal position is neutral in the sagittal plane, with 5 degrees of valgus and 5–10 of external rotation. Under some circumstances the position of fusion may need to be altered, e.g., in patients with a very stiff midfoot, when dorsiflexion of 5 degrees maybe preferred or, in patients with polio, where the ankle must be fused with some plantarflexion otherwise, due to quads weakness, they hyperextend at the knee and lose the power of propulsion.

An array of different surgical techniques, approaches and fixation modes is available to the operating surgeon. Arthroscopic ankle arthrodesis with internal fixation has been advocated for patients with minimal deformity. Using a combination of shavers and burrs the cartilage is removed down to cancellous bone and, under fluoroscopic guidance two or three compression screws (6.5 mm) are inserted. This technique avoids the need for extensile approaches. Larger deformities are more difficult to address via an arthroscopic technique and the learning curve is steep, but once mastered, increasing deformities can be treated with this method avoiding the wound complications that can be associated with open arthrodesis.

Open arthrodesis may be preferred for larger deformities. Compression and fixation can be achieved with either cannulated or solid compression screws (6.5/7/8 mm) or pre-countered plates (Figure 7.7).

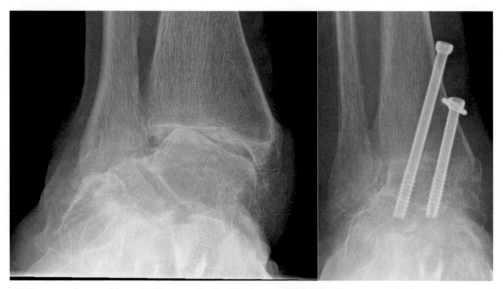

Figure 7.7 Severe valgus ankle arthritis in patient with rheumatoid arthritis, corrected via an arthroscopic ankle arthrodesis.

Ankle arthroplasty

The recent resurgence of total ankle arthroplasty (TAR) has occurred due to improved designs and better fixation methods. This has led to increased survivorship. Initial results using first generation ankle arthroplasties, consisting of a cemented highly constrained design, were not good with unacceptably high failure rates (22–75%) (29, 30). The second generation, with unconstrained components, permits a more natural range of motion and the results are already more promising with survival rates quoted at 84% at 8 years (31).

Ng's paper describes the ideal RA patient for a TAR as 'one who is moderately active, has a well-aligned ankle and heel, has a fair range of motion in the ankle joint and in who the disease is in remission' (31). Using this description, we can understand that not every patient is an 'ideal' candidate for a TAR and certain prerequisites need to be met in order to achieve a successful outcome.

As with any hindfoot surgery, an assessment of alignment is key and this should be done clinically and using radiographs. An aligned hindfoot reduces excessive 'edge loading' of the prosthesis thus preventing prosthesis breakage and loosening.

The postoperative range of motion is dependent upon the preoperative movement within the ankle and patients with very stiff ankles are unlikely to gain a great deal of movement following a TAR (32).

Contraindications specific to RA patients include uncontrolled disease with recurrent flare ups, poor skin quality, vasculitis, poor bone stock, soft tissue compromise with deltoid insufficiency and severe deformity within the coronal plane (greater than 10 degrees of varus or valgus). Radiological features that preclude a TAR from being performed include severe bone loss and large intraosseous cysts, as there is a higher risk of failure due to prosthesis subsidence (Figure 7.8).

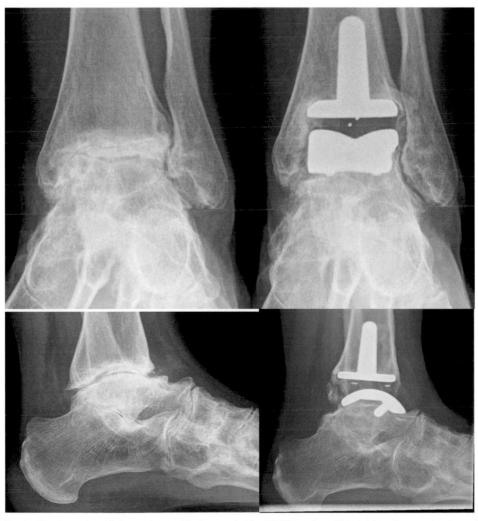

Figure 7.8 Neutrally aligned ankle in patient with rheumatoid arthritis and multi-joint involvement pre- and post-TAR.

Pantalar fusion

Due to the severe stiffness resulting from a pantalar arthrodesis, this should be avoided where possible in patients with RA. There are however some instances, where there is no alternative option. Indications may include patients with severe polyarthritis affecting the hindfoot and ankle with significant deformity and/or stiffness precluding TAR. Patients undergoing a pantalar fusion should be counselled regarding the significant alteration in gait that ensues with increased forefoot loading. Various stabilisation and compressive devices can be utilised including hindfoot nails and pre-contoured plates and screws. Fusion rates quoted range between 84% and 86% (33, 34).

Take home messages

- A multidisciplinary team approach is necessary and every patient should be considered from a more 'global', holistic perspective, including other joints that may be affected and the systemic effects of the disease and medications used.
- Although the approach to treatment varies and is dependent upon the presenting complaint, we advocate a treatment algorithm that involves a progression of options, which should commence with lifestyle modifications, orthotics and analgesia, leaving surgery as a last option.
- Indications for surgical intervention include deformity progression, and/or an inability to walk without pain following failure of nonoperative treatment modalities.
- A thorough examination of the entire limb should be performed to rule out proximal deformities, which should be addressed first.
- Goals for treatment in RA patients should be to obtain a pain-free plantigrade functional foot, which is 'shoeable'.
- Always remember to assess ligamentous and soft tissue integrity around the ankle when planning treatment of the hindfoot.

References

1. Gibofsky A. Overview of epidemiology, pathophysiology, and diagnosis of rheumatoid arthritis. Am J Manag Care 2012; 18(13):295–302.
2. Vainio K. Rheumatoid foot. Clinical study with pathological and roentgenological comments. Ann Chir Gynaecol Fenn Suppl 1956; 45(Suppl):1–107.
3. Jaakola JI, Mann RA. A review of rheumatoid arthritis in the foot and ankle. Foot Ankle Int 2004; 25:866–874.
4. Van der Heijde DM, van't Hof MA, van Riel PL, Theunisse LA, Lubberts E W, van Leeuwen MA, van Rijswijk MH, van de Putte LB. Judging disease activity in clinical practice in rheumatoid arthritis: first step in the development of a disease activity score. Ann Rheum Dis 1990; 49:916–920.
5. Kay J, Upchurch KS. ACR/EULAR 2010 rheumatoid arthritis classification criteria. Rheumatology 2012; 51(Suppl _6): vi5–vi9. https://doi.org/10.1093/rheumatology/kes279
6. Koopman, WJ. Prospects for autoimmune disease: research advances in rheumatoid arthritis. JAMA 2001; 285:648–650.
7. Trieb K. Management of the foot in rheumatoid arthritis. J Bone Joint Surg Br 2005; 87B(9):1171–1177. https://doi.org/10.1302/0301-620X.87B9.16288
8. D'Agostino MA, Ayral X, Baron G, Ravaud P, Breban M, Dougados M. Impact of ultrasound imaging on local corticosteroid injections of symptomatic ankle, hind-, and midfoot in chronic inflammatory diseases. Arthritis Care Res 2005; 53(2):284–292.
9. Michelson J, Easley M, Wigley FM, Hellman D. Foot and ankle problems in rheumatoid arthritis. Foot Ankle Int 1994; 15:608–613.
10. Coughlin JM, Saltzman LC, Anderson BR. Mann's Surgery of the Foot and Ankle. 9th Edition. Philadelphia. Elsevier Saunders. 2014, pp. 867–1007.
11. Amin A, Cullen N, Singh D. Rheumatoid forefoot reconstruction. Acta Orthop. Belg 2010; 76:289–297.
12. Stainsby GD. Pathological anatomy and dynamic effect of the displaced plantar plate and the importance of the plantar plate-deep transverse metatarsal ligament tie-bar. Ann R Coll Surg Engl 1997; 79:58–68.
13. Coughlin MJ. Rheumatoid forefoot reconstruction. A long-term follow-up study. J Bone Joint Surg 2000; 82-A: 322–341.
14. Politi J, Hayes J, Njus G, Bennett GL, Kay DB. First metatarsophalangeal joint arthrodesis: a biomechanical assessment of stability. Foot Ankle Int 2003; 24:332–337.
15. Shi K, Hayashida K, Tomita T, Tanabe M, Ochi T. Surgical treatment of hallux valgus deformity in rheumatoid arthritis: clinical and radiographic evaluation of modified Lapidus technique. J Foot and Ankle Surg 2000; 39:376–382.
16. Hanyu T, Yamazaki H, Murasawa A, Tohyama C. Arthroplasty for rheumatoid forefoot deformities by a shortening oblique osteotomy. Clin Orthop Related Research 1997; 338: 131–138.
17. Rahmann H, Fagg PS. Silicone granulomatous reactions after first metatarsophalangeal joint hemiarthroplasty. J Bone Joint Surg 1993; 75-B:637–639.
18. Loveday D, Jackson G, Geary N. The rheumatoid foot and ankle: current evidence. Foot Ankle Surg 2012; 18(2):94–102.
19. Vahvanen VA. Arthrodesis of the TC or pantalar joints in rheumatoid arthritis. Acta Orthop Scand 1969; 40(5):642–652.
20. Figgie MP, O'Malley MJ, Ranawat C, Inglis AE, Sculco TP. Triple arthrodesis in rheumatoid arthritis. Clin Orthop Relat Res 1993;292:250–254.
21. Maenpaa H, Lehto MUK, Belt EA. What went wrong in triple arthrodesis? An analysis of failures in 21 patients. Clin Orthop Relat Res 2001; 391:218–223.
22. Astion DJ, Deland JT, Otis JC, Kenneally S. Motion of the hindfoot after simulated arthrodesis. JBJS AM 1997; 79: 241–246.
23. Fogel GR, Katoh Y, Rand J, Chao EYS. Talonavicular arthrodesis for isolated arthritis: 9.5 year results and gait analysis. Foot Ankle Int 1982;3:105–113.
24. Harper MC, Tisdel CL. Talonavicular arthrodesis for the painful acquired flatfoot. Foot Ankle Int 1996; 17: 658–661.

25. Miehlke W, Gschwend N, Rippstein P, Simmen BR. Compression arthrodesis in the rheumatoid ankle and hindfoot. Clin Orthop 1997; 340:75–86.

26. Piriou P, Culpan P, Mullins M, Cardon JN, Pozzi D, Judet T. Ankle replacement versus arthrodesis: a comparative gait analysis study. Foot Ankle Int 2008; 29(1):3–9.

27. Trieb K, Wirtz DC, Dürr HR, König DP. Results of arthrodesis of the ankle joint. Z Orthop 2005; 143:221–226.

28. Winson IG, Robinson DE, Allen PE. Arthroscopic ankle arthrodesis. J Bone Joint Surg Br 2005; 87(3):343–347. https://doi.org/10.1302/0301-620X.87B3.15756

29. Kitaoka HB, Patzer GL. Clinical results of the Mayo total ankle arthroplasty. J Joint Surg 1996; 78A:1658–1664.

30. Kofoed H, Sorensen TS. Ankle arthroplasty for rheumatoid arthritis and osteoarthritis: prospective long-term study of cemented replacements. J Bone Joint Surg 1998; 80B: 328–332.

31. Ng YC Sean, Crevoisier X, Assal M. Total ankle replacement for rheumatoid arthritis of the ankle. Foot Ankle Clin N Am 2012; 17:555–564.

32. Coetzee JC, Castro MD. Accurate measurement of ankle range of motion after total ankle arthroplasty. Clin Orthop Relat Res 2004; 31:424–427.

33. Papa JA, Myerson MS. Pantalar and tibiotalocalcaneal arthrodesis for post-traumatic osteoarthritis of the ankle and hindfoot. J Bone Joint Surg 1992; 74A:1042–1049.

34. Acosta R, Ushiba J, Cracchiolo A. The results of a primary and staged pantalar arthrodesis and tibiocalcaneal arthrodesis in adult patients. Foot Ankle Int 2000; 21(3):182–194.

8 Pes plano valgus

Manuel Monteagudo, Pilar Martínez de Albornoz, and Maneesh Bhatia

Introduction

Pes Plano Valgus (PPV) is one of the commonest conditions referred to an outpatient foot and ankle clinic. Around 30% of flatfeet are not symptomatic, do not affect daily activities, and therefore, need no treatment. The prevalence of painful PPV in the UK is approximately 6%, and many cases may be undiagnosed (1).

Although initially believed to be the final common pathway due to posterior tibial tendon dysfunction (PTTD), the progression of the condition is multifactorial. Symptomatic PPV may develop from a pre-existing flatfoot or from a normal foot that flattens and becomes painful in adulthood (adult acquired flatfoot deformity – AAFD). The terms PPV, PTTD and AAFD are often used interchangeably in the literature. The common finding is the collapse of the medial arch of the foot with pain in the medial soft tissues including posterior tibial tendon (PTT) and progressive deformity in the midfoot and forefoot. PPV affects women more frequently than men, with peak age of 55 years (1). A pre-existing flatfoot is present in most patients, with other risk factors including obesity, diabetes, hypertension, treatment with steroids and impact sports (2). Physical examination is the key to diagnose PPV, but imaging studies are necessary to exclude arthritis as this finding may influence the choice of treatment. Despite classifications that help to guide the management, no two PPV cases are the same so every patient should be addressed in terms of the type of deformity and risk factors to individualise conservative and surgical treatment.

Historically several authors have shared their experience in PPV allowing us to understand pathomechanics, classifications and management (Table 8.1) (2, 3).

Table 8.1 Historical evolution of the description, management and classifications of pes plano valgus (2, 3)

Year	Author/s	Description
1936	Kulowski	First description of PTT tendinopathy in 3 patients
1950	Lapidus/Seidenstein	First description of PTT synovitis in 2 patients that underwent decompressive surgery
1953	Key	First description of PTT rupture
1969	Kettelkam/Alexander	First results of an open debridement of PTT with pes plano valgus in 4 patients
1974	Goldner	First results of FDL or FHL transfer for complete PTT rupture, together with spring ligament reefing
1982	Mann/Specht	Eight patients underwent surgery for PTT complete rupture
1982	Jahss	Another series of 10 patients with PTT rupture and pes plano valgus
1983	Johnson	Detailed description of signs and symptoms associated with PTT rupture
1986	Funk	Description of PTT tendinopathy in relation to accessory navicular
1989	Johnson/Strom	Three-stage classification of AAFD
2007	Bluman/Myerson	Fourth stage is added (affection of ankle joint)
2012	Raikin	RAM classification based on segments of foot

Abbreviations: AAFD, adult acquired flatfoot deformity; FDL, flexor digitorum longus; FHL, flexor hallucis longus; PTT, posterior tibialis tendon.

Pathogenesis of deformities in Pes plano valgus

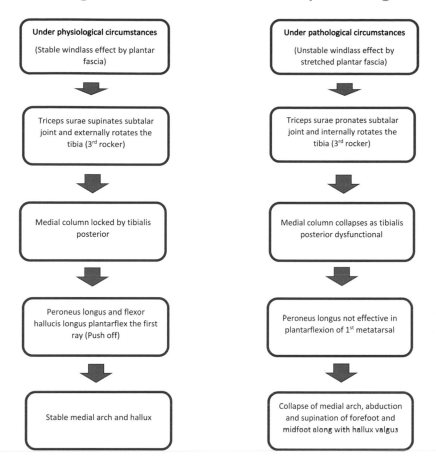

Visual gait analysis in the outpatient clinic is very valuable to analyse and understand the pathomechanics of PPV. During the first milliseconds of the first rocker of gait, the subtalar joint (STJ) pronates more than it physiologically should thus cause an abnormal loading of the medial soft tissues. Medial soft tissue overload causes structural stress and subsequent pain in the deltoid ligament, spring ligament (plantar calcaneonavicular), PTT, flexor digitorum longus (FDL) and flexor hallucis longus (FHL). Repeated abnormal subtalar pronation ultimately leads to structural damage resulting in partial or even complete rupture of the aforementioned medial structures (4). During the transition from the first to the second rocker of gait, foot dorsiflexor tendons are activated to restrict subtalar pronation so pain may also be present around the anterior and lateral leg and ankle. At the end of the second rocker, with the foot flat on the ground and the medial arch collapsed, all medial soft tissue structures are stressed and elongated whereas the lateral structures (lateral STJ and the peroneal tendons) are compressed. This lateral compression explains that why some patients complain of lateral subfibular pain.

When medial pain combines with lateral pain, patients experience circumferential peritalar pain that is a common finding in long-standing PPV. The plantar fascia also suffers from abnormal stretching and the physiological windlass mechanism is progressively lost. Loss of the windlass mechanism and tarsal pronation during the second rocker of gait does not allow the peroneus longus tendon to position with the adequate attack angle to plantarflex the first metatarsal. In this scenario, the peroneus longus works continuously to plantarflex the first metatarsal but is unable to do so. In the end this results in insertional tendinopathy of peroneus longus with tenderness upon palpation of the plantar proximal region of the first metatarsal. Prolonged flattening of the foot with subtalar pronation and midfoot/forefoot abduction results over time in fixed forefoot supination. This is the reason why hallux valgus deformity occurs in cases of severe PPV (Figure 8.1).

Many PPVs are asymptomatic as long as the compensatory mechanisms in the leg, ankle and foot work properly and the patient can heel raise. When all compensatory mechanisms are exhausted, sometimes due

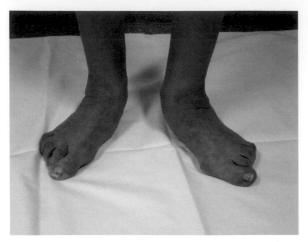

Figure 8.1 Associated pes plano valgus and hallux valgus deformity usually means apropulsive gait in a patient with long-standing deformity.

to the progressive degeneration of subtalar ligaments (cervical and interosseous talocalcaneal ligaments), gait becomes apropulsive and the patient needs the support of contralateral limb for the progression of gait. Gait speed and cadence slow down and stride length shortens. In this context of mechanical failure, transfer loading on adjacent segments is responsible for knee, hip and lumbar pain in these patients. All these findings may be identified during a thorough clinical examination.

Clinical examination

The commonest complaint of the patient is medial ankle and arch pain on activity. Some patients refer collapse of the foot when walking. Lateral pain due to fibular impingement may be present in severe deformities.

Clinical examination should start with a visual gait analysis with the patient barefoot and both knees and ankles visible. It is very important to rule out proximal deformities because PPV may be secondary to compensation of a varus knee. Feet should be observed from the front, side and behind to know which foot segments are involved in the deformity.

With the patient seated and feet hanging from the examination couch, palpation reveals pain mainly in the medial soft tissues around the ankle. The PTT may be swollen and tender in different segments or all the way from the retromalleolar region down to its insertion in the navicular. With the progression of the deformity, most medial structures are stretched resulting in tenderness around the spring ligament, the deltoid ligament, TPP, FDL and FHL. In severe deformities, compression of the peroneal tendons, the sinus tarsi and the lateral STJ also causes lateral ankle pain because of fibular impingement. In these cases the patient develops circumferential pain around the talus. Manual passive correction of hindfoot valgus and forefoot abduction deformities helps in the evaluation of forefoot supination. In cases of a fixed forefoot supination deformity, the forefoot cannot be brought to plantigrade position passively. This is an indication of plantarflexion osteotomy of the medial cuneiform as part of the reconstructive surgical plan.

The dynamic examination should include the heel rise/raise (bilateral and single) tests. Bilateral heel rise test helps to determine whether the hindfoot valgus is flexible (correction of subtalar valgus into varus on heel raise) or rigid (fixed valgus on heel raise). Inability to perform repeated single heel raise is suggestive of weakness of the tibialis posterior tendon. Various clinical signs and tests that are used for the assessment of PPV are summarised in Table 8.2 (2, 5, 6).

Table 8.2 Some of the signs/tests described for the clinical examination of pes plano valgus (2, 5, 6)	
Sign/test	**Description**
"Too many toes sign"	With hindfoot valgus and midfoot/forefoot abduction "too many toes" (2 or more) are seen when examiner looks at the patient's feet from behind
Single heel raise test	The patient is asked to perform heel raise on single limb stance. When compensatory mechanisms fail, the patient is unable to perform a single heel raise. On the other hand with weakness of TPP the patient cannot perform repeated single heel raises
Bilateral heel rise test	The patient is asked to perform bilateral heel rise on double limb stance. The examiner checks whether the heel on the affected side tilts into varus (flexible subtalar) or remains in valgus (rigid subtalar)
The first metatarsal rise sign	With patient standing and fully weight-bearing, the shank of the affected foot is taken with one hand and externally rotated, or the heel of the affected foot is taken with one hand and brought passively into a varus position. The head of the first metatarsal raises in the case of PTT dysfunction and remains on the ground in normal function
Abbreviations: PTT, posterior tibial tendon	

Role of imaging

Imaging studies should ideally include weight-bearing x-rays of both feet and ankles. The x-ray features of PPV include (Figure 8.2):

1. Loss of calcaneal pitch
2. Plantarflexion of talus leading to abnormal talar-first metatarsal angle (Meary's angle)
3. Obliteration of STJ space
4. Reduction of cuneiform height
5. Increased talocalcaneal angles
6. Talonavicular uncoverage

It is interesting to note that there might be a radiological-clinical dissociation in some patients with PPV (7). Until all compensatory mechanisms are lost the true degree of deformity may not be appreciated in the weight-bearing x-rays. Patients may have their "minute of glory" in the x-ray cabinet and get the flexor and invertor tendons to work to compensate for the arch collapse thus resulting in an almost "normal" image. Only when all the compensatory mechanisms are lost, x-rays reliably reflect the clinical condition (Figure 8.2). It is therefore not advisable to base surgical planning on the amount of talar displacement or talonavicular uncovering as these parameters may be affected by the motor reserve of the patient.

Ultrasound scan can be useful especially in the initial stage of tenosynovitis of tibialis posterior tendon, as an ultrasound guided steroid injection could be considered provided there is no tendon tear (Figure 8.3).

Magnetic resonance imaging (MRI) may reveal arthritis in the affected peritalar joints. The diagnosis of arthritis may influence the surgical decision-making (with arthrodesis usually being indicated in arthritis). The PTT runs behind the medial malleolus and changes its orientation almost 90° around the tip of the malleolus to finally insert in the navicular. This abrupt change of orientation is responsible for signal abnormalities in the MRI that results in many false-positive and false-negative interpretations of partial and/or complete ruptures. MRI findings have a poor correlation with surgical findings (8). So, PTT findings in MRI should not guide our surgical decision-making. MRI may also show medial osteochondral lesions of the talus that might be explained by the ischemic torsional effect of pronation to the deltoid artery, a branch of the posterior tibial artery. Most of these medial lesions are asymptomatic and need no specific treatment. Computerised tomography (CT) helps to better define arthritic changes and the state of neighbouring joints. Weight-bearing CT scan gives valuable information on the shape of the STJ and single-photon emission computed tomography (SPECT-CT) may be of help in defining latent cases

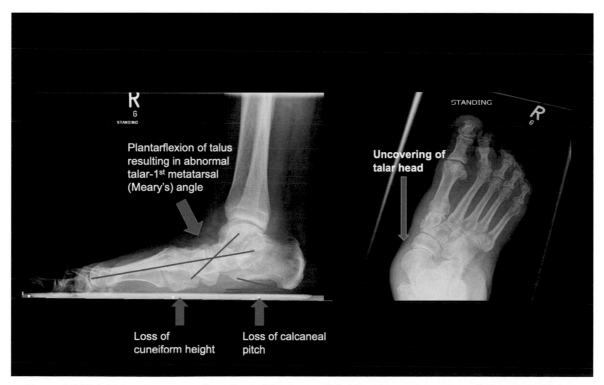

Figure 8.2 Weight-bearing x-rays of a patient with severe painful pes plano valgus when all the compensatory mechanisms are lost.

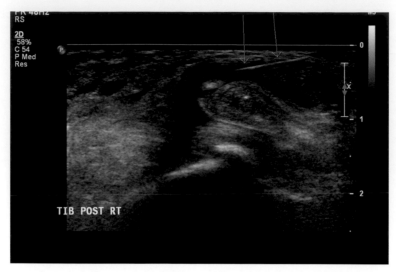

Figure 8.3 Ultrasound guided steroid injection for stage I disease.

of arthritis and activity of associated osteochondral lesions of the talus (9).

Classifications

The pioneering classification of PTTD was formulated in 1989 (Johnson and Strom) and divided the deformity into three stages (10). In 1997, Bluman and Myerson added the fourth stage when the deformity affected the tibiotalar joint (11). This modified classification has been widely used as it guides for the indication/type of surgical procedure based on staging (Table 8.3). In 2007, stage II was divided into IIA and IIB depending on the amount of talonavicular coverage (midfoot/forefoot

Table 8.3 Clinical stages and surgical interventions in adult pes plano valgus according to the classical classification by Johnson and Strom, modified by Bluman/Myerson and other authors. Surgical options include the most reported in the literature (10, 11)

Stage	Clinical findings	Surgical options
I	Medial foot and ankle pain, swelling, mild weakness, tendon length is normal. No deformity (pre-existing relative flatfoot often present)	Open tenosynovectomy +/− FDL transfer or tendoscopic debridement
IIA	Moderate flexible deformity (minimal abduction through the talonavicular joint, <30% talonavicular uncoverage) Medial or lateral pain or both. The "too many toes sign" is positive and the patient cannot perform repeated single heel rise The tendon is elongated and functionally incompetent	Medial displacement calcaneal osteotomy and FDL transfer or Medial displacement calcaneal osteotomy and Cobb procedure +/− Spring ligament repair +/− Achilles tendon lengthening/gastrocnemius recession
IIB	Severe flexible deformity with either abduction deformity through the talonavicular joint (>30%–40% talonavicular uncoverage) or subtalar impingement	Lateral column lengthening (Evans osteotomy) +/− plantarflexion osteotomy of medial cuneiform (Cotton osteotomy)
III	Fixed deformity (involving the triple-joint complex). Lateral pain at the calcaneal-fibular contact	Arthrodesis of hindfoot joints (single, double or triple)
IVA	Hindfoot valgus and flexible ankle valgus without significant ankle arthritis	Arthrodesis of hindfoot joints (single, double or triple) +/− deltoid reconstruction
IVB	Hindfoot valgus with rigid ankle valgus or flexible deformity with significant ankle arthritis	Triple arthrodesis with total ankle replacement or pantalar (tibiotalocalcaneal + talonavicular) fusion

Abbreviations: FDL, flexor digitorum longus; PTT, posterior tibial tendon.

Table 8.4 Clinical stages/deformity of pes plano valgus centred on the spring ligament (14)

Stage	Deformity
0	Spring ligament laxity but no TPP tendinopathy or plano valgus
1	Spring ligament laxity/failure with TPP tendinopathy but normal tendon length and no deformity
2	Spring ligament failure with TPP lengthening and flexible plano valgus deformity
3	Spring ligament failure with TPP lengthening and fixed plano valgus deformity

abduction) and stage IV (tibiotalar valgus) was also divided into IVA and IVB, depending on the presence of ankle stiffness and arthritis (3). Other authors classified the different PPV scenarios depending on PTT changes on MRI findings (12). Raikin et al. developed a new classification (The RAM classification) considering the deformity of the different segments rearfoot, ankle and midfoot (13). Recently, the spring (plantar calcaneonavicular) ligament has been identified as one of the structures that could suffer damage at the beginning of the arch collapse and some authors have set up a classification taking the spring ligament as the reference to explain the different clinical scenarios in PPV (Table 8.4) (14).

Conservative treatment

There is paucity of high-quality clinical research regarding conservative treatment of PPV especially regarding the role of physiotherapy in PTTD (15). Ultrasound-guided steroid injections can be considered in stage I (tenosynovitis) provided there is no tendon tear. Use of plaster cast or boot for 6 weeks in patients with acute symptoms of medial pain and swelling in stage I disease can be considered.

Orthoses are generally the most effective conservative intervention in the management of PPV. Around 80% of patients get notably better with the regular use of the correct devices (16). The ideal orthotic for PPV is custom-made medial heel wedge (measuring at least 10–12 mm) to counter hindfoot pronation during the first milliseconds of the first rocker (just after heel strike). Longitudinal medial arch support should not be greater than the medial heel wedge, otherwise it could result in a shearing effect around the talonavicular region leading to increased medial pain. When orthoses have a high longitudinal medial arch support and a low medial heel wedge, subtalar pronation during the first rocker of gait is abruptly stopped with an impact of the talonavicular region onto the medial arch

of the orthotic. That scenario would explain why some patients feel worse when wearing the (incorrect) orthoses. The modification of the supinatory gradient in the heel region produces an important impact in pain relief and better function for most patients. Orthoses are very effective in most patients regardless of the stage of the flatfoot deformity. They are more effective in flexible PPV than in rigid feet, but even in arthritic feet pain relief and better function may be expected.

Surgical treatment

When all conservative interventions fail to provide pain relief and the patient suffers from severe limitations for daily activities, surgical treatment may correct the deformity and dramatically change the shape and function of the foot and ankle (17).

PPV is a myriad of pathomechanical scenarios and decision-making regarding the type of surgery should be individualised for each patient. Clinical examination and imaging studies allow us to know whether the deformity is flexible (think of osteotomies) or rigid (think of arthrodesis).

Most patients with PPV present with a short triceps surae, and therefore, Achilles lengthening (percutaneous) used to be a popular surgical adjunct. However, Achilles lengthening may result in loss of calf power so in the last few years the threshold for Achilles lengthening is higher than before and is performed if residual equinus is present after the bony procedure. If there is tightness of gastrocnemius on Silfverskiöld test (Chapter 1), gastrocnemius recession is a good option.

Flexible pes plano valgus

The goal of surgery for a flexible but painful PPV is deformity correction to achieve a plantigrade foot. Ideally all passive (capsules, ligaments, joints) and active (tendons/muscles) structures should work harmonically and efficiently with the least energy consumption while maintaining maximum motion in the Chopart and STJs. The correction of the transverse and sagittal plane deformities allows for the restoration of tension in the plantar fascia and thereby restoring the windlass effect (anti-collapse effect). A flexible painful PPV may present different scenarios that need different surgeries for its reconstruction:

1. *Stage I* (Tenosynovitis of PTT, no deformity): Tenosynovectomy of the PTT either open (Figure 8.4A) or tenoscopic (Figure 8.4B and C) may be indicated (18, 19). In patients with high risk of deformity progression (rheumatoid arthritis, hypermobility, morbid obesity) a "prophylactic" medial displacement calcaneal osteotomy may be performed in addition to tenosynovectomy to prevent the progression of the deformity (20).

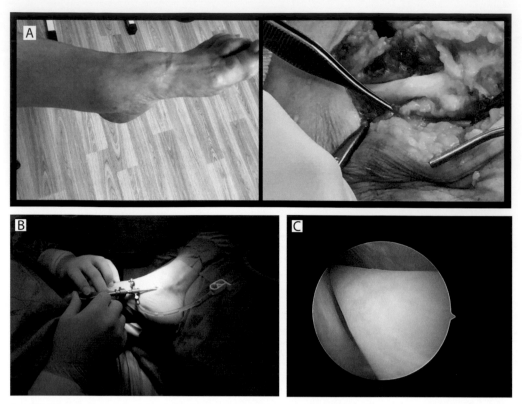

Figure 8.4 (A) Clinical photograph on left showing marked posteromedial swelling. Intraoperative picture of same patient showing florid tenosynovitis of PTT. (B) Tendoscopy of PTT showing first portal is placed close to the navicular insertion of the tendon. (C) Tendoscopy of PTT showing an intact tendon with mild synovitis as the most common finding in early stages of pes plano valgus.

2. *Stage IIA* (Isolated hindfoot valgus deformity and no associated deformities in the midfoot and forefoot): Medial displacement calcaneal osteotomy (Koutsogiannis effect) with 10 mm of medial slide is usually enough to produce a substantial change in the function of the triceps surae thereby converting valgus/pronation moment across the STJ into varus/supination moment. PTT tendoscopy may be associated to evaluate potential synovitis, plicae or partial rupture that might continue to be painful despite the unloading effect of the osteotomy. Injuries of the deltoid ligament, the spring ligament or the PTT may be repaired with open surgery (2). In cases of severe damage to the tendon (extensive partial or complete rupture Figure 8.5) the most common surgical technique associated to the bony procedure is the transfer of FDL – with or without a tenodesis effect – to the PTT and subsequent fixation to the navicular (2, 17).

Some authors find arthroereisis of the STJ to be useful for deformity correction in adult PPV by blocking

subtalar pronation with a sinus tarsi implant (21). It has the potential advantage of the mini invasive approach, but it reduces subtalar motion and it is not difficult to overcorrect into a varus hindfoot (badly tolerated and

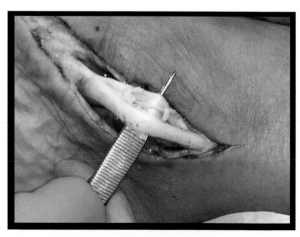

Figure 8.5 Intraoperative picture demonstrating partial longitudinal tear of PTT.

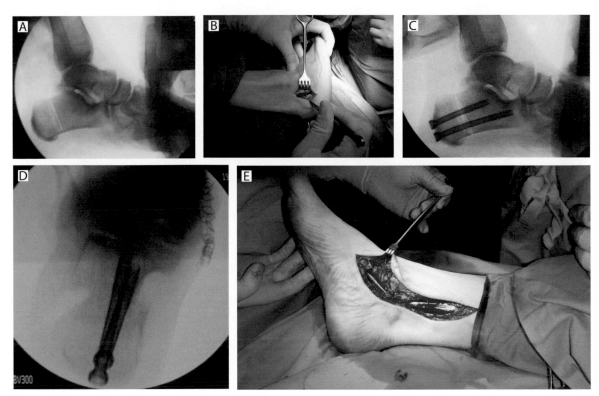

Figure 8.6 The most popular surgical intervention for painful flexible PPV combines calcaneal osteotomy and medial soft tissue reconstruction. (A) Posterior calcaneal osteotomy is performed. (B) Medial displacement of around 10 mm is needed to realign the valgus hindfoot. (C) Stable screw fixation is obtained with two 6.5 mm cannulated screws. (D) Intraoperative imaging shows the shifting of the calcaneal tuberosity medially. (E) FDL transfer to the PTT is shown with the transferred tendon fixed to the navicular.

very unusual complication with a calcaneal osteotomy). Other techniques have been reported for stage IIA but are less popular than FDL tendon transfer. These include: allograft reconstruction of PTT and the Cobb procedure, which involves the use of partial anterior tibial tendon graft which is rerouted through the medial cuneiform to the proximal stump of PTT (2, 20).

Surgical interventions for painful flexible PPV are presented in Figure 8.6.

3. *Stage IIB* (Hindfoot valgus deformity and abduction of the midfoot/forefoot with an altered talonavicular coverage): Lengthening of the lateral column by performing the Evans calcaneal osteotomy is indicated (Figure 8.7) (22). The Evans osteotomy and its variants have a triplanar effect. Supination of the forefoot should be evaluated following the Evans osteotomy. If the forefoot is easily passively corrected (flexible supination), the combination of medial sliding and lateral lengthening osteotomies of the os calcis may achieve the desired correction.

In case of fixed supination of the forefoot, the Cotton osteotomy is helpful to achieve a plantigrade foot (23). The Cotton osteotomy is a dorsal opening wedge osteotomy of the medial cuneiform and results in plantarflexion of the medial column (Figure 8.8). It is indicated if there is no significant arthritis of first tarsometatarsal (TMT) joint. However, if there is arthritis of first TMT joint then the Lapidus procedure (arthrodesis of first TMT joint) is indicated (24). Failure to obtain a plantigrade forefoot results in chronic insertional peroneus longus tendinopathy and lack of push off strength during the third rocker of gait. Restoration of windlass effect of the plantar fascia is the most important anti-collapse mechanism to obtain a strong foot and prevents the recurrence of the deformity.

Rigid pes plano valgus

4. *Stage III* (Fixed deformity involving hindfoot): Most rigid and painful PPVs have some degree of subtalar arthritis. In the presence of arthritis,

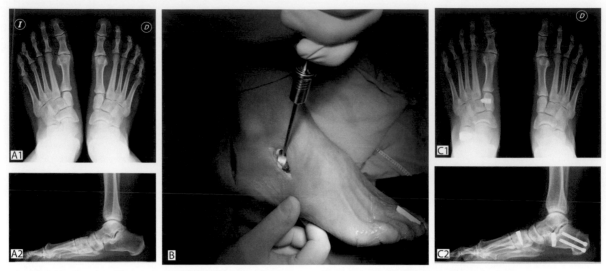

Figure 8.7 When hindfoot valgus combines with midfoot/forefoot abduction, a lateral column lengthening procedure is usually indicated. (A1 and A2) Weight-bearing x-rays of a patient with painful PPV and midfoot/forefoot abduction showing talonavicular uncoverage. (B) A double calcaneal osteotomy – medial displacement osteotomy and lateral column lengthening – is performed. A trial metal wedge is used to evaluate the amount of lengthening needed. (C1 and C2) Weight-bearing x-rays showing postoperative correction after reconstruction with medial displacement calcaneal osteotomy (10 mm and fixed with screws), lateral column lengthening osteotomy (9 mm Evans) and plantarflexion osteotomy of the medial cuneiform (8 mm Cotton) (both Evans and Cotton fixed with titanium porous wedges).

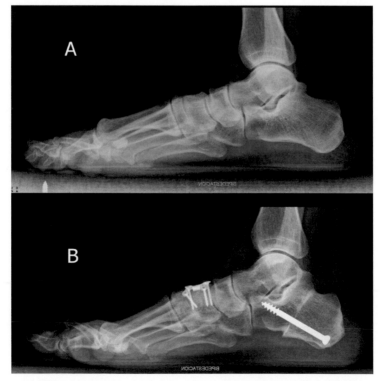

Figure 8.8 Plantarflexion effect of a Cotton osteotomy. (A) An elevation of the first metatarsal with respect to the second reveals forefoot supination. (B) After medial sliding calcaneal osteotomy, plantarflexion of the medial column has been achieved by a 7 mm plantarflexion Cotton osteotomy fixed with plate and screws.

osteotomies would not address the pain and stiffness. Arthrodesis is the procedure of choice for a rigid PPV deformity affecting the hindfoot coupled with arthritis of talonavicular joint (TNJ), STJ and/or calcaneocuboid joint (CCJ). Depending on the joints affected by arthritis an isolated STJ, a double (STJ and TNJ) or a triple (STJ, TNJ and CCJ) fusion may be indicated. In some patients, a combination of fusion and osteotomy may render a plantigrade and painless foot. Association of different fusions in different segments usually results in too much stiffness and a less functional foot.

If hindfoot valgus is coupled with midfoot/forefoot abduction and significant talonavicular uncoupling, a double tarsal arthrodesis with a medial approach allows for the shortening of the medial column and the reconstruction of the deformity (24). Calcaneocuboid fusion may be added in the rare presence of calcaneocuboid arthritis. If arthritis changes and collapse are located in other joints of the medial column (naviculocuneiform or first TMT joint), then selective fusion of the affected joint should be indicated to restore the height of the medial longitudinal arch and windlass effect of the plantar fascia.

Surgical interventions for painful rigid PPV are presented in Figure 8.9.

5. *Stage IV* (Tibiotalar joint arthritis and valgus in long-standing PPV): The choice of the surgical technique depends on the degree of arthritic changes in the ankle joint. If mild arthritic changes are present *(IVA)* then repair of the deltoid ligament with allograft or synthetic internal bracing may result in better alignment and function of the ankle. In cases of severe arthritis *(IVB)*, medial soft tissue repair may be associated

with ankle fusion, or pantalar fusion combining a tibiotalocalcaneal with a TN arthrodesis or total ankle replacement (24).

Outcomes of reconstructive surgery of PPV are usually very good with most patients getting better function and pain relief (12). Evaluation of results should be long term as the adaptation of the foot and ankle to a new spatial position and function takes more than a year in most cases. Outcomes are generally better in flexible PPV treated with osteotomies than in rigid feet treated with fusions (25). In a long-term follow-up study additional surgery was necessary in 16.8% of patients, with the removal of metalwork being the most common procedure (57.4%) followed by a conversion from failed osteotomies to triple fusions (16.7%) (25). Isolated flexible hindfoot valgus deformity (stage IIA) without midfoot/forefoot deformities treated with medial displacement calcaneal osteotomy and medial soft tissue repair is the type of PPV associated with the best functional results (2, 17, 20).

Take home messages

- Adult flatfoot deformity is a compendium of mechanical situations which share pathological tarsal pronation ending in a painful flattening of the foot with variable dysfunction.
- Diagnosis is essentially clinical combining visual gait analysis with physical examination. Imaging studies allow for the evaluation of peritalar arthritis and help us in the planning of surgical treatment.
- Conservative treatment with the use of orthoses with a medial heel and longitudinal medial arch support makes most patients better with pain relief and better overall function.
- Osteotomies and soft tissue reconstruction are the procedures of choice for the surgical reconstruction of a flexible pes plano valgus, whereas arthrodesis is preferred when the foot is rigid and/or arthritic.
- Long-term outcomes of reconstructive surgery are usually very good with most patients getting better function and pain relief. Osteotomies are associated with better results than fusions.

References

1. Kohls-Gatzoulis J, Woods B, Angel JC, Singh D. The prevalence of symptomatic posterior tibialis tendon dysfunction in women over the age of 40 in England. Foot Ankle Surg. 2009; 15(2):75–81.
2. Myerson MS. Adult acquired flatfoot deformity: Treatment of dysfunction of the posterior tibial tendon. Instr Course Lect. 1997; 46:393–405.
3. Abousayed MM, Tartaglione JP, Rosenbaum AJ, Dipreta JA. Classifications in brief: Johnson and Strom classification of

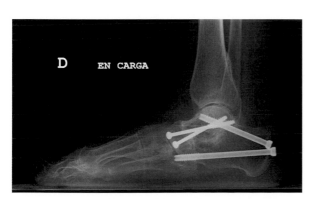

Figure 8.9 Long-standing PPV usually associates severe deformity with disabling arthritis. Triple tarsal arthrodesis combining subtalar, talonavicular and calcaneocuboid fusion is an indication for a rigid arthritic PPV.

adult-acquired flatfoot deformity. Clin Orthop Relat Res. 2016; 474(2):588–93.

4. Maceira E, Monteagudo M. Subtalar anatomy and mechanics. Foot Ankle Clin. 2015; 20(2):195–221.

5. Rodrigues-Fonseca J. Pe plano. Estudo dinâmico. Lab Bial Oporto. 1984.

6. Hintermann B, Gächter A. The first metatarsal rise sign: A simple, sensitive sign of tibialis posterior tendon dysfunction. Foot Ankle Int. 1996; 17(4):236–41.

7. Sutter R, Pfirrmann CW, Espinosa N, Buck FM. Three-dimensional hindfoot alignment measurements based on biplanar radiographs: Comparison with standard radiographic measurements. Skeletal Radiol. 2013; 42(4): 493–8.

8. Gianakos AL, Ross KA, Hannon CP, Duke GL, Prado MP, Kennedy JG. Functional outcomes of tibialis posterior tendoscopy with comparison to magnetic resonance imaging. Foot Ankle Int. 2015; 36(7):812–9.

9. de Cesar Netto C, Shakoor D, Dein EJ, Zhang H, Thawait GK, Richter M, Ficke JR, Schon LC, Weightbearing CT International Study Group, Demehri S. Influence of investigator experience on reliability of adult acquired flatfoot deformity measurements using weightbearing computed tomography. Foot Ankle Surg. 2019; 25(4):495–502.

10. Johnson KA, Strom DE. Tibialis posterior tendon dysfunction. Clin Orthop Relat Res. 1989; 239:196–206.

11. Bluman EM, Title CI, Myerson MS. Posterior tibial tendon rupture: A refined classification system. Foot Ankle Clin. 2007; 8(3):637–45.

12. Conti MS, Garfinkel JH, Ellis SJ. Outcomes of reconstruction of the flexible adult-acquired flatfoot deformity. Orthop Clin North Am. 2020; 51(1):109–20.

13. Raikin SM, Winters BS, Daniel JN. The RAM classification: A novel, systematic approach to the adult-acquired flatfoot. Foot Ankle Clin. 2012; 17(2):169–81.

14. Pasapula C, Cutts S. Modern theory of the development of adult acquired flat foot and an updated spring ligament classification system. Clin Res Foot Ankle. 2017; 5:247.

15. Ross MH, Smith MD, Mellor R, Vicenzino B. Exercise for posterior tibial tendon dysfunction: A systematic review of randomised clinical trials and clinical guidelines. BMJ Open Sport Exerc Med. 2018; 4:e000430.

16. Pascual-Huerta J, Ropa JM, Kirby KA, Orejana AM, García-Carmona FJ. Effect of 7 degree varus and valgus rearfoot wedging on rearfoot kinematics and kinetic during the stance phase of walking. J Am Podiatr Med Assoc. 2009; 99(5):415–21.

17. Deland JT. Adult-acquired flatfoot deformity. J Am Acad Orthop Surg. 2008; 16:399–406.

18. van Dijk CN, Knort N, Scholten PE. Tendoscopy of the posterior tibial tendon. J Arthroscopic Rel Surg. 1997; 13(6):692–8.

19. Monteagudo M, Maceira E. Posterior tibial tendoscopy. Foot Ankle Clin. 2015; 20(1):1–13.

20. Giza E, Cush G, Schon LC. The flexible flatfoot in the adult. Foot Ankle Clin. 2007; 12(2):251–71.

21. Viladot Voegeli A, Fontecilla Cornejo N, Serrá Sandoval JA, Alvarez Goenaga F, Viladot Pericé R. Results of subtalar arthroereisis for posterior tibial tendon dysfunction stage IIA1. Based on 35 patients. Foot Ankle Surg. 2018; 24(1):28–33.

22. Marks RM, Long JT, Ness ME, Khazzam M, Harris GF. Surgical reconstruction of posterior tibial tendon dysfunction: Prospective comparison of flexor digitorum longus substitution combined with lateral column lengthening or medial displacement calcaneal osteotomy. Gait and Posture. 2009; 29:17–22.

23. Kunas GC, Do HT, Aiyer A, Deland JT, Ellis SJ. Contribution of medial cuneiform osteotomy to correction of longitudinal arch collapse in stage IIb adult-acquired flatfoot deformity. Foot Ankle Int. 2018; 39(8):885–93.

24. Johnson JE, Yu JR. Arthrodesis techniques in the management of stage II and III acquired adult flatfoot deformity. Instr Course Lect. 2006; 55:531–42.

25. Goss M, Stauch C, Lewcun J, Ridenour R, King J, Juliano P, Aynardi M. Natural history of 321 flatfoot reconstructions in adult acquired flatfoot deformity over a 14-year period. Foot Ankle Spec. 2020; 1938640020912859.

9 The cavovarus foot

Rick Brown and Rajesh Kakwani

Introduction

The foot is an amazing piece of engineering. It is a complex three-dimensional structure held in shape by the delicate balance of the intrinsic and extrinsic muscles. It not only allows the transfer of weight but also allows the shock absorption, flexibility to adapt to uneven ground and an effective gait.

The medial longitudinal arch of the foot can vary from a flat to a high-arched foot. Cavus foot is found in around 10–20% of the population and is as common as the flatfoot (1, 2). In the early stage, the "high arched" or cavus foot is flexible and can be managed with corrective orthotics or perhaps the transfer of appropriate tendons. When the deformity is fixed, the foot will require an accommodative insole or realignment bony surgery.

Biomechanics

A very simple analogy

Imagine yourself driving a chariot with 4 horses. If all the 4 horses are of equal strength (balanced) you will move ahead in a straight line. If your left 2 horses are stronger than the right 2 horses, you will move around in circles, anticlockwise. Similarly, if the right 2 horses are stronger, you will move in clockwise circles.

A very similar issue happens in the cavus foot, when the invertors and plantar flexors are stronger than the evertors and dorsiflexors, respectively, and hence the foot deforms into inversion and plantarflexion.

Mechanical stability of the foot

It is important to acknowledge the various antagonistic muscles around the foot and ankle; this helps us understand the pathophysiology of the development of the cavus foot.

Sagittal plane balance

The first ray is plantarflexed by the peroneus longus and is dorsiflexed by the tibialis anterior. Imbalance between these two, i.e., weak tibialis anterior and a normal or relatively stronger peroneus longus can lead to a plantarflexed first ray.

In the sagittal plane, the dorsiflexion of the foot is mainly by the tibialis anterior, the extensor hallucis longus (EHL) and extensor digitorum longus, whereas the plantarflexion of the foot is mainly by the gastrocsoleus complex. Weakness of the tibialis anterior and a relatively overpowered gastrocsoleus complex can lead to a foot drop type of deformity and contracture of the gastrocsoleus complex.

Hindfoot coronal plane balance

Inversion of the hindfoot is predominantly powered by the tibialis posterior and, to a certain extent, to the tibialis anterior. The eversion of the foot is mainly by the peroneus brevis, with a small contribution from the peroneus longus. Again, weakness of the peroneus brevis and a relatively stronger tibialis posterior can lead to a varus deformity of the hindfoot.

Forefoot

The dynamic stabilisers of the metatarsophalangeal joints are the intrinsic muscles. Weakness of the intrinsic muscles, relatively strong long flexors and extensors of the toes can lead to clawing of the toes. This is very similar to the deformities seen in the hand, with an ulnar claw hand caused by a weakness in the intrinsics of the hand. In most cases, probably all the muscles of the leg and the foot are weak but it is the relatively stronger muscles, which drive the deformity. Cavus foot deformity can be either forefoot driven or hindfoot driven or a combination of both.

The foot as a tripod

The standing foot is often considered to be a tripod, where the body weight is distributed between the heel, first metatarsal head and the fifth metatarsal head. In this analogy, if the first ray is plantarflexed (forefoot driven deformity) then for the tripod stool to stand, the hind foot must be twisted into a varus direction. Therefore, the plantarflexed first ray is said to have driven the cavovarus foot deformity. This also forms the basis of the Coleman's block test to be discussed in this chapter.

Implications of the biomechanical deformity

In a forefoot driven cavovarus foot, early clinical problems can be from overloading of the first metatarsal head area, resulting in a plantar callosity, sesamoid disease or early hallux rigidus. During mid-stance, the plantarflexed first ray requires a compensatory hindfoot varus moment. A hindfoot in excessive varus locks the subtalar joint, which in turn, reduces the shock absorbance of the foot (achy foot), that can eventually lead to early degeneration of the hindfoot joints.

Aetiology

The pes cavus encompasses a wide spectrum of foot shapes with an elevated medial longitudinal arch; mainly associated with hindfoot varus, ankle equinus and forefoot adduction and plantarflexion. Almost two-thirds of adults with a symptomatic cavus foot have an underlying neurological condition (3). The rest of patients with a heightened arch are generally labelled as idiopathic. Some neurologists would argue that these patients probably have an undiagnosed, inconsequential, underlying subtle neurological condition (Tables 9.1 and 9.2).

The commonest neurological cause of the cavus foot is hereditary motor and sensory neuropathy (HMSN), of which Charcot-Marie-Tooth (CMT) disease is the most common. However, neurological conditions can affect any level of the central or peripheral nervous system that controls the muscle power. This necessitates a thorough examination of the spinal and neurological system in patients with cavus feet.

The probability of a patient with bilateral cavovarus feet being diagnosed with CMT disease is around 78% (4). There are various types of CMT disease and each type presents in a different manner. Knowing the precise sub-type guides the prognosis, which allows the

Table 9.2 Neurological causes of cavus foot

Level of defect	Example
Cortex	Cerebral palsy, Stroke
Cerebellum	Friedreich's ataxia
Spinal column	Syrinx, Spinal tumour
Terminal spine	Spina bifida, Spinal dysraphism
Ventral root ganglia	Polio
Peripheral nervous system	HMSN, Polyneuritis
Muscle disease	Muscular dystrophy

surgeon to predict the benefit and outcome of the surgical procedure (Table 9.3).

The autosomal dominant demyelinating condition of CMT disease type 1 presents in the teenage years but can present earlier in childhood in 25% of patients. Usually the patient's parents complain of lesser toe deformities and subtle fatigue or weakness. The diagnosis can be confirmed with lower velocity on nerve conduction tests.

CMT type 2 develops slower, with most patients seeking help in their 20s or 30s with profound weakness, calf atrophy and decreased peripheral sensation.

The muscle involvement is generally distal to proximal affecting the intrinsic muscles of the foot, the tibialis anterior and the peroneus brevis. This can lead to relatively stronger posterior tibial and peroneus longus muscles driving the deformities, causing heel inversion and plantarflexion of the first ray, respectively. The relatively stronger long extensors and the loss of stabilisation of the intrinsics cause hyperextension of the metatarsophalangeal joints, producing a pistoning effect on the metatarsal heads and dorsal subluxation of the metatarsophalangeal joint. The relatively powerful long flexor of the toes causes the clawing of the toes. Plantarflexed metatarsal heads lead to metatarsalgia

Table 9.1 Categories of the causes of cavus foot

Neurological
Congenital 　• CTEV 　• Arthrogryposis
Trauma
Idiopathic

Table 9.3 Sub-types of Charcot-Marie-Tooth disease

CMT 1	AD. Demyelination due to duplication of gene 17. 50% of all cases
CMT 2	Abnormalities in the axon of the peripheral nerve cell
CMT 3	Severe demyelinating neuropathy
CMT 4	AR. Demyelinating motor & sensory neuropathies
CMT X	X linked dominant. Mutation of connexin 32 gene on X chromosome

type of symptoms and amplify the forefoot equinus (5, 6). The plantarflexed first ray, as explained earlier, forces the hindfoot into varus. The hindfoot initially remains flexible, but gradually becomes rigid over time. With the hindfoot varus, the Achilles tendon becomes a secondary inverter of the foot, and hence acts as a deforming force, becoming contracted over time (5, 6).

Clinical features

The commonest presenting features in patients with cavus foot are (Table 9.4):

- Chronic fatigue or ache (90%)
- Lesser toe problems (62%) – i.e., clawing of the toes, rubbing of the toes against the shoe
- Metatarsalgia (52%)
- Chronic ankle instability and a giving way sensation of the foot (31%)
- Lateral border pain in the foot (11%)
- Hindfoot pain (9%)
- Ulceration (only 1%)

The clinical examination needs to be focused on:

1. Evaluation of the degree of deformity
2. Neurological assessment of the leg
3. Evaluation of the underlying cause

Footwear

The patient's shoes are inspected for asymmetrical lateral wear of the shoe. The insoles need to be inspected to assess and determine whether they cater to the patient's deformity appropriately.

Standing position

A systematic examination is essential with an assessment of the hindfoot alignment and the height of the arch.

Looking from the front: The peek-a-boo sign with prominence of the heel along the medial border of the foot, prominence of the fifth metatarsal base region and any obvious clawing of the toes.

Looking from behind: The varus attitude of the heel is noted.

Gait

Patients generally have a slight foot drop. They commonly recruit the long toe extensors to allow the forefoot to clear the ground. This causes an exaggeration of the clawing of the toes. Some patients may have a varus thrust every time the hindfoot bears weight during the stance phase of gait.

Special tests: Coleman's block test (7)

Coleman's block test (Figure 9.1) gives an indication whether the deformity is forefoot driven. For balancing purposes, the authors would recommend using equal height blocks under both feet simultaneously. Initially the whole foot is placed over the blocks. The hindfoot varus is noted at this stage. The first ray is then placed outside the block, so that it is allowed to plantarflex. Looking from behind, an assessment is made whether the hindfoot varus is corrected to physiological valgus, after the first ray is allowed to plantarflex. If positive, this suggests that the deformity is forefoot driven and the hindfoot is still flexible.

Sitting down position

Inspection is important for callosities under the metatarsal heads, as well as, at the level of the base of the fifth metatarsal (Figure 9.2). Palpation for any focal bony tenderness may suggest a possible stress fracture from overloading. Silfverskiöld's test would assess for any gastrocnemius tightness. The passive range of movement of the ankle, subtalar and midfoot joints are documented. The passive correctability of the deformity is also assessed. The stability of the lateral ankle

Table 9.4 Clinical features of cavus foot	
Hindfoot	**Forefoot**
Equinus deformity	Metatarsalgia
Chronic ankle instability	Lateral border pain
Dorsal bony prominence	Fifth metatarsal stress fracture
Peroneal tendon damage	Plantar ulceration
Medial ankle pain	Clawed hallux
Foot drop	Hammering of lesser toes
	Sesamoid pathology

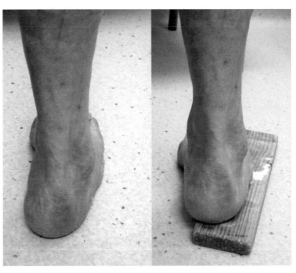

Figure 9.1 Coleman block test.

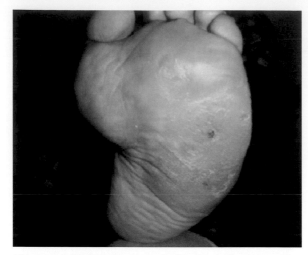

Figure 9.2 Clinical photograph showing callosities under the fifth metatarsal head and base.

ligaments is confirmed using anterior drawer and varus stress tests.

Neurological examination

Documentation of the power of all the muscles of the leg (tibialis anterior, tibialis posterior, peroneus longus, peroneus brevis, gastrocsoleus complex, EHL and extensor digitorum longus) is extremely important, with a particular focus on tibialis anterior. Reduced proprioception is believed to be the first sensory modality to be affected in the sensory examination.

Evaluation of the underlying causes

The examination of the *spine* includes documentation of any cutaneous manifestations of spinal dysraphism.

The *hands* are examined for any first web space wasting: commonly seen in patients with CMT disease.

Now is the time to stop and think in order to consider what is the underlying cause of the cavo-varus foot deformity. It helps to know that there are five most common tendon imbalances, seen in Table 9.5.

Investigations

Weight-bearing radiographs of the foot and ankle would demonstrate an increased calcaneal pitch, generally more than 30° (Figure 9.3). The talus-first metatarsal (Meary's) angle may be disrupted with an abnormal plantarflexed first ray by more than 4° (Figure 9.4). The CORA (centre of rotation of alignment) of the deformity is calculated with the weight-bearing lateral view of the foot (+/– weight-bearing CT scan if available), that would help surgical planning to try and correct the deformity at the level of the CORA. A flat domed talus is a common finding on the lateral radiographs. The posterior facet of the subtalar joint, as well as, the Chopart joints are clearly viewed in the lateral radiograph due to the rotation of the hindfoot (Figures 9.3 and 9.4). The distal fibula appears enlarged and posteriorly located. The weight-bearing lateral view demonstrates the increased navicular and medial cuneiform height. Lastly, the heel alignment view confirms the degree of heel varus.

The functional distribution of weight under the foot can be investigated by observing the ink distribution with the Harris McBeath foot pad (Figure 9.5). Alternatively, objective pressure studies can be measured with a pedobarograph, which may help design an orthotic. Formal gait analysis is not usually needed, although it may aid the decision of whether to transfer a tendon in the more complex neurological patients.

Table 9.5 Tendon imbalances in cavovarus deformity		
Deformity	**Weak**	**Strong**
Equinus	Tibialis anterior	Gastrocnemius
Adduction/ varus	Peroneus brevis	Tibialis posterior
Plantarflexed first ray	Tibialis anterior	Peroneus longus
Toe deformities	Small muscles of the foot	Long flexors
Claw hallux	Intrinsic muscles of the foot	Extensor hallucis longus and flexor hallucis longus

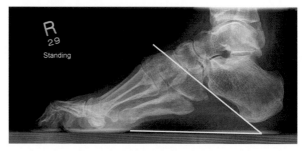

Figure 9.3 Weight-bearing lateral radiograph of cavus foot showing increased calcaneal pitch.

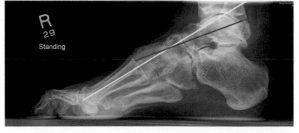

Figure 9.4 Weight-bearing lateral radiograph of cavus foot showing abnormal talar-first metatarsal (Meary's) angle.

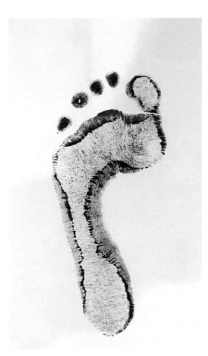

Figure 9.5 The Harris McBeath foot pad demonstrating weight-bearing pattern.

Nerve conduction studies help confirm the diagnosis and guide prognosis. Additionally, an MRI scan of the whole spine and the brain would help the neurological workup.

An opinion from a neurologist helps guide regarding the probability of the deformity progressing in the future.

Management

Aim: A pain-free plantigrade shoe-able foot

Non-surgical management

1. Physiotherapy with gastrocnemius stretching exercises, strengthening of all the weak muscles and joint range of movement exercises. Although the muscle strength can be maintained in certain cases with physiotherapy, it can be a slow-losing battle in more severe conditions as the neurological condition slowly deteriorates.
2. Footwear modification in the form of wide toe box shoes to accommodate the lesser toe deformities. Adding a slight heel raise to the rearfoot can help increase the available ankle joint dorsiflexion by plantarflexing the talus.
3. Orthotics: Insoles in the form of the University of California Berkeley Laboratory (UCBL) shoe insert to maintain the heel in neutral to slight valgus, arch support with a cut-out under the first metatarsal head to allow plantarflexion of

the first ray can be used in flexible deformity. A total contact orthosis may help distribute the forces on the forefoot over a larger plantar surface area. This can be improved by adding a metatarsal dome/bar in patients with metatarsalgia symptoms. A lateral hindfoot and midfoot wedge generally helps with symptomatic relief in milder cases. Keeping the lateral side of the post unbevelled provides a more stable platform and improves the resistance of the post to inversion forces. As the deformity worsens, adjustments of the insoles are required as increasing corrective forces are needed. Caution regarding use of strong rigid orthotics in patients with alteration in skin sensation to avoid pressure necrosis. Bracing of the ankle is helpful in patients with chronic ankle instability. Foot drop cases may need an ankle foot orthosis in the form of a foot drop splint.

4. In some units the neurologist may aim to control the deformity and delay the need for surgical intervention by weakening the overpowering muscle using botulin toxin injections, as part of the spasticity treatment.

When to operate?

The main indication to operate is when nonoperative management no longer controls the patient's symptoms. However, knowledge of the prognosis and the current muscle strength of the imbalanced muscles can allow prediction that the deformity will inexorably worsen. In this case, it is reasonable to operate prophylactically.

Children and adolescents also merit prophylactic surgery to prevent abnormal forces across the growing bones, leading to dysmorphic bones and a lifelong deformity.

Operative management

When considering operative treatment, the goal is to establish the **pain-free stable plantigrade foot**, but with **preservation of as many joints as possible.**

A wide range of potential operations are described in literature which can be daunting.

Every patient needs a bespoke plan for his/her surgical management.

The management can be logically divided into **three main principles** (Figure 9.6):

1. Restore the alignment of the heel under the leg.
2. Recreate a plantigrade foot with correction of the deformity at the CORA.
3. Balance the forces.

Additional procedures may be needed in certain cases such as release of the gastrocnemius fascia/plantar fascia release, etc.

A) Restoration of heel alignment

    Lateral displacement calcaneal osteotomy+/-
subtalar joint fusion or triple fusion

B) Recreation of plantigrade foot

    Dorsiflexion 1st metatarsal osteotomy Or midfoot fusion

    The Jones procedure

    Lesser toe interphalangeal joint fusion+/-The Hibbs tenosuspension procedure

C) Balancing the forces

    Tibialis posterior tendon transfer

    Peroneus longus to brevis transfer

    Split Tibialis anterior transfer

D) Additional procedures

    Modified Bostrom's reconstruction

    Achilles tendon lengthening or Strayer's release or gastrocnemius recession

    Plantar fascia release

Figure 9.6 An algorithm for cavovarus deformity correction.

Each of the discussed categories may need a combination of soft tissue/bony procedures.

Restoration of the alignment of the heel under the leg

Coleman's block test would give an indication regarding the correctability of the hindfoot. However, the Coleman's test is not binary and a hindfoot that is still flexible, but stiffening may require a calcaneal osteotomy at the time of the surgery. The clinical findings guide the ability of the surgeon to predict the future course of the condition. If there is only partial correction and the condition is deteriorating, most patients prefer a definitive procedure rather than frequent returns to the operating table. In order to preserve the subtalar joint in patients with a flexible hindfoot valgus, the malalignment is addressed by a lateralising calcaneal osteotomy (Figure 9.7). This can be a sliding cut performed by open surgery with a saw or by minimally invasive technique

using a burr. For more severe or complex deformities, the surgeon needs to consider that the deformity is correctable in three dimensions. In a calcaneovarus deformity, the increased calcaneal pitch can be reduced by incorporating a vertical component in the sliding of the posterior fragment attached to the Achilles tendon. For a severe deformity or where the lateral skin is under tension or compromised, a lateral based closing wedge osteotomy as described by Dwyer (8), or a 'Z' osteotomy with wedges (6) can be performed.

In patients where the hindfoot joints are degenerate and the source of pain, the hindfoot varus malalignment can be straightened by a subtalar or a triple fusion. The most severe, rigid, degenerate cavovarus deformities may require removal of trapezoidal bone blocks in a Lambrinudi (9) type of triple fusion (Figure 9.8). The long-term results of corrective triple fusion are not great. Wetmore and Drennan (10) followed 16 patients with HSMN who underwent 30 triple fusion procedures for 21 years. Unfortunately, only 7% continued to report

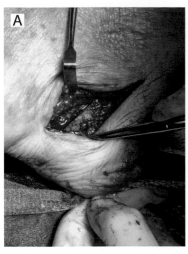
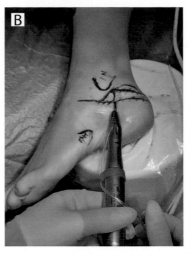
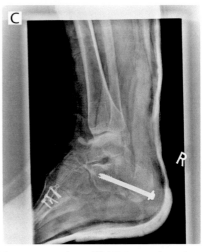

Figure 9.7 Photographs of two different methods of calcaneal osteotomy (A) Open procedure; (B) Minimum invasive technique); (C) Radiograph of a lateralising calcaneal osteotomy.

excellent relief of symptoms, and either ankle or midfoot arthritis affected 47%.

Joint preservation is key principle for patients with this lifelong condition.

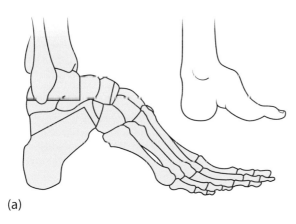

(a)

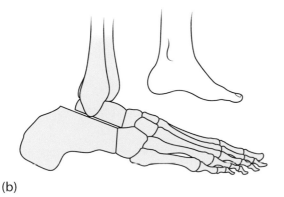

(b)

Figure 9.8 Lambrinudi type of triple fusion.

Recreating the plantigrade foot

The most common cavovarus deformity is due to an excessively plantarflexed first ray. This can be addressed with a closing wedge dorsiflexion type of osteotomy of the base of the first metatarsal. An oblique dorsally based wedge osteotomy can be cut in an oblique direction for maximal stability, which can be held with a screw, staple or a plate, as preferred (Figure 9.9). The degree of correction is chosen on the operating table in order to balance the weight distribution across all five metatarsal heads over a flat surface (simulated floor) with the heel in neutral. For a child, operating in the region of the first metatarsal base is best avoided until after the closure of the physis.

A severe rigid midfoot cavus deformity without any significant hindfoot varus may require a wedge osteotomy. The deformity is more easily corrected by cutting a trapezoidal bone block (Figure 9.10), which shortens the longitudinal arch to relax the adjacent structures. This is a difficult operation to perform: to make the bone cuts at the CORA of the deformity, whilst keeping away from the joints at the same time. In practice avoiding damage to a midfoot joint is nearly impossible. There is no correct level to perform this osteotomy, but the cancellous bone of the midfoot is more likely to unite than the metatarsals.

Clawing of the toes

Clawing of the great toe can be rebalanced by the Jones procedure, which involves transfer of EHL to the first metatarsal neck and stabilisation of the interphalangeal joint by fusion in a straight position. The tendon transfer of EHL to the first metatarsal neck augments the foot dorsiflexor power, as well as, the correction of

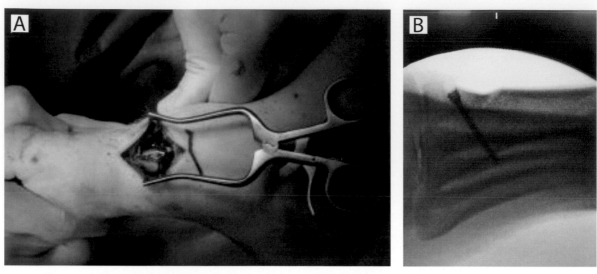

Figure 9.9 (A) 1st metatarsal dorsiflexion osteotomy (B) X-ray of 1st metatarsal dorsiflexion osteotomy.

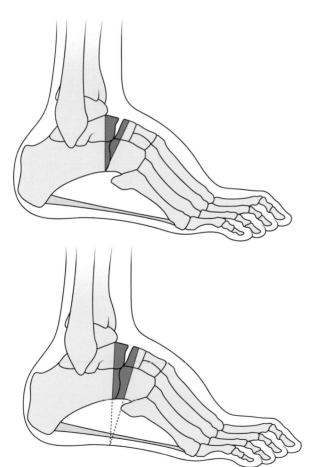

Figure 9.10 Wedge excision of bone block to correct rigid midfoot cavus.

the plantarflexed first ray. Hammering of the lesser toes can be corrected by a similar tenosuspension procedure of the long toe extensor tendon to the metatarsal neck, as described by Hibbs (11). Follow-up of this procedure by Vlachou et al. in 2008 (12) showed an 87% excellent to satisfactory improvement in both toe symptoms and metatarsalgia.

Balancing the forces

After the alignment and structure of the foot has been corrected, the forces acting across the foot must be balanced. This is perhaps the most important part of the art of cavovarus foot correction. It can involve correcting a weak tendon, which has been overpowered by a normal tendon; or a normal tendon overpowered by an excessively strong tendon.

The most common tendon transfer procedures are performed to balance the forces are:

Peroneus longus to brevis transfer

Dividing the peroneus longus will reduce the plantarflexion of the first ray, and technically it is very easy to attach this to the adjacent peroneus brevis tendon. This augments the hindfoot eversion force.

Tibialis posterior tendon transfer (Figure 9.11)

Most patients with a pes cavus have a foot drop and a weak tibialis anterior muscle. The power in the tibialis posterior is relatively stronger causing plantarflexion and inversion of the hindfoot. Some cases may necessitate the transfer of the tibialis posterior

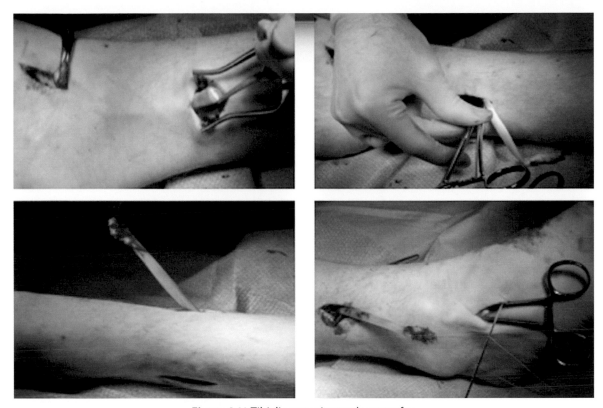

Figure 9.11 Tibialis posterior tendon transfer.

to the dorsum of the foot through the interosseous membrane. This augments the dorsiflexion force and removes the inversion force. Some surgeons are concerned that after harvesting a full tibialis posterior tendon, this could result in the foot collapsing into a pes planus. They advocate transfer of the flexor digitorum profundus to the stump of the tibialis posterior, or to perform split tibialis posterior tendon transfers, taking just 50% of the tendon to the dorsolateral aspect of the midfoot.

Attaining a balanced foot is essential to reduce the risk of recurrence of the deformity (13).

Additional procedures

Modified Broström's procedure (in chronic ankle instability with permanent damage to the lateral ligaments)

In patients with pes cavus having the hindfoot drifting into varus, the ankle is vulnerable to inversion injury and can lead to permanent damage to the lateral ligaments. Surgical management of this symptom involves a lateralising calcaneal osteotomy as described earlier, with repair of the anterior talofibular ligament using a modified Broström's type of procedure. The authors would recommend augmenting the lateral ligament repair with a synthetic augment such as the internal brace® suture.

Achilles lengthening

Often a patient will have tightness of the gastro-soleus mechanism. If the Silfverskiöld's test shows this to be due to a gastrocnemius contracture, then a release of the medial head of the gastrocnemius, at the popliteal skin crease, will suffice in most cases. Alternatively, this could be performed in the mid-calf area by the Strayer fractional lengthening technique. In practice more often the Achilles contracture involves the soleus muscle and requires a distal lengthening in the mid-substance of the Achilles tendon. This can be a formal 'Z' lengthening to regain significant length. However, a less invasive lengthening by the Hoke method (14) can give reasonable benefit with less surgical trauma. An important principle is to minimise surgical trauma and shorten the consequent postoperative recovery. It is disadvantageous to make the calf muscles weaker in these patients, who initially presented with a deformity due to muscle weakness.

Plantar fascia release

Paediatric patients may need an additional extended plantar fascia release (Figure 9.12) as described by

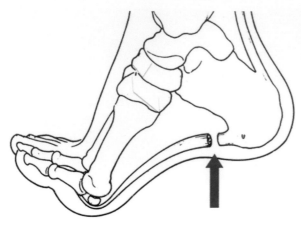

Figure 9.12 Diagram of the Steindler release in children.

Steindler (15), which involves the division of the plantar fascial and the abductor hallucis fascia. These structures usually reconnect and tighten as the child grows.

Take home messages

- Obtain an accurate diagnosis, which can aid the prediction of the likely prognosis and expected rate of deterioration.
- Ensure nonoperative treatments have been optimised, as they are often sufficient.
- Choose the specific bespoke surgical treatment according to the specific presenting complaint. Preserve as many joints as possible.
- Correct the bony alignment close to the centre of rotation of the abnormality (CORA).
- Assess the power of the tendons around the foot and surgically balance the muscles acting across the foot.

References

1. Sachithanandam V, Joseph B. The influence of footwear on the prevalence of flat foot. A survey of 1846 skeletally mature persons. J Bone Joint Surg Br 1995; 77(2):254–7.
2. Aminian A, Sangeorzan BJ. The anatomy of cavus foot deformity. Foot Ankle Clin 2008; 13:191–8.
3. Brewerton DA, Sandifer PH, Sweetnam DR. "Idiopathic" pes cavus: an investigation into its aeitiology. Br Med J 1963; 2:659–61.
4. Nagai MK, Chan G, Guille JT, Kumar SJ, Scavina M, Mackenzie WG. Prevalence of Charcot-Marie-Tooth disease in patients who have bilateral cavovarus feet. J Pediatr Orthop 2006; 26(4):438–43.
5. Aminian A, Sangeorzan BJ. The anatomy of cavus foot deformity. Foot Ankle Clin 2008; 13(2):191–8.
6. Ortiz C, Wagner E, Keller A. Cavovarus foot reconstruction. Foot Ankle Clin 2009; 14(3):471–87.
7. Coleman SS, Chesnut WJ. A simple test for hindfoot flexibility in the cavovarus foot. Clin Orthop Relat Res 1977; (123):60–2.
8. Dwyer FC. Osteotomy of the calcaneum for pes cavus. J Bone Joint Surg Br 1959; 41-B(1):80–6.
9. Lambrinudi C. New operation on drop foot. BrJ Surg 1927; 15:193–200.
10. Wetmore RS, Drennan JC. Long-term results of triple arthrodesis in Charcot-Marie-Tooth disease. J Bone Joint Surg [Am] 1989; 71-A:417–22.
11. Hibbs RA. An operation for claw foot. J Am Med Assoc 1919; 73:1583–5.
12. Vlachou M, Dimitriadis D. Results of triple arthrodesis in children and adolescents. Acta Orthop Belg 2009; 75:380–8.
13. Li S, Myerson M. Failure of surgical treatment in patients with cavovarus deformity: why does this happen and how do we approach treatment? Foot Ankle Clin 2019; 24(2):361–70.
14. Hoke M. An operation for stabilizing paralytic feet. J Orthop Surg (Hong Kong) 1921; 3:494.
15. Steindler et al. Plantar muscle release with tendon transfers and cuneiform osteotomy fusions gave more predictable better outcomes. Surg Gynec Obstet 1928; 523–62.

10 Inferior heel pain

Dishan Singh, Shelain Patel, and Karan Malhotra

Introduction

Inferior heel pain is a common foot and ankle complaint. It is prevalent in people of all ages, with the prevalence of disabling pain almost 8% in patients aged over 50 years. Approximately 12% of all UK foot and ankle referrals relate to heel pain, 7.5% of which may be attributed to plantar fasciitis (1). Plantar fasciitis may also be seen in approximately 12.5% of young military recruits.

There are several causes of inferior heel pain, which often originates from the calcaneum, surrounding nerves and surrounding soft tissues. The aetiology is often unclear but is likely multifactorial. Recognised risk factors include raised body mass index (BMI) >30 kg/m², prolonged standing/impact, pronated forefoot/midfoot and limited ankle dorsiflexion. It is important to note that the studies identifying these various risk factors have established association, but not causation. Symptoms are often self-limiting but may become chronic in up to 10% of cases (2). It is likely many patients with refractory symptoms are misdiagnosed and prescribed the incorrect treatment for their specific condition, and therefore obtaining the correct diagnosis is critical.

Plantar fasciitis is the most common diagnosis attributed to inferior heel pain, but there are myriad other conditions that can present with similar symptoms. It is important to take a detailed history and perform a thorough examination prior to attributing a cause, and in cases where there are atypical symptoms further investigation is warranted. A further description of signs and symptoms specific to each differential diagnosis are listed in the appropriate sections; however, it is important to ascertain level of activity, changes in the nature of the pain over time, duration of pain and when it is worse, any aggravating and relieving factors, and the exact location of the pain (Figure 10.1). Indeed, the acronym SOCRATES, commonly taught in UK medical schools, is applicable when assessing inferior heel pain (Table 10.1). Clinical examination should look for scars, foot posture and alignment, Achilles/gastrocnemius tightness and site of tenderness.

Symptoms atypical for plantar fasciitis are listed in Table 10.2. A retrospective review found that 24% of cases with persistent inferior heel pain and 29% of cases with atypical symptoms had alternative diagnoses. The same series found that patients with night pain had calcaneal oedema in 71% of cases, and patients with acute pain had plantar fascia tears in 44% of cases (3). It may therefore be important to investigate cases with atypical or recalcitrant symptoms, and MRI is the preferred modality as it can assess both the bony and soft tissue elements.

Broadly speaking, the differentials of inferior heel pain may be divided into four categories as shown in Figure 10.2. These include problems with the bone (calcaneus), surrounding nerves, surrounding soft tissues and the plantar fascia itself. These are elaborated upon in the relevant sections in this chapter.

This chapter aims to provide an overview on the various causes of inferior heel pain, the relevant anatomy, history and investigations, and the treatment options available. The structure of the chapter serves as a guide for the reader to develop their surgical sieve and apply this knowledge in their everyday orthopaedic practice.

Bony causes of inferior heel pain

Calcaneal stress fractures

A stress fracture is an overuse injury, which occurs when the bone is repetitively loaded at an intensity below its ultimately tensile strength. However, microfractures of the trabecular structure still occur, and if these are not allowed to heal, they propagate, producing a fatigue or stress fracture. This fracture line may not travel the whole length of the bone.

The history of a stress fracture is one of pain on activity, particularly running or walking longer distances. This is in contra-distinction from the classically described 'pain on first step' associated with

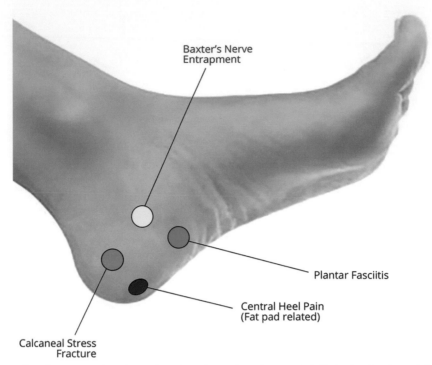

Figure 10.1 Illustration demonstrating the various locations of tenderness in inferior heel pain and the likely diagnosis.

plantar fascial pathology. The pain in a stress fracture is worse with activity and throughout the day and improves with rest. Associations include recent change in activity, long-distance running, raised BMI, recent change in footwear and low bone density. Vitamin D deficiency is commonly cited as a risk factor, but there is no evidence that it is an independent risk factor for calcaneal fractures (4).

Clinical examination will demonstrate tenderness over the body of the calcaneum as illustrated in Figure 10.1. This pain can be particularly elicited by performing a '*squeeze test*' where the examiner applies pressure to the calcaneum from both the medial and lateral sides simultaneously (Figure 10.3). Radiographs may demonstrate a radiolucent line or sclerosis in chronic/well established cases, but MRI is more sensitive (almost 100% sensitivity) for early/less florid lesions. MRI findings include periosteal and/or adjacent soft tissue oedema,

Table 10.1 Pertinent features of history to elicit in inferior heel pain (SOCRATES)

Acronym	Feature
Site	Where is the site of maximal tenderness (Figure 10.1)
Onset	Sudden or gradual, progressive or improving
Character	Burning, cramping, dull, etc.
Radiation	Localised, travels along the sole of the foot
Associations	Paraesthesia, temperature changes, numbness
Time/Duration	Worse in the morning, worse on activity, duration of symptoms
Exacerbating/Relieving factors	Better on rest, better with analgesia, better with splint
Severity	e.g., VAS score

Table 10.2 Features of inferior heel pain, atypical for plantar fasciitis

Some atypical features of inferior heel pain	
Atypical feature	**Alternative diagnosis**
Night pain	Tumour/infection
Bilateral symptoms in young patient	Systemic inflammatory condition
Neuritic symptoms	Nerve compression
Acute pain	Plantar fascial tear
Weakness	Radiculopathy
Central-proximal location	Related to heel fat pad

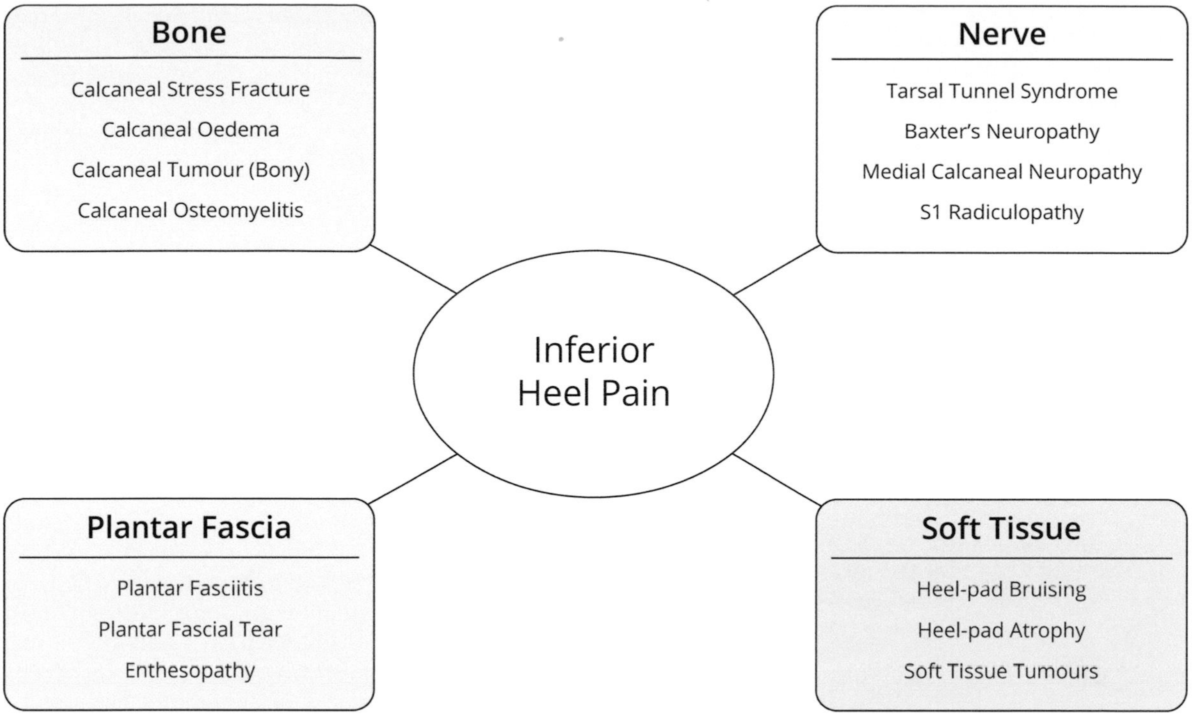

Bone

Calcaneal Stress Fracture

Calcaneal Oedema

Calcaneal Tumour (Bony)

Calcaneal Osteomyelitis

Nerve

Tarsal Tunnel Syndrome

Baxter's Neuropathy

Medial Calcaneal Neuropathy

S1 Radiculopathy

Inferior Heel Pain

Plantar Fascia

Plantar Fasciitis

Plantar Fascial Tear

Enthesopathy

Soft Tissue

Heel-pad Bruising

Heel-pad Atrophy

Soft Tissue Tumours

Figure 10.2 Illustration demonstrating the main differentials in inferior heel pain.

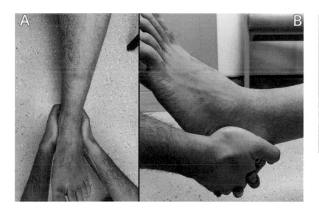

Figure 10.3 Clinical photograph demonstrating the squeeze test from above (A) and to the side (B). Side-to-side compression of the calcaneum elicits pain in the setting of a calcaneal stress fracture.

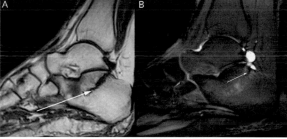

Figure 10.4 (A) T1- and (B) T2-weighted MRI images of the calcaneus. White arrows depict stress fracture line.

bone marrow oedema on T2 sequences and a hypodense fracture line visible on the T1 sequences (Figure 10.4).

In majority of cases treatment is supportive with rest and activity modification to allow healing over 6–8 weeks. In cases of severe symptoms, immobilisation with a splint, boot or plaster cast may be required. Footwear modification and orthotics may help to prevent recurrence but return to the precipitating activity should be gradual. Investigations should be carried out to detect any precipitating factors, which may be treated such as osteoporosis or metabolic bone disease.

Calcaneal oedema

Calcaneal bone marrow oedema can occur at the site of insertion of the plantar aponeurosis (Figure 10.5) or at the calcaneal tuberosity. It may be related to repetitive stress (i.e., as a precursor to a stress fracture) or calcaneal enthesopathy, but can also occur without this as part of an inflammatory process, metabolic disorder or generalised idiopathic bone marrow oedema syndrome.

Clinical features of this condition include night pain and MRI findings are of high signal on T2-weighted and fat-suppressed images. Treatment is with rest and

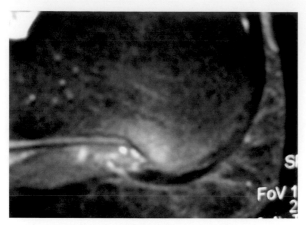

Figure 10.5 T2-weighted MRI demonstrating bone oedema at the insertion of the plantar aponeurosis.

cushioning orthotics; one paper describes potential benefit of shockwave therapy in this setting (5).

Infection

Infection is a potential cause of pain in the calcaneus, which should not be overlooked. Although infection can occur in any patient, some patients are more at risk: diabetics, immunocompromised, previous trauma, and children. The calcaneus consists anatomically of largely cancellous bone with a thin cortical shell. During ambulation it takes a significant load (> 1.5 × body weight with each step), which can result in micro-disruption of the cortical surface and thus create potential channels for infection.

Night pain is often a feature and blood tests will often demonstrate raised inflammatory markers. In cases where the history is greater than 3 weeks radiographs may demonstrate periosteal reaction. More chronic cases may demonstrate a focal sclerotic lesion or bony destruction. Bone scan is sensitive but has been largely superseded by MRI as the imaging modality of choice. MRI is sensitive and can detect very early infection, abscesses and surrounding soft tissue involvement. Gadolinium enhanced scans may be useful where abscess or sinus tracts are suspected.

Treatment for acute osteomyelitis is with antibiotics. The most common organism is *Staphylococcus aureus*, but polymicrobial infections are common and *Pseudomonas aeruginosa* is often seen when ulcers are/have been present. It is therefore imperative to obtain a microbiological sample to target therapy. In a child with pyrexia a blood culture may yield an organism; however, in majority of cases image guided biopsy or open debridement will be required. Multiple samples (at least five samples) will improve the accuracy. Depending on the organism involved, a prolonged course of antibiotics may be required, often for at least 4–6 weeks intravenously, although this should be discussed with the local microbiology/infectious diseases team.

Treatment of chronic recalcitrant osteomyelitis is multidisciplinary and will depend on factors such as patient comorbidities, surgeon preference and experience, vascular status and soft tissue availability. Treatment options include require lifelong suppression, debridement with or without local flap for soft tissue coverage, subtotal calcanectomy, total calcanectomy or below knee amputation. Bone preservation techniques are often associated with poor infection control and poor patient satisfaction. On the other hand, partial or total calcanectomy has a complication rate of up to 40%, although if patients avoid complications, they may remain ambulatory.

Bone tumours

Tumours are an important, albeit rare differential for heel pain. They may be benign or malignant. Malignant tumours may be associated with red flag symptoms such as unremitting or night pain, weight loss or constitutional symptoms. Radiographs and MRI are the mainstay of initial diagnosis when a tumour is suspected.

A full description of bony tumours is beyond the scope of this chapter, but benign lesions may include unicameral bone cysts, aneurysmal bone cysts, enchondromas, osteoid osteoma, osteoblastoma, fibrous dysplasia and intraosseous lipomas. The most common malignant tumour remains metastatic, but primary cancers include chondrosarcoma, Ewing's sarcoma and osteosarcoma.

Tumours need to be staged and graded and treatment will depend on chemo- and radio-sensitivity, location, spread and nature of the tumour. Tumours suspected of being malignant should not be biopsied locally, but should be referred to the regional tumour centre for further investigation and management.

Neurological causes of inferior heel pain

Tarsal tunnel syndrome

Tarsal tunnel syndrome is a condition where the posterior tibial nerve or its branches become compressed. The tarsal tunnel contains the tibialis posterior, flexor digitorum longus, posterior tibial artery and veins, tibial nerve, and flexor hallucis longus. These structures run in a fibro-osseous tunnel from the medial malleolus to the midfoot. From proximal to distal the '*floor*' of the tunnel is formed by the posterior aspect of the medial malleolus, the talus, the sustentaculum tali and the calcaneal body. Proximally, the '*roof*' of the tunnel is formed by the flexor retinaculum. At its termination the tarsal tunnel narrows and merges with the fascia of the abductor hallucis muscle. The tibial nerve lies posterior

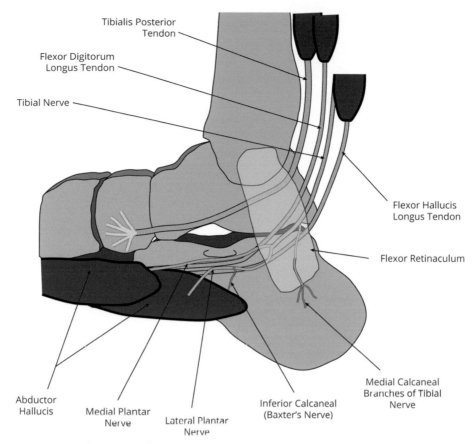

Figure 10.6 Boundaries and contents of tarsal tunnel (for clarity, the artery and vein have not been drawn). The illustration depicts one possible anatomical variant of tibial nerve branching.

to the artery and branches into the medial and lateral plantar nerves and the medial calcaneal nerve. This trifurcation has a variable location, but usually occurs proximal to or within the tarsal tunnel. The medial and lateral plantar branches enter the foot deep to the abductor hallucis (Figure 10.6).

Within or adjacent to the tarsal tunnel, the tibial nerve of its branches may become compressed. The nerve is particularly vulnerable within the tunnel as it forms an enclosed space and so any space occupying lesion or mass can cause compression; most commonly this is in the form of a ganglion, although it could be a bony prominence/exostosis. An example of a space occupying lesion causing compression in the tarsal tunnel is shown in Figure 10.7.

The symptoms of tarsal tunnel syndrome may often be vague and poorly localised, but may include paraesthesia, dysesthesia or numbness in the medial or lateral sole of the foot in addition to inferior heel pain. Symptoms may worsen throughout the day and may be reported as cramping in nature. Pain may also radiate proximally.

Objectively, there may be reduced sensation in the sole of the foot, and a Tinel's sign may be elicited at the tarsal tunnel, although these findings are very variable. Symptoms may also be provoked by performing the *'dorsiflexion-eversion test'* where the ankle is passively and maximally everted whilst holding the metatarsophalangeal joints in maximal extension. MRI to examine the tarsal tunnel and electrophysiological studies may aid in confirming tarsal tunnel syndrome, if caused by a space occupying lesion.

In the setting of a space occupying lesion, conservative management is unlikely to be effective. Surgical intervention may be indicated when conservative measures have failed. Space occupying lesions may be excised, although ganglia may respond to aspiration and injection with corticosteroid. In other causes, tarsal tunnel decompression may be performed. This should be performed under tourniquet to allow adequate visualisation of the nerve and its branches. The procedure involves release of the flexor retinaculum and should be extended to the superficial and deep fascia of the abductor hallucis muscle. Endoscopic and ultrasound

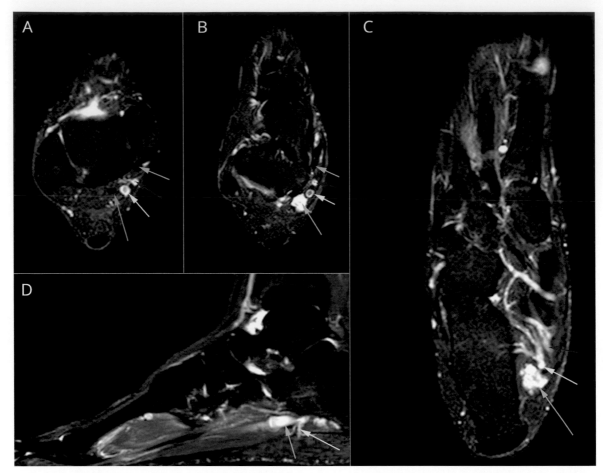

Figure 10.7 Axial (A, B and C) and sagittal (D) MRI STIR sequences demonstrating a space occupying lesion in the tarsal tunnel. Sub-figures a, b and c progress from proximal to distal. In this case it is a vascular dilatation which begins behind the medial malleolus and extends into the plantar aspect of the foot. The arrows on the various images represent: FHL tendon (green arrow), FDL (grey arrow), posterior tibial artery (red arrow), tibial nerve/its branches (yellow arrow) and the space occupying lesion (cyan arrow).

guided releases have also been described. Postoperative course and response is highly variable and recurrence frequent.

Baxter's neuropathy

As described in the section "Tarsal tunnel syndrome", the medial and lateral plantar nerves enter the foot deep to the abductor hallucis muscle. The lateral plantar nerve, however, passes through the muscle belly itself on its way to the lateral side of the foot (Figure 10.6). The first branch of the lateral plantar nerve (the inferior calcaneal nerve) supplies motor innervation the abductor digiti quinti and sensation to the area of insertion of the plantar fascia. The course of this nerve is illustrated in Figure 10.8 and proposed sites of compression are marked with circles labelled 1, 2 and 3, respectively (6).

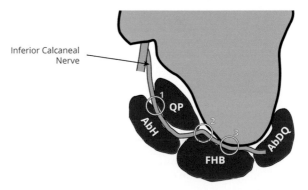

Figure 10.8 Coronal cross-section demonstrating the path of the inferior calcaneal (Baxter's) nerve. (Abbreviations: AbDQ, abductor digiti quinti; AbH, abductor hallucis; FHB, flexor hallucis brevis; QP, quadratus plantae. The circles represent the three proposed sites of compression of the nerve.)

The pain may be felt inferiorly and medially, superior to the pain in plantar fasciitis, although this is not always the case and symptoms are variable as it may be associated with plantar fasciitis. There may be associated weakness in the abductor digiti quinti. MRI may be aid in diagnosis by demonstrating acute or chronic denervation (atrophy) of the abductor digiti quinti. Nonoperative treatment includes orthotics and/or injection of corticosteroid. If these modalities fail surgical decompression may prove successful.

Medial calcaneal nerve entrapment

As depicted in Figure 10.6, the medial calcaneal branches of the tibial nerve pierce the flexor retinaculum before providing sensory innervation to the medial aspect of the calcaneum. The anatomy is variable, but they usually originate in the tarsal tunnel. This may result in altered sensation or pain on the medial side of the heel although this is a rare entity. There may be an association with plantar fasciitis. Conservative management with orthotics and activity modification is the mainstay of treatment, but occasionally surgery may be required. Surgical options include release or neurotomy. In the latter case the stumps are buried to prevent recurrence. Ultrasound guided radiofrequency ablation has also been described with some success (7).

Disc herniation

Patients with neuritic symptoms may have irritation of the S1 nerve root due to disc or spinal pathology. This is because the S1 dermatome includes the inferior heel. Other features suggestive of this diagnosis include back pain, previous history of disc herniation, symptoms of sciatica and associated hypoesthesia/paraesthesia in the region. Clinical signs, which may be present, include a positive sciatic stretch test, reduced ankle jerk reflex and reduced power in ankle plantarflexion. However, the gastrocnemius-soleus complex is innervated by the S1 and S2 nerve roots, so some power and/or reflex may be present. Diagnosis is confirmed by MRI of the lumbosacral spine.

Inferior heel pain arising from the plantar fascia

The plantar fascia originates from the plantar tuberosity of the calcaneus with a contribution of fibres from the gastrocnemius-soleus complex of the calf. As seen in Figure 10.9, it splits into three thick fibrous bands (lateral, central and medial) that extend distally. The term plantar aponeurosis is used in some texts interchangeably with plantar fascia whilst other texts refer to only the central band as the aponeurosis. The lateral

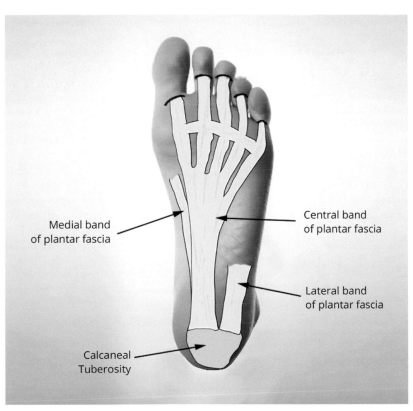

Medial band of plantar fascia

Central band of plantar fascia

Lateral band of plantar fascia

Calcaneal Tuberosity

Figure 10.9 Schematic of the plantar fascia showing its origin and constituent bands.

band is known as the calcaneo-metatarsal ligament and inserts onto the base of the fifth metatarsal covering the plantar aspect of the abductor digiti quinti. The central band is the thickest and strongest band and arises from the medial process of the calcaneal tuberosity posterior and superficial to the origin of the flexor digitorum brevis. It divides near the metatarsal heads into five processes (one for each toe), which each has a superficial and deep layer. The superficial layer inserts into the skin of the transverse groove to separate the toes from the sole. The deeper layer divides into two slips which attach either side of their respective toe flexor tendon sheath. The medial band covers the plantar aspect of the adductor hallucis and blends with the dorsomedial fascia of the foot. The primary function of the plantar fascia is to maintain the medial longitudinal arch and the windlass mechanism where extension of the metatarsophalangeal joints leads to hindfoot inversion.

Heel spurs are present in up to 25% of the population. Importantly whilst they may be seen in patients presenting with plantar fascia pathology, they are an incidental finding and not the cause of pain or a sign of pathology. The spur is instead usually a point of attachment for the flexor digitorum brevis which is deep to the plantar fascia. Removal of the spur is therefore not indicated in patients with isolated plantar fascia pathology.

Plantar fasciitis

Plantar fasciitis is the most common condition affecting the plantar fascia, although the term is a misnomer since histological examination in symptomatic patients show degeneration rather than inflammation. Excessive, repetitive strain at the origin leads to microtears of the fascial enthesis with subsequent inhibition of normal reparative processes causing fibre disorientation, increased mucoid ground substance, angiofibroblastic hyperplasia and calcification (8). This excessive load means fasciitis is thus more frequently observed in three patient groups: obese patients, runners and people whose occupation involves prolonged standing. A tight posterior muscular chain (hamstrings and gastrocnemius-soleus complex) has also been observed more frequently in patients with plantar fasciitis. These conditions contribute to greater forefoot loading which increases strain on the plantar fascia through the windlass mechanism.

History and examination are usually sufficient to reach the diagnosis, although the availability of ultrasound and MRI means they are increasingly relied upon for confirmation. Females are more commonly affected than men, while the mean age of presentation in the sixth decade. Within the obese population, the degree of obesity strongly predicts the degree of disability. Pain classically occurs on the medial aspect of the inferior heel and may radiate around the heel or down the path

of the plantar fascia. Rarely, the pain is on the medial arch. Pain is typically worse in the morning since the plantar fascia and Achilles tendon have tightened whilst the foot adopts an equinus position during sleep. Activity tends to improve pain through the day before it worsens at the end of the day or after rigorous exercise.

Examination typically identifies tenderness on the medial origin of the plantar fascia which is exacerbated by dorsiflexion of the hallux. Silfverskiöld test should be performed to assess gastrocnemius-soleus tightness, and comprehensive examination should be completed to exclude the other differential diagnoses of inferior heel pain.

Plain radiographs are unhelpful for diagnosing plantar fasciitis. Ultrasound and MRI are helpful though not mandatory for confirming the diagnosis. The normal thickness of the plantar fascia is between 2.3 and 4.3 mm with a thickness of 4 mm or greater on imaging consistent with plantar fasciitis in the correct clinical setting (9). Imaging may also reveal perifascial oedema, calcaneal bone marrow oedema and a plantar fascia tear.

Plantar fasciitis is usually self-limiting, resolving over a period of up to 18 months in 95% of individuals, but early recognition and treatment can improve symptoms within 6 weeks (10). No established treatment algorithm exists, although common initial treatment themes are used including oral medications, exercises, activity modifications and orthotics. Beyond this, there is great variability between clinicians on how to treat recalcitrant cases.

Oral analgesia and anti-inflammatory medication will provide some symptomatic relief, but no good evidence exists which quantifies the benefit. Activity modifications include removing the precipitating cause so in occupational standers, this would involve sitting more during work whilst runners should reduce running and other impact activity. Weight loss will help patients who are obese (11).

Heel cushions can improve pain by reducing direct impact on the heel. Prefabricated or custom orthoses are occasionally advised, although a recent systematic review and meta-analysis has found that they are no better than sham or other conservative treatment for treating heel pain (12). Night splints work by keeping the foot dorsiflexed during sleep and thus reduces plantar fascia tightness, which occur with equinus. They are bulky and generally not well tolerated but can be useful in patients with early morning pain, and particularly when used as part of a multimodal programme (13, 14).

Exercises are universally prescribed and should form part of the initial treatment since they are low cost and are successful in three quarters of patients within 2 months of commencement. They can either be stretching exercises of plantar fascia, gastrocnemius-soleus complex and hamstrings or strengthening of the intrinsic musculature of the foot, which has recently shown to have similar if not better outcomes (15, 16).

Extracorporeal shockwave therapy (ESWT) works through the application of high energy waves to the plantar fascia. There is no defined number or intensity of waves, nor frequency of sessions which increases the heterogeneity of studies which have investigated this modality. It is theorised to work in two ways: firstly neurogenically where it promotes excessive axonal activation that affects pain pathways, and destroys unmyelinated sensory fibres; and secondly by creating a pro-inflammatory environment through the secretion of growth factors that repair tissue, angiogenic growth factors that improve vascularity and increasing nitrous oxide levels that cause vasodilatation. A recent meta-analysis of thirteen trials consisting of 1,185 patients found that ESWT conferred superior outcomes to many other therapies (17).

There are many options for injection therapy. The most widely used is corticosteroid, which confers excellent improvements within the first 3 months after treatment, although the effect is lost by 6 months and it carries a recurrence risk unless combined with a stretching regime (18–20). They should be injected deep to the fascia to lessen the risk of fat pad atrophy and ultrasound guidance may aid accurate placement. Plantar fascia rupture is also a risk of corticosteroid administration and this will be discussed here.

Platelet-rich plasma (PRP) injections theoretically lead to pro-inflammatory cytokine synthesis. There is interest in this injection therapy since it avoids the risk of fat pad atrophy and is not known to increase the risk of plantar fascia rupture which is seen with corticosteroids. Wide variability exists within the PRP preparations from different manufacturers however, which means that there should be caution when generalising positive or negative outcomes. The mid-term effects appear to be comparable to corticosteroids for pain and function (18, 21).

Botulinum toxin injections have been shown in a recent randomised study into the gastrocnemius muscle to produce improvement of symptoms of plantar fasciitis at 1 year as compared to placebo (22). This may suggest an alternative treatment strategy to surgical gastrocnemius recession. Other injection techniques that have limited evidence and are thus not recommended unless performed as part of a prospective study are dry needling, autologous blood and prolotherapy.

Plantar fasciitis resolves nonoperatively in the vast majority of cases. Surgical management should thus be reserved for patients whose symptoms persist beyond 12–18 months despite exhausting nonoperative measures. This includes weight loss for obese individuals since surgery would not be expected to be successful unless the precipitating stressor is removed.

Surgical strategies include plantar fasciotomy, lengthening the gastrocnemius-soleus complex or both these techniques. Release of the medial head of the gastrocnemius has been shown in some studies to have a beneficial effect on symptoms, but no randomised studies have been carried out. Fasciotomy can be accomplished through percutaneous, open and endoscopic techniques. Releasing a maximum of 50% of the plantar fascia is suggested, since the risk of medial arch collapse and lateral column overload increases beyond this value (23, 24). Broadly speaking all three techniques are associated with significant improvements in the modern literature. Lengthening the gastrocnemius-soleus complex can be accomplished at various levels along the myotendinous unit. A recent randomised trial identified comparable outcome scores between open plantar fasciotomy and posteromedial gastrocnemius recession, although the latter technique was associated with a faster recovery (25).

Plantar fascia tear

Tears usually present with a sudden onset of pain in the heel or medial arch of the foot, and subsequent difficulty in toe-off or standing. Local corticosteroid administration to the plantar fascia is a known risk factor and it most commonly occurs after running or other similar sporting activity. Radiographs may show a reduced calcaneal pitch due to flattening of the medial arch although ultrasound or MRI will more reliably confirm the diagnosis (Figure 10.10). Treatment involves temporary immobilisation in a plaster cast or removable boot for up to 6 weeks or until symptoms improve.

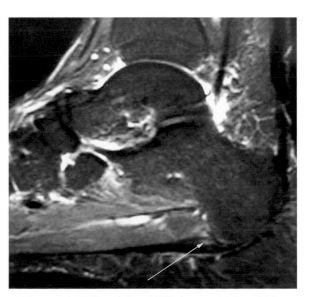

Figure 10.10 T2-weighted MRI demonstrating thickened plantar fascia with a small tear (indicated by white arrow).

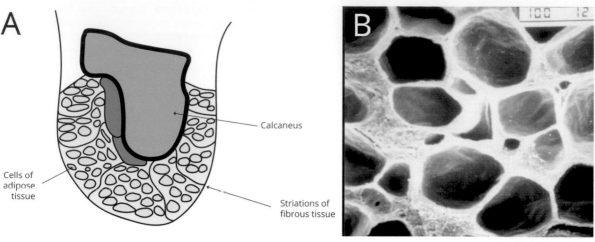

Figure 10.11 Illustration (A) depicting the calcaneus and the surrounding heel pad (coronal section). On the microscopic level (B) the fat is arranged in between fibrous septae, forming a highly effective cushioning structure.

Plantar fascia enthesopathy

This is a confusing term given that plantar fasciitis is a disorder of the origin of the plantar fascia. However, it is distinguished as 'plantar fascia enthesopathy' since this condition does not arise from repetitive trauma but as part of systemic inflammatory arthropathies, e.g., ankylosing spondylitis, psoriatic arthritis, reactive arthritis and Reiter's syndrome. Patients will still present with inferior heel pain, but a careful history including bilateral presentation and stigmata of other diseases will aid diagnosis. Blood tests for inflammatory markers and a rheumatology screen may help. Management should be undertaken by a rheumatologist.

Other soft tissue causes of inferior heel pain

Heel pad bruising/atrophy

The heel pad is a specialised anatomical structure designed to withstand repeated stress and distribute load. It consists of silos of adipose tissue surrounded by fibrous septae, which are anchored to the calcaneus (Figure 10.11). Loss of integrity of the septae can result in spreading of the fat and loss of cushioning function. This can happen on account of trauma or corticosteroid injections. The result is bruising, pain, and eventually atrophy and displacement.

The pain is often located centrally in the heel and posterior to the site of pain from the plantar fascia (central heel pain, as illustrated in Figure 10.1). The mainstay of treatment is conservative with a focus on relief of symptoms through insoles and cushioning. Silicone heel cups may be used in this setting and may contain the fat pad (Figure 10.12A). Another reported conservative option is

'Low-Dye Taping' although the benefit is questionable (Figure 10.12B). Surgical options are few.

Soft tissue tumour

Local soft tissue tumours may present with inferior heel pain and should form part of the differential diagnosis. MRI and ultrasound scanning may help to diagnose these conditions in atypical cases. They may be associated with localised swelling or skin changes, although this is not always the case.

These tumours may be benign or malignant. Benign tumours include foreign body reaction and epidermal inclusion cysts and plantar fibromatosis. However, plantar fibromatosis usually occurs more distally along the plantar fascia, and therefore is unlikely to be a cause for inferior heel pain. The most common malignant soft tissue tumour in the foot is synovial sarcoma.

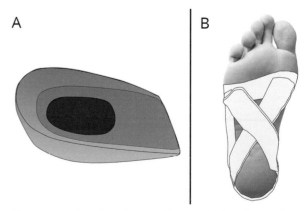

Figure 10.12 Heel cup (A) and figure-of-8 low-dye taping (B) which may be used in symptomatic relief of inferior heel pain.

Where there is concern of malignancy or doubt in diagnosis local biopsy should not be attempted; the case should be referred to the regional tumour/sarcoma centre for specialist advice and further management.

Take home messages

- Inferior heel pain is a common presenting complaint with a variety of causes.
- Careful history and examination are required to ascertain the cause.
- In cases of atypical or persistent symptoms further investigation (such as with MRI) is warranted.
- Causes of inferior heel pain may include pathology of the bones, nerves, plantar fascia or surrounding soft tissues.
- Most patients with plantar fascial pathology will respond to nonoperative therapy, but a select few may require more invasive therapy; however, it is not clear which patients will most benefit from surgical treatment and what the best method of treatment is.

References

1. Thomas MJ, Whittle R, Menz HB, Rathod-Mistry T, Marshall M, Roddy E. Plantar heel pain in middle-aged and older adults: population prevalence, associations with health status and lifestyle factors, and frequency of healthcare use. *BMC Musculoskelet Disord*. 2019;20(1):337.
2. Lapidus PW, Guidotti FP. Painful heel: report of 323 patients with 364 painful heels. *Clin Orthop Relat Res*. 1965;39:178–86.
3. Chimutengwende-Gordon M, O'Donnell P, Singh D. Magnetic resonance imaging in plantar heel pain. *Foot Ankle Int*. 2010;31(10):865–70.
4. Malhotra K, Baggott PJ, Livingstone J. Vitamin D in the foot and ankle: a review of the literature. *J Am Podiatr Med Assoc*. 2020;110(3):Article_10.
5. Maier M, Steinborn M, Schmitz C, Stäbler A, Köhler S, Pfahler M, Dürr HR, Refior HJ. Extracorporeal shock wave application for chronic plantar fasciitis associated with heel spurs: prediction of outcome by magnetic resonance imaging. *J Rheumatol*. 2000;27(10):2455–62.
6. Moroni S, Zwierzina M, Starke V, Moriggl B, Montesi F, Konschake M. Clinical-anatomic mapping of the tarsal tunnel with regard to Baxter's neuropathy in recalcitrant heel pain syndrome: part I. *Surg Radiol Anat*. 2019;41(1):29–41.
7. Counsel PD, Davenport M, Brown A, Ooi CC, Comin J, Marks P, Connell DA. Ultrasound-guided radiofrequency denervation of the medial calcaneal nerve. *Clin J Sport Med*. 2016;26(6):465–70.
8. Snider MP, Clancy WG, McBeath AA. Plantar fascia release for chronic plantar fasciitis in runners. *Am J Sports Med*. 1983;11(4):215–9.
9. Mahowald S, Legge BS, Grady JF. The correlation between plantar fascia thickness and symptoms of plantar fasciitis. *J Am Podiatr Med Assoc*. 2011;101(5):385–9.
10. Wolgin M, Cook C, Graham C, Mauldin D. Conservative treatment of plantar heel pain: long-term follow-up. *Foot Ankle Int*. 1994;15(3):97–102.
11. Boules M, Batayyah E, Froylich D, Zelisko A, O'Rourke C, Brethauer S, El-Hayek K, Boike A, Strong AT, Kroh M. Effect of surgical weight loss on plantar fasciitis and health-care use. *J Am Podiatr Med Assoc*. 2018;108(6):442–8.
12. Rasenberg N, Riel H, Rathleff MS, Bierma-Zeinstra SMA, van Middelkoop M. Efficacy of foot orthoses for the treatment of plantar heel pain: a systematic review and meta-analysis. *Br J Sports Med*. 2018;52(16):1040–6.
13. Sheridan L, Lopez A, Perez A, John MM, Willis FB, Shanmugam R. Plantar fasciopathy treated with dynamic splinting: a randomized controlled trial. *J Am Podiatr Med Assoc*. 2010;100(3):161–5.
14. Lee WC, Wong WY, Kung E, Leung AK. Effectiveness of adjustable dorsiflexion night splint in combination with accommodative foot orthosis on plantar fasciitis. *J Rehabil Res Dev*. 2012;49(10):1557–64.
15. Rathleff MS, Molgaard CM, Fredberg U, Kaalund S, Andersen KB, Jensen TT, Aaskov S, Olesen JL. High-load strength training improves outcome in patients with plantar fasciitis: a randomized controlled trial with 12-month follow-up. *Scand J Med Sci Sports*. 2015;25(3):e292–300.
16. Thong-On S, Bovonsunthonchai S, Vachalathiti R, Intravoranont W, Suwannarat S, Smith R. Effects of strengthening and stretching exercises on the temporospatial gait parameters in patients with plantar fasciitis: a randomized controlled trial. *Ann Rehabil Med*. 2019;43(6):662–76.
17. Sun K, Zhou H, Jiang W. Extracorporeal shock wave therapy versus other therapeutic methods for chronic plantar fasciitis. *Foot Ankle Surg*. 2020;26(1):33–8.
18. Chen YJ, Wu YC, Tu YK, Cheng JW, Tsai WC, Yu TY. Autologous blood-derived products compared with corticosteroids for treatment of plantar fasciopathy: a systematic review and meta-analysis. *Am J Phys Med Rehabil*. 2019;98(5):343–52.
19. Ugurlar M, Sonmez MM, Ugurlar OY, Adiyeke L, Yildirim H, Eren OT. Effectiveness of four different treatment modalities in the treatment of chronic plantar fasciitis during a 36-month follow-up period: a randomized controlled trial. *J Foot Ankle Surg*. 2018;57(5):913–8.
20. Johannsen FE, Herzog RB, Malmgaard-Clausen NM, Hoegberget-Kalisz M, Magnusson SP, Kjaer M. Corticosteroid injection is the best treatment in plantar fasciitis if combined with controlled training. *Knee Surg Sports Traumatol Arthrosc*. 2019;27(1):5–12.
21. Jain SK, Suprashant K, Kumar S, Yadav A, Kearns SR. Comparison of plantar fasciitis injected with platelet-rich plasma vs corticosteroids. *Foot Ankle Int*. 2018;39(7):780–6.
22. Abbasian M, Baghbani S, Barangi S, Fairhurst PG, Ebrahimpour A, Krause F, Hashemi M. Outcomes of ultrasound-guided gastrocnemius injection with botulinum toxin for chronic plantar fasciitis. *Foot Ankle Int*. 2020;41(1):63–8.
23. Brugh AM, Fallat LM, Savoy-Moore RT. Lateral column symptomatology following plantar fascial release: a prospective study. *J Foot Ankle Surg*. 2002;41(6):365–71.
24. Cheung JT, An KN, Zhang M. Consequences of partial and total plantar fascia release: a finite element study. *Foot Ankle Int*. 2006;27(2):125–32.
25. Gamba C, Serrano-Chinchilla P, Ares-Vidal J, Solano-Lopez A, Gonzalez-Lucena G, Gines-Cespedosa A. Proximal medial gastrocnemius release versus open plantar fasciotomy for the surgical treatment in recalcitrant plantar fasciitis. *Foot Ankle Int*. 2019:1071100719891979.

11 Ankle arthritis

C Senthil Kumar, Robert Clayton, and Mansur Halai

Introduction

Functional limitations in patients with ankle arthritis are often substantial. When compared to hip arthritis, a Level 1 study revealed that ankle arthritis had significantly worse mental component summary scores, role-physical scores and general health scores.[1] Therefore, the mental and physical disability associated with end-stage ankle arthritis should not be underestimated. This chapter will cover the pathophysiology of ankle arthritis and the spectrum of its management.

Aetiology

The ankle joint, more than any other joint, is subjected to the highest forces per square centimetre and is the most commonly injured. Yet the incidence of age-related symptomatic ankle arthritis is approximately nine times lower than that of the hip and knee.[2] The exact prevalence of ankle arthritis is difficult to define, but various National Joint Registries will reflect hip/knee replacements being performed 30 times more than that for the treatment of ankle arthritis. Of those patients with ankle arthritis, trauma remains the most common cause, with reports of up to 75% (Table 11.1).[3] Primary arthritis (possibly secondary to malalignment) occurs in approximately 10% of patients. The remaining causes include arthritis secondary to inflammatory joint disease (5%), haemochromatosis (3%), haemophilia, talar osteonecrosis and sepsis.

As the leading cause, trauma deserves more elaboration. Direct cartilage injury will be proportional to the energy imparted and the comminution of the articular surface (e.g., pilon fractures). A frequent citation reports rates of symptomatic ankle arthritis from rotational Weber A, B and C fractures of 4%, 12% and 33%, respectively.[4] Furthermore, the presence of a fractured posterior malleolus resulted in a greater likelihood of developing arthritis. Accurate reduction of these fractures with internal fixation is critical, as it has been reported that even 1 mm of increased lateral talar shift will decrease the tibiotalar contact area by 42%,

decreasing joint congruity and increasing focal tibiotalar contact pressure, leading ultimately, to cartilage breakdown and arthritis.[5]

Pathophysiology

The articular cartilage at the ankle joint has distinct characteristics that play a role in both protection and susceptibility to arthritis. Ankle articular cartilage is relatively uniform in thickness, (1–1.7 mm), whereas knee cartilage has been shown to have a large variation in thickness from 1 to 6 mm.[6] An inverse relationship was also found between cartilage thickness and its compressive modulus, i.e., thin ankle cartilage has a high-compressive modulus. In contrast to the hip, the tensile strength of the talar cartilage decreases only slightly with age.[7] Furthermore, loading leads to increased congruity.

The cartilage of the ankle joint is made up of chondrocytes and extracellular matrix (ECM), which is made up of collagen. Initially, the damage to the cartilage causes activation of the innate immune system via pattern-recognition receptors (PPRs), to which the family of toll-like receptors (TLRs) also belong to. PPRs are found on macrophages, chondrocytes and fibroblast-like synoviocytes (FLS). PPRs recognise signals, which indicate either the presence of pathogens or signals that indicate tissue damage, known as pathogen-associated molecular patterns (PAMPs) and alarmins, respectively. Alarmins and PAMPs are collectively termed damage-associated molecular patterns (DAMPs).[8] DAMPs cause the activation of the synovium and chondrocyte-derived inflammatory mediators and adipose-derived inflammatory mediators, which together consist of cytokines (TNFα and interleukins), growth factors (TGFβ), chemokines and prostaglandins. Further, the ankle does not produce matrix metalloproteinase 8 (MMP8) mRNA, an enzyme which is expressed by normal knee cartilage and which causes cartilage degradation.

The local inflammation caused by the tissue damage, DAMPs and inflammatory mediators results in angiogenesis and vascular leak of plasma proteins, complement, cytokines and adipokines into the synovial fluid

Table 11.1 The aetiology of ankle arthritis

Aetiology	Specific factors/causes
Trauma	Damage to articular surface Residual joint incongruity/instability Avascular necrosis of fractured talus/ distal tibia
Mechanical axis malalignment	Primary Secondary malalignment of hip, knee, tibia, foot
Ligamentous instability	Lateral insufficiency Deltoid insufficiency Syndesmotic insufficiency Ehlers-Danlos syndrome
Inflammatory	Rheumatoid arthropathy Psoriatic arthropathy Ankylosing spondylitis Crystalline arthropathy (gout, pseudogout)
Sepsis	Joint sepsis sequelae Osteomyelitis
Haemorrhagic	Haemophilia Haemochromatosis (excess iron deposition) Recurrent traumatic haemarthroses
Neuropathic	Alcohol excess Charcot diabetic neuropathy Amyloidosis
Tumour	Benign (polyvillonodular synovitis) Malignant
Ochronosis	Deficiency of homogentisic acid oxidase leading to accumulation of homogentisic acid in cartilage
Gaucher disease	Deficiency of glucocerebrosidase leading to accumulation of glucocerebroside causing bone necrosis/fracture

due to the increased permeability of the vasculature. The inflammation affects the nerve endings within the bone, causing the characteristic pain patients experience with osteoarthritis. The plasma proteins also work as DAMPs, promoting further inflammatory mediator release, leading to chronic inflammation which culminates in ankle arthritis.[9] This is summarised in Figure 11.1.

Investigations and classification

Estimation of the severity of arthritis is important for determining the treatment approach. In terms of diagnosis, the National Institute for Health and Care Excellence (NICE) Osteoarthritis guidelines state that a patient can be diagnosed clinically, without any investigation, if they fit the following three criteria:

- 45 years of age or older
- 30 minutes of early morning joint stiffness
- joint pain due to activity[10]

Radiologically, weight-bearing anteroposterior and lateral radiographs are recommended. Additional radiographs to assess the midfoot and forefoot joints may also be required in some patients. Tanaka modified the Takakura classification for the assessment of ankle arthritis as shown in Table 11.2.[11]

- Stage 1: early sclerosis and formation of osteophytes without narrowing of the joint space
- Stage 2: narrowing of the medial joint space
- Stage 3A: obliteration of the medial joint space with subchondral bone contact limited to the medial malleolus
- Stage 3B: subchondral bone contact extending to the roof of the dome of the talus
- Stage 4: obliteration of the entire joint space, resulting in bone contact throughout the ankle.

This classification is particularly useful when monitoring the progression of arthritis, but fails to guide surgical management. It also does not account for the state of the surrounding joints, contractures of the Achilles' tendon, or other deformities. A more recent classification by the Canadian Orthopaedic Foot and Ankle Society (COFAS) has been proven to be valid and reproducible.[12] It does not take into account systemic comorbidities, but takes into account the deformity and arthritis of the surrounding hindfoot joints (Table 11.3). It is reliable when measuring postoperative outcomes as well as suggesting treatment strategies.

Comparative views of the contralateral normal or less affected ankle may help quantify the reduced joint space, although this is less commonly used. Magnetic resonance imaging (MRI) tends to be more useful when a discrete osteochondral lesion is suspected to be the underlying cause of pain, or the tendons need to be investigated (see Figure 11.5). Computed tomography (CT) is useful when there is a question about bone stock, for example, with a talar cyst. Increasingly, single-photon emission computed tomography (SPECT-CT) is performed to evaluate the extent of degenerative changes and their biological activities. This radiographic modality may also help assess for any osteoarthritic changes in neighbouring joints of the hindfoot and midfoot. Standing CT scanning is a new imaging modality which, for the first time, allows three-dimensional load-bearing imaging of the ankle and foot. This will also often include the contralateral foot for comparison.

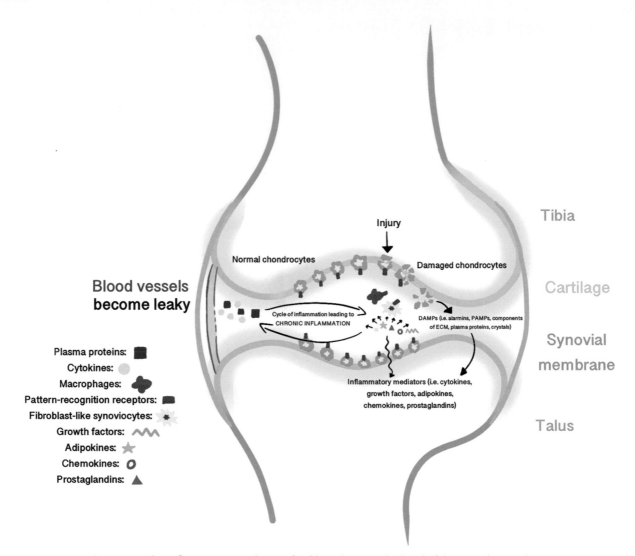

Figure 11.1 The inflammatory pathway of ankle arthritis at the level of the articular cartilage.

Table 11.2 The Tanaka modification of the Takakura radiological classification of ankle arthritis[11]

Stage	Description on AP radiograph
1	Osteophytes and early sclerosis. No joint space narrowing.
2	Narrowed medial joint space. No subchondral contact.
3a 3b	No remaining medial joint space. Subchondral bone contact over talar dome.
4	Obliteration of joint space with complete bone contact.

Non-surgical management

Essentially, these interventions aim to reduce weight-bearing forces through the ankle joint. These include weight reduction, avoidance of impact sports such as running and the use of a walking aid. Ankle braces or Ankle-Foot-Orthoses (AFOs) can be used, with the aim of rendering the ankle joint more rigid (see Figure 11.2). These are often not tolerated in the long term, but can be useful for short-term relief in early-stage arthritis. Physiotherapy can be useful to keep the other joints supple and to maintain strength, both of which will help to improve the outcome of any future operative treatments.

Beyond over-the-counter analgesics, COX-2 inhibitors are available but remain controversial due to their

Table 11.3 The Canadian Orthopedic Foot and Ankle Society (COFAS) pre- and postoperative classification system for end-stage ankle arthritis[12]

	Type 1	Type 2	Type 3	Type 4
Preoperative classification	Isolated ankle arthritis	Ankle arthritis with intra-articular varus or valgus deformity, ankle instability and/or a tight heel cord	Ankle arthritis with hindfoot deformity, tibial malunion, midfoot ab- or adductus, supinated midfoot, plantar-flexed first ray, etc	Types 1-3 plus subtalar, calcaneocuboid. or talonavicular arthritis
Postoperative classification	AA or TAR with no procedure requiring a second incision except syndesmosis fusion	AA or TAR with a soft-tissue procedure requiring a separate incision	AA or TAR with an additional osteotomy including midfoot arthrodesis	AA or TAR with an additional hindfoot arthrodesis
Concurrent procedures	None, hardware removal	Deltoid ligament release, ligament reconstruction, tendo Achilles lengthening, gastrocnemius recession, tendon transfer, capsule release, forefoot reconstruction, metatarsal osteotomy, dissection of neurovascular structures, plantar fascia release, syndesmosis reconstruction	Fibular osteotomy, calcaneal osteotomy, tibial osteotomy, midtarsal arthrodesis	Arthrodesis: triple, subtalar, talonavicular, calcaneocuboid

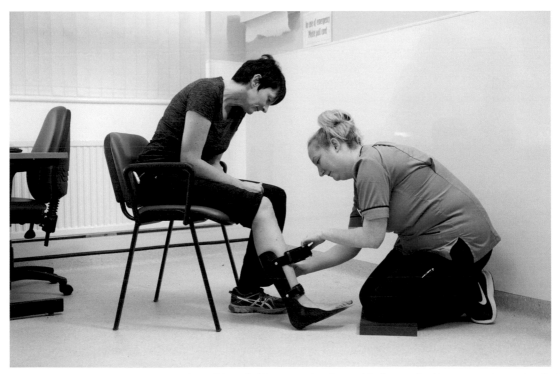

Figure 11.2 Non-operative treatment for ankle arthritis: example of an ankle foot orthosis commonly used to limit sagittal plane movements.

side effects. Intra-articular corticosteroid injections are recommended by NICE, with short-term benefits being demonstrated up to 3 months. Many surgeons recommend the use of ultrasound guidance, or fluoroscopy with the use of a radio-opaque dye, so as to ensure accurate placement, of the injection. Although the risks are low, when consenting a patient for a steroid joint injection, the following risks should be mentioned: infection, failure to improve pain, the likelihood of benefit being short-lived, a transient worsening of symptoms and fat atrophy causing altered pigmentation of the skin.[13] Although there is no concrete evidence, most surgeons recommend no more than three injections per year, leaving a 'steroid holiday' of 3 months before any planned operations.

Despite their initial popularity, the use of hyaluronic acid joint injections has decreased since NICE stated their questionable efficacy. Platelet-rich plasma (PRP) injections have shown some initially promising results, but more robust studies are required, and therefore their routine use cannot be recommended presently. It will be interesting to see the results of the Dutch multicentred randomised trial which will compare PRP to saline injections.[14] Stem cell injections are at an early stage of development and may become a viable therapeutic option in the future.

Surgical management

If symptoms of ankle arthritis are refractory to non-operative treatment, surgical options can be considered, in a holistic manner. These options vary in their invasiveness from arthroscopy and osteotomy to arthrodesis and arthroplasty.

Ankle arthroscopy

Ankle arthroscopy has some specific indications in the early stages of ankle arthritis. These include anterior impinging tibiotalar osteophytes, isolated osteochondral lesions and loose bodies (see Figure 11.3).

a) b)

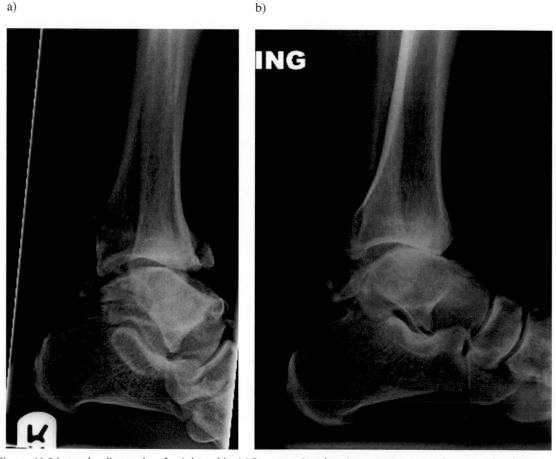

Figure 11.3 Lateral radiographs of a right ankle. (a) Preoperative showing anterior osteophytes on the distal tibia and anterior talus, (b) postoperatively illustrating elimination of these osteophytes, which has been performed arthroscopically.

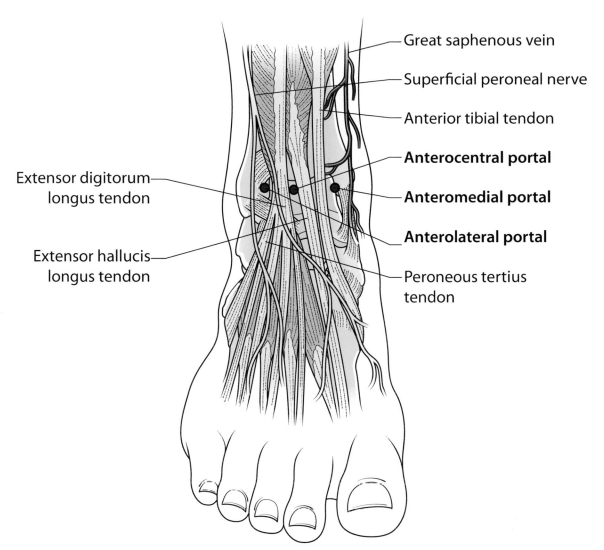

Great saphenous vein

Superficial peroneal nerve

Anterior tibial tendon

Anterocentral portal

Anteromedial portal

Anterolateral portal

Peroneous tertius tendon

Extensor digitorum longus tendon

Extensor hallucis longus tendon

Figure 11.4 Diagram illustrating the pertinent surface anatomy of the standard anterior portals used in ankle arthroscopy.

Prospective studies have supported arthroscopic debridement, especially for stage 1 and 2 arthritis, with up to 75% of patients gaining functional improvement.[15]

Certain nuances come with experience of ankle arthroscopy. The anatomical path of the superficial peroneal nerve should be marked out to avoid iatrogenic damage with the lateral portal, the most common complication. This can be aided by supinating the foot and plantarflexing the fourth toe, which will make the nerve more palpable, and often visible, just medial to the peroneus tertius, (see Figure 11.4). A custom traction device is often utilised to distract the ankle joint although in some cases, traction can impede the vision of the anterior 'kissing' osteophytes, as the ankle capsule will be taut. The advantage of a small joint arthroscope is its maneuverability, at the expense of a smaller field of vision. One should follow a stepwise inspection of the tibiotalar joint, the gutters and the syndesmosis. Arthroscopic pictures (see Figure 11.5) can help counsel the patient on the severity of their disease and be a useful adjunct in the consenting process if further surgery is warranted.

Distal tibial osteotomy

Malalignment of the weight-bearing axis of the hindfoot can, over a period of time, lead to increased point loading resulting in arthritis of the ankle. Distal tibial osteotomy can be a useful joint sparing procedure in a younger patient; the most common procedure is the supramalleolar osteotomy, such as a medial opening

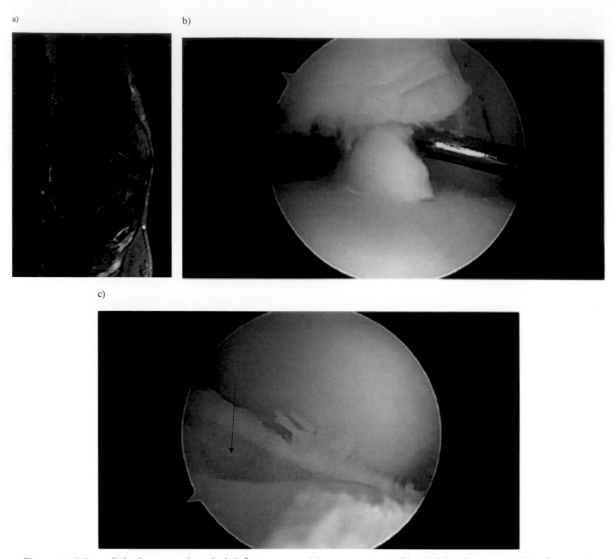

Figure 11.5 A medial talar osteochondral defect seen on (a) preoperative MRI and (b) arthroscopy. (c) Arthroscopic picture taken intraoperatively after debridement and microfracture (arrow).

wedge osteotomy to correct an extra-articular varus ankle deformity (see Figure 11.6). The high tibial osteotomy performed for the varus knee can also restore alignment at the ankle joint. To make a detailed measurement of the correction required, long leg plain radiographic standing views are required or, more frequently, CT scanograms. A standing CT scan of the entire leg (hip, knee, ankle) will also aid in the assessment of multiplanar deformities.

Calcaneal osteotomies have an important role when the deformity is distal to the ankle joint. These displacements are especially important when considering an ankle arthroplasty. After osteotomy, the posterior tuberosity can be shifted medially for a valgus deformity and laterally for varus heel deformities. Neutral alignment of the hindfoot is crucial for the longevity of any future ankle replacement or arthrodesis.[16]

Ankle distraction arthroplasty

As the term suggests, this treatment distracts the ankle joint, typically up to 1 cm, using a circular frame. The aim is to allow the articular cartilage to regenerate whilst correcting deformity. It will appeal to younger, active patients who may want to be able to bear weight during the treatment (see Figure 11.7). Limited numbers of studies have shown its benefit with approximately 50% not requiring further surgery at 8 years.[17] Disadvantages to be aware of when considering this treatment are potential future surgery and the psychological burden of prolonged frame treatment.

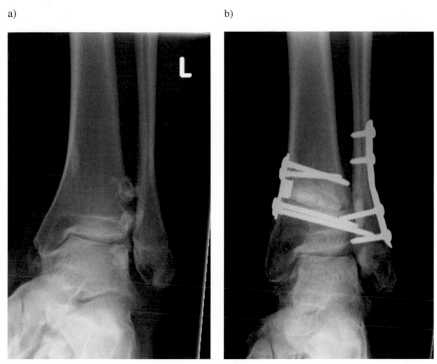

Figure 11.6 Supramalleolar distal tibial osteotomy. (a) Anteroposterior standing radiograph of X ankle showing a varus ankle deformity. (b) The same ankle after a distal medial tibial opening wedge osteotomy and grafting to correct the hindfoot alignment.

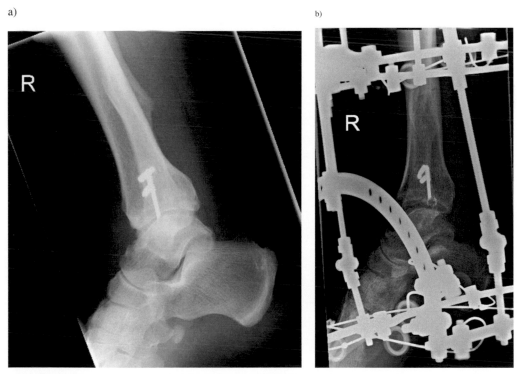

Figure 11.7 A lateral plain radiograph of a left ankle showing an Ilizarov frame assisted distraction ankle arthroplasty. (a) Preoperative and (b) with frame in position.

Ankle arthrodesis

When considering all treatments, this is the gold standard for end-stage ankle arthritis. Rates of over 90% union can be achieved with a consistent reduction in pain. Arthrodesis is commonly offered to patients under 50 years of age, manual workers or, if the deformity is too large (>30° coronal plane) for ankle replacement.

In the presence of ankle arthrodesis with a normally functioning subtalar joint complex, the mechanics of gait are minimally affected – there is a slight decrease in stride length and cadence. The oxygen consumption during steady-state walking is increased by 3% and gait efficiency is 90%. In contrast, arthrodesis of the hip has a greater deleterious effect on gait with oxygen consumption increasing by 32% and gait efficiency decreasing to 53% of normal.[18] With an arthrodesed ankle, walking fast or running is difficult for some patients because the full functional capacity of all three rockers is required during these activities.

The ideal position for ankle after fusion is a neutral, plantigrade foot, with 5° valgus and 5° external rotation. There should be some posterior translation of the talus under the tibia. This is important as a vaulting gait pattern can result from anterior talar translation (secondary to a shorter lever arm from the gastro-soleus complex). Similarly, a plantarflexed arthrodesis will result in

hyperextension of the knee leading to laxity of the medial collateral ligament and posterior capsule of the knee.

The ankle can be fused through a traditional open approach or arthroscopically. The latter has the advantages of a quicker hospital stay, reduced time to fusion and less blood loss, whilst achieving similar radiological and clinical outcomes.[19] Because open procedures are usually reserved for more complex cases, one must be cognisant that, due to the inherent selection bias, comparisons between open and arthroscopic arthrodeses have limited value.

Arthroscopic ankle fusion is useful when there is a higher risk of wound breakdown (diabetics, immunocompromise or previous ankle trauma). Many surgeons view it as the gold standard technique in patients with good bone stock and minimal deformity. Some limited coronal deformity and talar translation can be corrected with arthroscopic fusion. Nevertheless, we recommend an open technique if there is a larger, irreducible deformity or if bone grafting is required. The surgeon should be familiar with arthroscopy and its setup as described earlier. Important tips include meticulous joint preparation down to bleeding subchondral cancellous bone, including the medial gutter. Careful clearance of anterior osteophyte is essential to avoid fusion in plantarflexion. We suggest the use of at least two parallel cannulated 6.5 mm screws (Figure 11.8)

a)

b)

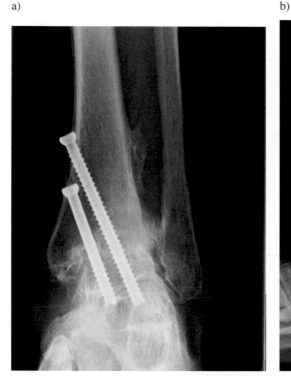
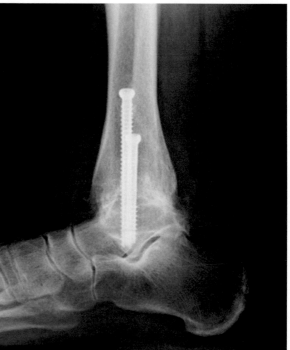

Figure 11.8 (a) Anteroposterior and (b) lateral radiographs of a left ankle showing arthroscopic fusion of the tibiotalar joint with two cannulated 6.5 mm screws.

and to aim the screw slightly medially in the talus. A third screw in the sagittal plane can aid torsional control. Several studies have commented that lateral gutter preparation is not required. A common reason for anxiety is the transparency and gap seen on fluoroscopy after the compression screws are sited. This is normal. The theory is that the cocktail of growth factors and immunomodulators enclosed in the joint will aid the fusion and this space reliably fills in with bone by 3 months.[20]

Open arthrodesis is frequently used for the treatment of post-traumatic ankle arthritis as these patients often have a deformity, voids requiring grafting and previous internal fixation metalwork to remove. The two most common approaches are the anterior (in between tibialis anterior and extensor hallucis longus) or the lateral transfibular approach.

The lateral approach can be advantageous, as the resected fibula can be used for autograft and access to the subtalar joint is easily performed for a more extensive tibio-talo-calcaneal fusion. However, as the outcomes of arthroplasty improve, there is an increasing consideration to convert an arthrodesed ankle to total ankle arthroplasty (TAA), and therefore having intact malleoli is a prerequisite for this. Some surgeons use the *antero-lateral approach*, which does not require a fibular osteotomy.

The anterior approach which often employs a plate, supplemented with a cannulated screw has been demonstrated to increase construct rigidity and decrease micromotion, at the expense of a heavier metallic footprint (see Figure 11.9). If there is risk of wound breakdown due to previous surgery on the anterior aspect of ankle, a trans-Achilles' tendon posterior approach, with the patient in the prone position, allows excellent access to the ankle and subtalar joints.

For all arthrodeses, a period of immobilisation is required (usually 6–8 weeks). While many surgeons recommend 6 weeks non–weight-bearing, some surgeons now recommend early weight-bearing, particularly after arthroscopic fusion with parallel screws where weight-bearing can promote compression at the arthrodesis. We recommend risk assessment for prophylaxis to prevent venous thromboembolism for this period. The risk of non-union is between 5–10% and the following risk factors have been consistently identified: poorly controlled diabetes, smoking, vitamin D deficiency, poor fixation construct and an ipsilateral subtalar fusion.[21] The latter is due to the greater lever arm on the ankle joint and partial disruption of the blood supply to the talus following a subtalar arthrodesis. Paradoxically, patients should be warned of adjacent joint arthritis following ankle arthrodesis, with the possible requirement for subsequent fusion surgery.

a)

b)

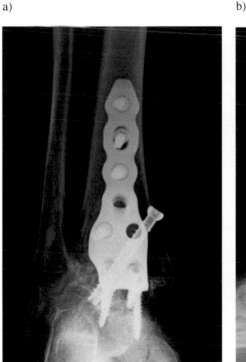
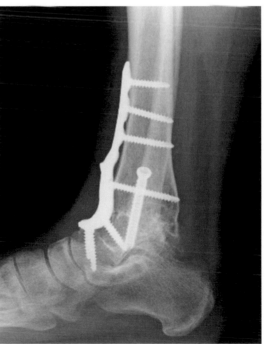

Figure 11.9 Open ankle fusion. (a) Anteroposterior and (b) lateral view showing fusion achieved with a plate and an additional cannulated screw in the coronal plane.

Ankle arthroplasty

Surgeons are increasingly favouring TAA for end-stage ankle arthritis, a fact that corresponds with advancements in implant design and instrumentation. Advances in prosthesis design, instrumentation to assist accurate implantation and surgical techniques have led to greatly improved outcomes when compared to earlier series. Furthermore, a recent analysis from the COFAS multicentre database suggests that patients with a significant deformity or ipsilateral peritalar arthritis who undergo an arthroplasty have statistically improved outcomes when compared to ankle fusion.[22]

As design and technique refinements continue to progress with TAA, traditional contraindications have been successfully challenged such that now, there is a larger group of 'relative' contraindications. These include coronal plane deformity of >15°, obesity, diabetes mellitus, previous ankle sepsis and smoking. These factors have to be accounted for when making a holistic decision. One must remember that a poor surgical candidate for TAA would similarly be a poor candidate for ankle arthrodesis. Major complications following an arthrodesis are generally easier to manage than a major complication following a TAA, and this fact should be discussed with a potential patient preoperatively.

Like our colleagues in hip and knee arthroplasty, foot and ankle surgeons are successfully performing TAAs in more complex preoperative deformities (see Figure 11.10). These should be assessed preoperatively

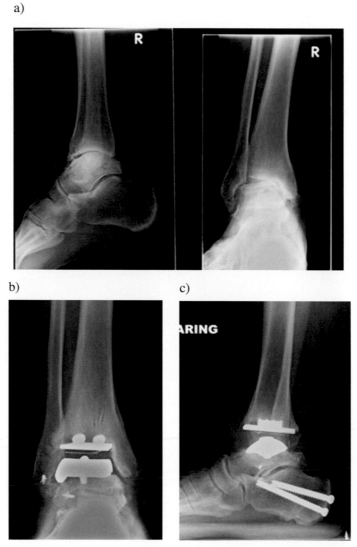

Figure 11.10 Varus coronal plane ankle deformity. (a) Preoperative anteroposterior and lateral radiographs showing post-traumatic arthritis. (b) Postoperative anteroposterior and (c) lateral radiographs showing a neutrally aligned total ankle replacement.

with weight-bearing radiographs. When examining the AP radiograph, one evaluates the coronal plane talar deformity, ankle joint congruity, post-traumatic changes and the orientation of the malleoli. Congruent deformities are characteristically more rigid and may require an extra-articular correction such as a supra-malleolar osteotomy. In cases with a varus tilt of the talus, the medial malleolus may be dysplastic due to long-term talar malalignment, potentially requiring a translational osteotomy or a prophylactic screw to prevent a postoperative fracture. In cases with a valgus tilt of the talus, the fibula can be dysplastic due to the excessive laterally directed forces from the talus and calcaneal impingement resulting in stress fractures. If this is significant, fibular realignment osteotomy may be required. On the lateral radiograph, the talar position is evaluated. Classically, it is posteriorly translated in valgus alignment and anteriorly translated in varus deformities. Indeed, there are TAA implants available with a bias in their sagittal profile to counter this. CT is indicated when there are concerns about bone quality, cystic voids or rotational malalignment. Standing CT may yield additional information for preoperative planning purposes.

MRI is rarely required but can be useful in the assessment of cases where avascular necrosis or ligamentous damage is suspected or present.

Except for one laterally inserted TAR, the arthroplasty is performed through the anterior surgical approach. If there is a previous incision it is best to utilise this unless it would jeopardise the operative exposure. If the area has had a previous skin graft or myocutaneous flap, we recommend preoperative advice from a plastic surgeon. The main intraoperative complications of TAA include iatrogenic fracture when performing the bony cuts and component malposition. Often, we find that one is focused on the resection height of the tibia and less emphasis is paid to the rotation. Both are of equal importance and should be checked regularly throughout the operation. Liberal use of intraoperative fluoroscopy, especially whilst on the learning curve, and using pins to protect the malleoli is recommended.

Postoperatively, reported wound complication rates in the region of 10% are not uncommon. These high frequencies should not come as a surprise because the anterior ankle, unlike the hip, has thin skin over very superficial tendons and precarious blood supply. However, careful attention to soft tissue handling, avoiding the use of self-retainers and other excessive retraction and with meticulous wound closure, far lower rates of wound complications should be routinely achievable. Previous trauma or immunosuppression, combined with lengthy surgical procedures, could theoretically further increase the potential for postoperative wound issues which, in turn, could lead to poorer outcomes. We recommend limiting the tourniquet time to under 2 hours because studies have shown that longer operative times correspond with increased wound breakdown.[23] If there is a complex deformity to correct, adjunctive procedures such as calcaneal or supramalleolar osteotomy, subtalar, or midfoot fusion or lateral ligament reconstruction may be required. Consideration will need to be given as to whether to carry out a single or a staged procedure.

Subsidence of implants and loosening, deep peri-prosthetic infection or instability due to component malpositioning are the main longer term postoperative complications. Lesser adjunctive procedures such as gutter debridement, bone grafting of cysts or polyethylene exchange may also be required. Currently, larger reports show a major complication rate of 15% after 5 years. However, one must also emphasise to their patient that there is approximately a 20% chance that a secondary procedure, to optimise the TAA, becomes necessary at a later date. This is usually due to disease progression in adjacent joints. Only a few prostheses have long-term results published from non-designer centres; cumulative Joint Registry data from around the world indicate a survival rate of 0.81 (95% CI, 0.74–0.88) at 10 years.[24]

Arthroplasty versus arthrodesis

There is a plethora of Level 3 and 4 evidence showing comparable outcomes for arthroplasty versus arthrodesis, albeit with a higher rate of revision or secondary operation in the former (15%). This is confirmed by a recent meta-analysis, which revealed no significant difference between the two for clinical outcomes and patient satisfaction.[25] Perhaps one of the most eagerly awaited results in orthopaedics is that from the total ankle replacement versus ankle arthrodesis (TARVA) trial. TARVA is a randomised, un-blinded, parallel-group trial between these two treatments across multiple centres in the UK.[26] The primary outcome is the Manchester-Oxford Foot Questionnaire walking/standing domain score at 1-year post-surgery. Secondary outcomes include measures of pain, social interaction, physical function, quality of life and range of motion. It is hoped that the TARVA analysis will provide the first robust Level 1 evidence on the relative effectiveness of these two treatments.

Take home messages

- The ankle articular cartilage is more resistant to arthritis compared to the hip/knee due to its uniformly thin profile and specific inflammatory characteristics.
- Trauma is the most common cause of ankle arthritis.
- Weight reduction, braces and injections are the mainstay of non-operative management.

- Arthroscopic debridement surgery can be effective in deferring more radical surgery but only in early-stage ankle arthritis.
- Arthrodesis is the gold standard surgical treatment. It can be performed arthroscopically, if there is minimal deformity and normal bone stock.
- Ankle arthroplasty can offer similar outcomes to arthrodesis, but with a higher chance of revision or secondary procedures. It is particularly indicated when there is ipsilateral hindfoot arthritis.

References

1. Barg A, Pagenstert GI, Hügle T, Gloyer M, Wiewiorski M, Henninger HB, & Valderrabano V. Ankle osteoarthritis: etiology, diagnostics, and classification. Foot Ankle Clin 2013; 18(3):411–26.
2. Cushnaghan J, Dieppe P. Study of 500 patients with limb joint osteoarthritis. I. Analysis by age, sex, and distribution of symptomatic joint sites. Ann Rheum Dis 1991; 50:8–13.
3. Valderrabano V, Horisberger M, Russell I, Dougall H, & Hintermann B. Etiology of ankle osteoarthritis. Clin Orthop Relat Res 2009; 467:1800–6.
4. Lindsjo U. Operative treatment of ankle fracture-dislocations. A follow-up study of 306/321 consecutive cases. Clin Orthop Relat Res 1985; (199):28–38.
5. Ramsey PL, Hamilton W. Changes in tibiotalar area of contact caused by lateral talar shift. J Bone Joint Surg Am 1976; 58:356–7.
6. Shepherd DE, Seedhom BB. Thickness of human articular cartilage in joints of the lower limb. Ann Rheum Dis 1999; 58(1):27–34.
7. Wan L, de Asla RJ, & Rubash HE, Li G. Determination of in vivo articular cartilage contact areas of human talocrural joint under weight-bearing conditions. Osteoarthritis Cartilage 2006; 14(12):1294–301.
8. Sokolove J, Lepus CM. Role of inflammation in the pathogenesis of osteoarthritis: latest findings and interpretations. Ther Adv Musculoskelet Dis 2013; 5(2):77–94.
9. Ding L, Buckwalter JA, & Martin JA. DAMPs synergize with cytokines or fibronectin fragment on inducing chondrolysis but lose effect when acting alone. Mediators Inflamm 2017; 2017:2642549.
10. National Institute for Health and Care Excellence. Osteoarthritis: care and management clinical guideline [CG177]. https://www.nice.org.uk/guidance/cg177/chapter/1-Recommendations#pharmacological-management; 2014
11. Tanaka Y, Takakura Y, Hayashi K, Taniguchi A, Kumai T, & Sugimoto K. Low tibial osteotomy for varus-type osteoarthritis of the ankle. J Bone Joint Surg Br 2006; 88(7):909–13.
12. Krause FG, Di Silvestro M, Penner MJ, Wing KJ, Glazebrook MA, Daniels TR, Lau J, & Younger ASE. The postoperative COFAS end-stage ankle arthritis classification system: interobserver and intraobserver reliability. Foot Ankle Spec 2012; 5(1):31–6.
13. Juni P, Hari R, Rutjes AWS, Fischer R, Silletta MG, Reichenbach S, & da Costa BR. Intra-articular corticosteroid for knee osteoarthritis. Cochrane Database Syst Rev 2015; (10):CD005328.
14. Paget L, Bierma-Zeinstra S, Goedegebuure S, Kerkhoffs G, Krips R, Maas M, Moen MH, Reurink G, Stufkens S, de Vos RJ, Weir A, & Tol JL. Platelet-rich plasma injection management for ankle osteoarthritis study (PRIMA): protocol of a Dutch multicentre, stratified, block-randomised, double-blind, placebo-controlled trial. BMJ Open 2019; 9(10):e030961.
15. Tol JL, Verheyen CP, & van Dijk CN. Arthroscopic treatment of anterior impingement in the ankle. J Bone Joint Surg Br 2001; 83(1):9e13.
16. de Keijzer DR, Joling BSH, Sierevelt IN, Hoornenborg D, Kerkhoffs GMMJ, & Haverkamp D. Influence of preoperative tibiotalar alignment in the coronal plane on the survival of total ankle replacement: a systematic review. Foot Ankle Int 2020; 41(2):160–9.
17. Bernstein M, Reidler J, Fragomen A, & Rozbruch SR. Ankle distraction arthroplasty: indications, technique, and outcomes. J Am Acad Orthop Surg 2017; 25(2):89–99.
18. Waters RL, Barnes G, Husserl T, Silver L, & Liss R. Comparable energy expenditure after arthrodesis of the hip and ankle. J Bone Joint Surg Am 1988; 70(7):1032–7.
19. Townshend D, Di Silvestro M, Krause F, Penner M, Younger A, Glazebrook M, & Wing K. Arthroscopic versus open ankle arthrodesis: a multicentre comparative case series. J Bone Joint Surg Am 2013; 95(2):98e102.
20. Winson IG, Robinson DE, & Allen PE. Arthroscopic ankle arthrodesis. J Bone Joint Surg 2005; 87(3):343–7.
21. Moore KR, Howell MA, Saltrick KR, & Caranzariti AR. Risk factors associated with non-union after elective foot and ankle reconstruction: a case control study. J Foot Ankle Surg. 2017; 56(3):457–62.
22. Penner M, Wing K, Glazebrook M, & Daniels T. The effect of deformity and hindfoot arthritis on midterm outcomes of ankle replacement and fusion: a prospective COFAS multi-centre study of 890 patients. AOFAS Annual Meeting Abstracts 2018. Foot Ankle Int 2018; 39(2S):76S–121S.
23. Gross CE, Hamid KS, Green C, Easley ME, DeOrio JK, & Nunley JA. Operative wound complications following total ankle arthroplasty. Foot Ankle Int 2017; 38(4):360–6.
24. Bartel AF, Roukis TS. Total ankle replacement survival rates based on Kaplan-Meier Survival Analysis of National Joint Registry Data. Clin Podiatr Med Surg 2015; 32(4):483–94.
25. Li Y, He J, & Hu Y. Comparison of the efficiency and safety of total ankle replacement and ankle arthrodesis in the treatment of osteoarthritis: an updated systematic review and meta-analysis. Orthop Surg 2020; 12(2).372–7.
26. Muller P, Skene SS, Chowdhury K, Cro S, Goldberg AJ, Dore CJ, & TARVA Study Group. A randomised, multi-centre trial of total ankle replacement versus ankle arthrodesis in the treatment of patients with end stage ankle osteoarthritis (TARVA): statistical analysis plan. Trials 2020; 21(1):197.

12 Ankle instability

Zoe Lin and Daniel Marsland

Introduction

In the United States, 3.1 million ankle sprains were recorded over a 4-year period (1). An 'ankle sprain' is one of the most common presenting complaints to the Emergency Department. The majority of injuries (85%) are lateral ankle sprains (LASs). Whilst most sprains resolve with simple measures, the rate of long-term disability is high, associated with a significant socio-economic burden due to time off work and inability to play sport (2). In one study, almost 40% of patients had residual complaints at 6.5 years following injury (3). Furthermore, up to 40% of patients develop chronic lateral ankle instability (CLAI) after a LAS (4). This has led some to say, *'There is no such thing as simple sprain!'* (5).

Ankle sprains can be broadly classified according to the anatomical region: lateral, syndesmotic and medial. Lateral injuries can also be classified as low or high ankle sprains. High ankle sprains refer to disruption of the syndesmosis and should be differentiated from low ankle sprains (lateral ligament complex) because they are higher energy injuries and are associated with prolonged disability. Medial ankle ligament injuries (deltoid) usually occur in combination with syndesmosis injuries, or ankle fracture-dislocations (6), and less frequently in isolation.

In this chapter, we provide an overview covering the management of both acute and chronic lateral ligament injuries, syndesmosis injuries and medial ankle sprains.

Anatomy and mechanism of injury

Although the anatomy of the ankle has been covered in depth in Chapter 2, key structures are summarised in Table 12.1.

Ligament injuries can range from a mild sprain (ligament oedema) to partial or complete rupture. The anterior talofibular ligament (ATFL) is the weakest of the lateral ligaments and functions as the primary restraint to inversion in plantarflexion and also resists anterior displacement of the talus. The calcaneofibular ligament (CFL) crosses the subtalar joint and is the primary restraint to inversion in neutral and dorsiflexion. A LAS usually results from an inversion injury (Figure 12.1). Inversion and plantarflexion cause injury to the ATFL or, if severe, to both the ATFL and CFL. Pure inversion with the ankle in neutral may injure the CFL in isolation. Small avulsion fractures from the distal fibula are common (there is a common origin of the ATFL and CFL).

The syndesmosis is made up of the fibula which fits within the incisura of the distal tibia and is a strong fibrous joint tightly bound by four ligaments: the anterior inferior tibiofibular ligament (AITFL); the interosseous ligament (IOL); the interosseous membrane (IOM) and the posterior inferior tibiofibular ligament (PITFL). It is important to note that the PITFL is the strongest syndesmotic ligament and that it inserts onto the posterior malleolus. The syndesmosis resists external rotation of the fibula and lateral talar translation. Injuries are usually high energy and can be partial (stable) or complete (unstable). They typically occur due to external rotation, whilst the foot is pronated and the ankle is in dorsiflexion (Figure 12.2). As the fibula rotates externally, the syndesmosis fails in sequence, initially anteriorly at the AITFL, followed by the IOL and membrane and then posteriorly through either rupture of the PITFL or fracture (avulsion) of the posterior malleolus (7). Rotation of the fibula can also result in a proximal fibula fracture (Maisonneuve injury) associated with the disruption of the IOM. ATFL sprains commonly occur in association with syndesmosis disruption.

The medial ankle ligaments are very strong and consist of the deltoid ligament complex (superficial and deep ligament components) and also the calcaneonavicular (spring) ligament (8). The superficial deltoid ligament (four components) crosses the ankle and subtalar joint and resists valgus tilting of the talus whilst the deep deltoid ligament (two components), which crosses the ankle joint only, resists external rotation. Most deltoid ligament injuries occur in association with high energy ankle fractures or syndesmotic injuries, when the talus is forced into either external rotation (foot supinated or pronated) or abduction (foot pronated).

Table 12.1 Summary of three main ligamentous complexes involved in ankle sprains and mechanism of injury

	Components	Function	Mechanism of injury
Lateral ligament complex (Low ankle sprain)	1. Anterior talofibular ligament (ATFL) 2. Calcaneofibular ligament (CFL) 3. Posterior talofibular ligament (PTFL)	• ATFL – limits anterior translation of talus • CFL – limits inversion at ankle and subtalar joints • ATFL/CFL most commonly injured • PTFL rarely injured	• Inversion +/− plantarflexion • Rupture of the ATFL and/ or CFL and sometimes avulsion fracture from the common origin of the ATFL/CFL from the tip of the distal fibula • Figure 12.1
Syndesmosis (High ankle sprain)	1. Anterior-inferior tibiofibular ligament (AITFL) 2. Posterior-inferior tibiofibular ligament (PITFL) 3. Inferior transverse ligament (ITL) 4. Interosseous membrane (IOM) 5. Interosseous ligament (IOL)	• Controls fibular rotation relative to tibia in the axial plane • Limits fibular translation relative to tibia on dorsi/plantarflexion • The PITFL is the strongest of the syndesmotic ligaments and inserts on to the posterior malleolus	• High energy external rotation and dorsiflexion of the ankle with the foot in pronation • Fibula externally rotates followed by sequential failure of the AITFL, IOL and then the PITFL or posterior malleolus • Figure 12.2
Medial ligament complex (Often injured in association with a syndesmosis injury and/or ankle fracture-dislocation)	1. Superficial deltoid ligaments (TSL, TNL, STTL and TCL) 2. Deep deltoid ligaments (PTTL and ATTL) 3. Spring ligament (calcaneonavicular ligament)	• Superficial deltoid ligament limits abduction • Deep deltoid ligament limits external rotation	• High energy external rotation or abduction of the ankle • Superficial deltoid often completely avulses from the medial malleolus as a sleeve • Figure 12.2

Abbreviations: ATTL, Anterior tibiotalar ligament; PTTL, Posterior tibiotalar ligament; STTL, Superficial posterior tibiotalar ligament; TCL, Tibiocalcaneal ligament; TNL, Tibionavicular ligament; TSL, Tibiospring ligament.

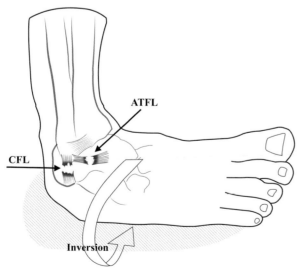

Figure 12.1 Inversion and plantarflexion injury causing rupture of the lateral ligaments.

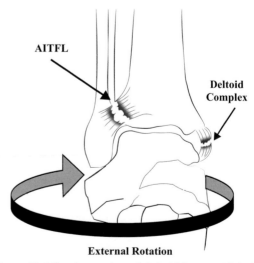

Figure 12.2 Syndesmosis and deltoid ligament injuries often occur together from high energy external rotation injuries.

Acute ankle injuries – associated injuries and conditions

It is important to identify and treat any acute concurrent injuries and also detect less common pathology that may masquerade as an 'ankle sprain'.

Fractures

Three types of fractures are known to commonly be associated with severe hindfoot inversion injuries: fractures of the 5th metatarsal base (Figure 12.3); fractures of the anterior process of the calcaneum (Figure 12.4) and fractures of the lateral process of the talus. Most of these fractures can be managed non-operatively. It is important to examine patients for bony tenderness according to the Ottawa ankle rules so that fractures are not missed.

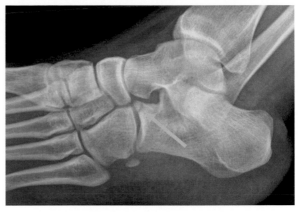

Figure 12.4 Radiograph showing an avulsion fracture from the anterior process of the calcaneum, due to pull off by the bifurcate ligament.

Osteochondral lesions (OCLs) of the talus

Approximately 66% of severe LAS are associated with an acute OCL, which most frequently occurs on the medial talar dome and less commonly on the lateral talar dome (Figure 12.5) (9). The presence of an OCL is associated with a higher risk of chronic pain (9) and can potentially progress to advanced osteoarthritis in the long term. Medial ankle tenderness may suggest an OCL is present but since most sprains do not warrant early MRI, the diagnosis of OCL is usually made late. An OCL should be

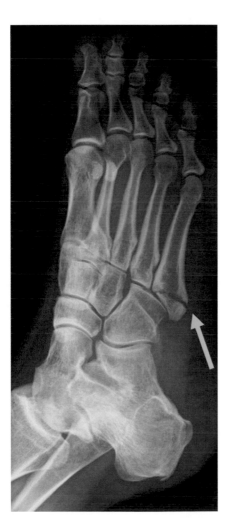

Figure 12.3 Radiograph showing a base of 5th metatarsal fracture following an inversion injury. Patients with this injury should also be examined for a coexisting LAS.

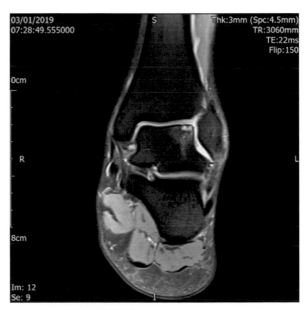

Figure 12.5 A lateral talar dome OCL in a soccer player who developed persistent pain after a LAS 18 months prior to presentation.

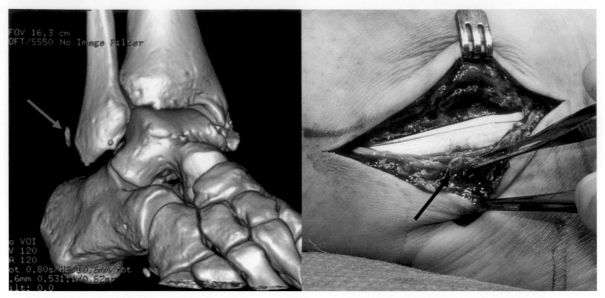

Figure 12.6 Peroneal tendon dislocation after a soccer injury. A 'fleck' sign (marked by arrows) indicates a superior peroneal retinaculum avulsion fracture from the fibula and is pathognomonic for peroneal tendon dislocation, shown in the corresponding intraoperative photograph.

suspected in patients who have persistent deep ankle pain more than 12 weeks after injury.

Peroneal tendon dislocation

Peroneal tendon dislocation is rare but commonly presents as an 'ankle sprain' and is often missed at initial presentation. It typically occurs when the peroneal tendons contract rapidly during eversion and forced dorsiflexion of the foot, leading to rupture of the superior peroneal retinaculum, and subsequent tendon subluxation or dislocation. Clinical features include extensive bruising over the posterior border of the distal fibula. Snapping of the tendons may be evident or there may be frank dislocation. Resisted foot eversion is usually adequate to determine whether the tendons are stable. A 'fleck' sign on radiographs or CT is a bony avulsion from the superior peroneal retinaculum, pathognomonic for peroneal tendon dislocation (Figure 12.6). MRI or dynamic ultrasound assessment may be necessary to confirm the diagnosis.

Tarsal coalition

Tarsal coalition classically presents in children aged 8–15 years, often with a history of 'recurrent ankle sprains' and symptom of pain (Figure 12.7). Although the rates of LAS are high in 10–19 year olds (1), the diagnosis of tarsal coalition should also be considered in this age group, especially if there is increased hindfoot valgus and/or a stiff subtalar joint. The pain from tarsal coalition occurs due to peroneal tendon spasm against

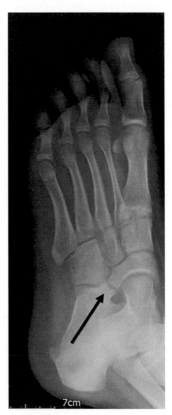

Figure 12.7 Example of a calcaneonavicular tarsal coalition in a 13-year-old female, referred with 'recurrent ankle sprains'.

a stiff valgus hindfoot, hence the term 'peroneal spastic flatfoot', but is often misinterpreted as an ankle sprain. Plain radiographs are usually adequate to diagnose a bony coalition, but CT or MRI may also be necessary if there is a high index of suspicion.

Acute lateral ankle sprain (LAS)

LAS is extremely common and approximately 50% occur whilst playing sport (1). Certain risk factors are known to predispose to an acute LAS and are classified as either intrinsic or extrinsic. Intrinsic factors are those specific to the patient and include limited ankle dorsiflexion, reduced proprioception, hindfoot varus and poor postural control on a single leg balance test (2). Female sex, increased height and a lower BMI are associated with an increased risk of LAS (2, 10), although a raised BMI may cause more severe injuries. Extrinsic factors relate to the type of sport in particular rugby, aeroball, basketball, volleyball, field sports and climbing (2).

Clinical features

Patients often describe an inversion injury associated with early swelling over the lateral ankle. Usually, patients can bear weight; inability to bear weight in association with extensive bruising and discolouration suggests a ligament rupture.

Clinical examination of an acute ankle injury should initially follow the Ottawa ankle rules to rule out a fracture. There is often tenderness over the lateral ligaments. The optimal time to assess a LAS is on day 5 after the injury when the pain has diminished, with 96% sensitivity and 85% specificity to detect ligament rupture (11). An anterior drawer test is performed with the ankle in slight plantarflexion (Figure 12.8) and considered positive when there is laxity, a soft end point and a dimple is seen just anterior to the tip of the fibula (when compared to the un-injured side) (11). The absence of visible discolouration and a negative anterior drawer sign at this stage reliably indicates that the ATFL is intact (11). To assess CFL, a talar tilt test is performed with the ankle in neutral (Figure 12.9).

Although subjective, a LAS can be graded according to severity:

- **Grade 1:** Mild sprain (stretching of the lateral ligament/s) – There is minimal swelling and pain, the patient is able to bear weight without significant pain, there is mild tenderness over ATFL, and the anterior drawer and the talar tilt tests are negative.
- **Grade 2:** Moderate sprain (partial tear of the lateral ligament/s) – There is tenderness over the lateral ligament complex; there is moderate bruising and pain, and the anterior drawer test is positive with moderate laxity and a detectable end point.

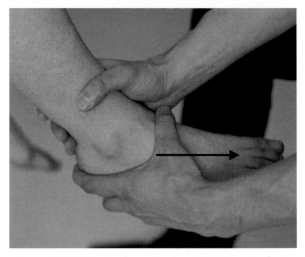

Figure 12.8 Anterior drawer to test ATFL integrity, best done on day 5 after injury. The foot should be placed in 10 degrees of plantarflexion and the heel then drawn forward.

- **Grade 3:** Severe sprain (complete rupture of the lateral ligament/s) – There is extensive bruising, discolouration and swelling, along with significant pain and tenderness; the patient is unable to bear weight, and the anterior drawer and/or talar tilt test is positive with laxity and soft end point.

Investigations

Plain radiographs of the foot and ankle are warranted if a fracture or syndesmosis injury is suspected. In most cases MRI is not necessary for an acute LAS, unless a

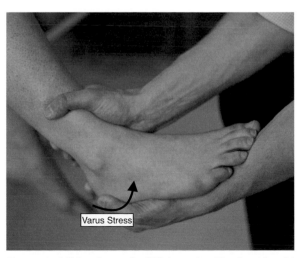

Varus Stress

Figure 12.9 Talar tilt test for CFL integrity. The foot should be placed in neutral and then varus applied to the heel.

syndesmosis injury is suspected. Elite athletes warrant early MRI in order to grade the injury, and to aid accurate prediction of return to play and to guide management.

Management

First line treatment for a LAS is non-operative. Functional bracing using a semi-rigid ankle brace for the first 4–6 weeks is the gold standard and better than an elastic bandage or kinesio tape (12). Self-directed exercise therapy combined with the use of a functional brace improves recovery and also reduces the risk of functional instability (2). For pain management, data from meta-analyses show that a short period of immobilisation in a boot or cast for less than 10 days reduces pain and swelling and improves functional outcomes (2). Longer periods of immobilisation however are detrimental to recovery. Supervised exercise therapy is indicated to treat ankle stiffness, especially as restricted dorsiflexion increases the risk of further sprains (2).

Surgical reconstruction for acute lateral ligament rupture has good outcomes but is unnecessary for most patients, as functional treatment is successful in up to 70% of cases (13). Treatment however should be tailored to the individual patient. Data from randomised controlled trials have shown that acute surgical reconstruction reduces the rate of a recurrent LAS and may also speed up return to play (14). Therefore, in professional athletes with acute high-grade lateral ligament injuries, arthroscopic washout of the joint and acute lateral ligament reconstruction can be recommended.

Depending upon the grade of injury, return to full work duties and sport can be expected by 3–4 weeks for a simple sprain. For partial or complete lateral ligament ruptures, return to normal activities can be expected by 6–8 weeks (2).

Anterolateral soft tissue ankle impingement

Pain following a LAS is most often due to ankle impingement. Soft tissue anterolateral impingement results from the formation of scar tissue after an ATFL tear. The thickened ligament is then prone to repetitive mechanical irritation, resulting in synovitis. Injury to the lower fibres of the AITFL (Bassett's ligament) can also result in thickening and subsequent impingement of the anterior syndesmosis. Initial treatment should include physiotherapy and a short course of non-steroidal anti-inflammatory drugs (NSAIDs). An ultrasound guided corticosteroid injection has high success rates, and in one study reported excellent pain relief in 74% of patients, with 46% of patients are pain free at 2 years (15). Arthroscopic debridement is effective for those patients who fail non-operative measures.

Chronic lateral ankle ligament injury (CLAI)

CLAI is defined as persistent pain, swelling and/or giving way in combination with recurrent ankle sprains for at least 12 months after the initial injury (16) and it occurs in up to 40% of patients following a LAS (4). Patients who are at increased risk of developing instability following a first time LAS are those who are slow to recover, including an inability to jump or land at 2 weeks, increased laxity at 8 weeks, and those with poor postural control (4).

Clinical features

Patients often have a long history of recurrent sprains prior to presentation. There may be a subjective feeling of insecurity and inability to 'trust' the ankle. Patients tend to look down at the ground when walking because of a lack of confidence when walking on uneven terrain. Medial or deep ankle pain should raise the possibility of an associated OCL. Anteromedial ankle pain is also commonly caused by bony impingement from a long-standing anteromedial talar neck spur, common in athletes. Pain from the posterolateral ankle suggests peroneal tendinopathy, which can result from tendon overload in an attempt to compensate for an unstable ankle (Figure 12.11).

It is important to establish the nature of previous treatment including the use of a brace, taping, physiotherapy and whether functional rehabilitation has been optimised. Hobbies and sports aspirations are also important to note.

Clinical examination should start with the patient standing to check hindfoot alignment. A cavovarus foot can lead to insufficiency of the lateral ligaments. Instability in association with a cavovarus foot should be carefully assessed, as an isolated lateral ligament reconstruction, without addressing the underlying deformity, may result in early failure. Pertinent components of the preoperative workup should establish whether hindfoot deformity is fixed or flexible, including a Coleman block test to assess for forefoot driven hindfoot varus.

Patients with CLAI often have poor postural control on a single leg balance test. The patient may also struggle to do a single leg heel raise due to calf and peroneal weakness. The presence of local swelling suggests a recent sprain. Palpation should include the medial joint (OCL, bony impingement), the anterior syndesmosis (anterolateral impingement from a thickened AITFL), ATFL (impingement or recent sprain) and peroneal tendons (tendinopathy).

A knee to wall test helps identify limited dorsiflexion. Weakness of eversion indicates that the peroneal tendons are weak, most commonly because rehabilitation has not been optimised but sometimes due to tendinopathy.

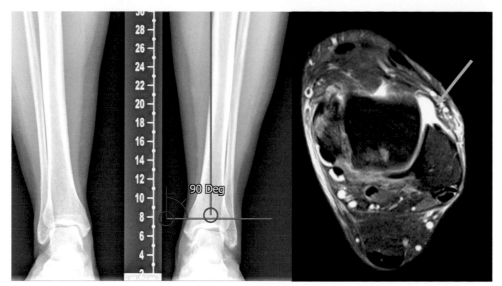

Figure 12.10 Weight-bearing radiographs demonstrating talar tilt due to incompetence of the ATFL, in a 42-year-old female with a history of CLAI. A subsequent MRI demonstrated a thin, wavy ATFL (arrow).

As described for a LAS, anterior drawer and talar tilt tests for ATFL and CFL integrity are important, but are more subjective and less accurate compared to when used to examine for acute injury. Patients should also be screened for joint hypermobility syndrome.

Investigations

Standing radiographs are useful to check alignment, and for talar tilt (Figure 12.10). Long leg radiographs are sometimes necessary to assess for varus deformity proximal to the ankle and to measure the angle of the tibial plafond relative to the mechanical axis (Figure 12.10). A hindfoot alignment view (Saltzman) may be helpful in assessing calcaneal alignment. MRI is the most useful investigation which allows assessment of the lateral ligaments, articular cartilage and peroneal tendons (Figure 12.11). Ultrasound, in the correct hands, is as sensitive as MRI in assessing ligament and tendon pathology and has the advantage of also facilitating the use of guided diagnostic (or therapeutic)

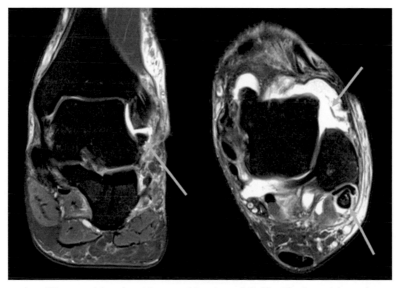

Figure 12.11 MRI scan in a 50-year-old male with a combination of CLAI, a fibula ossicle and peroneal tendinopathy (arrows) due to chronic overload. This patient required a lateral ligament reconstruction, excision of ossicle and peroneal tendon debridement and repair.

injections. CT is a useful adjunct for preoperative planning for bony impingement and OCLs. Inversion stress radiographs are considered positive if there is greater than 15 degrees talar tilt compared with normal ankle but are very rarely required and unnecessarily expose the clinician to radiation.

Management

Initial treatment of CLAI includes strengthening of the peroneal muscles (dynamic stabilisers) to optimise eversion strength. Exercise therapy, proprioceptive training (3) and ankle taping or a lace up brace have been shown to reduce the risk of recurrent sprains, especially in athletes (12). Full eversion power signifies a complete rehabilitation attempt and should be achieved prior to consideration for surgery.

If non-operative measures fail, then surgical reconstruction is warranted. Numerous surgical techniques have been described to treat CLAI and are classified as anatomical or non-anatomical reconstructions. Anatomical reconstructions have superior long-term outcomes compared with non-anatomical reconstructions (17), and the gold standard is considered the Broström-Gould lateral ligament reconstruction. It involves shortening and reattachment of the stretched ATFL and CFL (Broström component), with augmentation, using the extensor retinaculum and fibular periosteal flap (Gould component). Further augmentation using an extracapsular suture tape is also gaining popularity.

Non-anatomical reconstructions, such as the Evans tenodesis (sectioning the peroneus brevis tendon proximally followed by transfer to the distal fibula), have poor long-term outcomes with high rates of residual laxity and secondary osteoarthritis, chronic pain and reduced dorsiflexion (17). Other non-anatomical reconstructions have been associated with excessive stiffness and the feeling of the ankle being 'too tight'.

Senior author's preferred surgical technique – Modified Broström-Gould ligament reconstruction (anatomical reconstruction and augmentation with extensor retinaculum)

1. The patient is positioned supine with a large sandbag under the ipsilateral buttock – the heel is level with the end of the table. This position allows initial ankle arthroscopy to address intra-articular pathologies such as anteromedial talar neck spurs (bony impingement), or OCLs.
2. Preoperative examination under anaesthesia is performed including anterior drawer and talar tilt tests. The superficial peroneal nerve is marked using the '4th toe flexion' sign (Figure 12.12), especially if arthroscopy is planned.

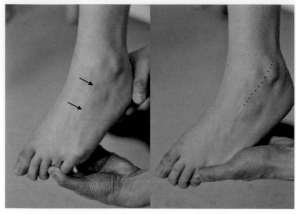

Figure 12.12 The 4th toe flexion sign allows identification of the superficial peroneal nerve prior to arthroscopy.

3. A curvilinear incision is made just distal to the lateral malleolus (Figure 12.13). If peroneal tendon surgery is required, or revision surgery is being performed using a tendon graft then a longitudinal incision is preferred, centered over the distal fibula, extending towards the base of the 4th metatarsal.
4. Dissection through fat is performed. The superior edge of the extensor retinaculum is identified and separated from the deep tissues.
5. The distal tip of the lateral malleolus is identified, followed by identification of the peroneal tendons. The CFL lies deep to the tendons.
6. The common origin of the ATFL and CFL is at the anterior distal tip of the lateral malleolus. Using sharp dissection, the common origin is detached from the distal lateral malleolus, protecting the peroneal tendons throughout. If an ossicle is present it is excised. The periosteum over the footprint of the common origin of the ATFL and CFL is then elevated, lifting a layer proximally. The footprint is then nibbled down to bleeding cancellous bone to promote healing and reattachment of the ligament reconstruction. Two suture anchors are then inserted (preferably absorbable rather than metal in case subsequent MRI is required).
7. The sutures from each suture anchor are then passed, respectively, through the ATFL and CFL using a Kessler type configuration, and carefully sited ensuring that an adequate 'bite' of each ligament is achieved. As the sutures are tied, the foot is positioned in eversion and 5 degrees of plantarflexion. *Note – if the patient has joint hypermobility syndrome or a revision Broström-Gould is being performed, the reconstruction is augmented with an extracapsular suture tape secured with interference screws, between the talus and lateral malleolus.*

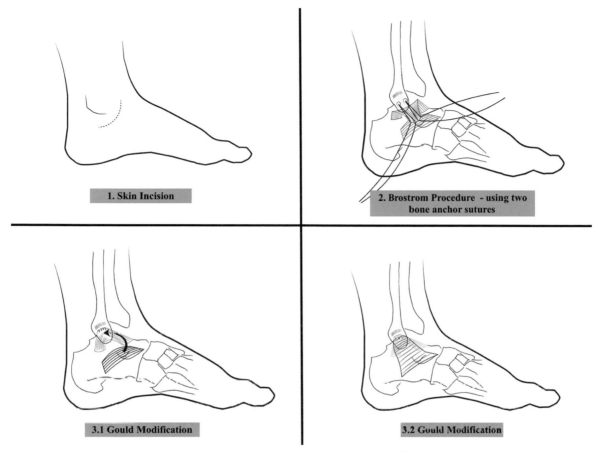

1. Skin Incision

2. Brostrom Procedure - using two bone anchor sutures

3.1 Gould Modification

3.2 Gould Modification

Figure 12.13 Schematic drawings to show the Broström-Gould anatomical lateral ligament reconstruction.

8. The Gould first component of the reconstruction involves suturing the elevated periosteal layer of the lateral malleolus down over the repair, using a 'pants over vest' technique. The second component, which may have an important proprioceptive function, is to advance the proximal edge of the previously identified extensor retinaculum over the repair and then to secure it down to the fibula via the suture anchors.

9. Following skin closure and dressings, a below-knee plaster of Paris backslab is applied.

10. The following postoperative instructions are used in most cases:
    i. Chemical venous thromboembolism prophylaxis for 2 weeks.
    ii. Review in clinic at 2 weeks, convert to a boot – partial weight-bearing for 2 weeks, then full weight-bearing for further 2 weeks. Allow inline active range of movement exercises out of boot from 2 weeks, working hard on dorsiflexion, but avoiding plantarflexion.
    iii. Wean out of boot from week 6. Apply taping from week 6–9 and start functional/balance work, particularly peroneal and calf muscle strengthening.
    iv. No restrictions from week 9 onwards as long as physiotherapy milestones have been met. Aim for return to sport by 12 weeks.

Long-term outcomes following the Broström-Gould procedure are reported to be excellent, with revision rates of 1.2% at a mean of 8.4 years follow up (18). Long-term rates of osteoarthritis are also low and one study of 310 ankles reported that only 3% of patients developed osteoarthritis at 11 years follow up (19). As surgical techniques have advanced, arthroscopic lateral ligament reconstruction has emerged as a safe technique, and early evidence shows equivalent short-term outcomes compared with an open Broström reconstruction.

Revision and salvage surgery for failed lateral ligament reconstruction

For those patients who have a failed lateral ligament reconstruction, surgical options include a revision Broström-Gould, augmented with an extracapsular

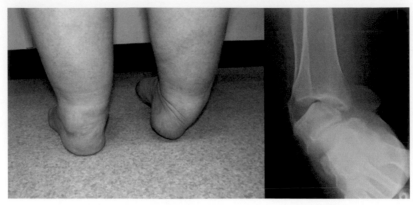

Figure 12.14 Severe CLAI in a 53-year-old woman following a failed revision lateral ligament reconstruction using peroneus brevis tendon autograft. In low demand patients with multiple comorbidities, salvage surgery should be considered. This woman subsequently underwent an ankle fusion.

suture tape. However, if the residual soft tissues are inadequate for reconstruction, then an anatomic reconstruction using tendon autograft (e.g., peroneus longus tendon) or allograft may be necessary, reconstructing both the ATFL and CFL. In case of severe instability and multiple failed reconstructions, especially in lower demand middle-aged patients, an ankle fusion should be considered (Figure 12.14).

Ankle arthritis and osteochondral lesions (OCLs) associated with chronic lateral ankle instability (CLAI)

The significance of talar OCLs in association with CLAI remains uncertain. OCLs often occur at the time of an acute LAS and are associated with long-term pain (3). Alternatively, due to CLAI, possibly due to altered biomechanics, repetitive microtrauma may occur over time causing cumulative damage to the articular cartilage, and subsequent development of an OCL. In one study reporting the treatment of OCL, the presence of CLAI was associated with a greater number of OCLs, larger lesions and inferior ability to do sport (20). In contrast, other research has reported outcomes following Broström-Gould repair that are the same, regardless of whether an OCL is present (21). Despite the lack of clear evidence, it is preferable to treat both the OCL and CLAI at the same sitting.

The relationship between CLAI and the development of arthritis remains unclear. Ankle arthritis affects 1% of the population and in a study of 390 patients with end-stage ankle arthritis, 16% had ligamentous instability (22). Typically, with instability, there is varus deformity, and incompetent lateral ligaments may have

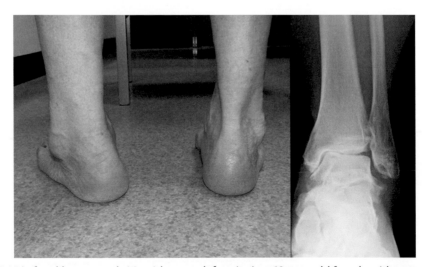

Figure 12.15 Left ankle osteoarthritis with varus deformity in a 60-year-old female with untreated CLAI.

implications if a total ankle replacement is being considered. Ankle fusion in this setting offers a more reliable solution. Whether early lateral ligament reconstruction protects against the development of an OCL and osteoarthritis remains unknown (Figure 12.15).

Syndesmosis injury

Up to 25% of ankle sprains involve the syndesmosis, especially common in the athletic population. High energy pronation-external rotation injuries with a dorsiflexed ankle tend to be complete injuries (unstable), compared with inversion-type syndesmosis injuries which are partial (stable). Injuries are associated with prolonged disability and pain, especially if diagnosed late (8, 23). Purely ligamentous syndesmosis injuries are classified according to the West Point ankle grading system (Table 12.2). Grade 1 injuries are stable and the AITFL is sprained in isolation. Grade 2 injuries are subclassified as either stable (2A) or dynamically unstable (2B). For grade 3 injuries, there is frank diastasis of the syndesmosis and all components of the syndesmosis are disrupted.

Clinical features

Patients may describe a high energy injury, often, whilst playing contact sport or sport with rigid footwear (skiing, ice hockey). An inability to bear weight suggests an unstable injury. Acutely, there is often a localised 'egg' like swelling over the anterior syndesmosis, with tenderness. Medial tenderness suggests possible deltoid ligament disruption and a higher grade of injury. Signs of instability include a positive squeeze test (Figure 12.16), cross-leg test, tenderness that extends along the IOM more than 6 cm proximal to the ankle and a positive external rotation test (24). The senior author prefers to perform the external rotation test with the patient prone (Figure 12.17), much like the dial test for posterolateral corner instability in the knee, as the proximal tibia is stabilised on the bed and also side-to-side comparison is possible. A positive test is when pain is felt in the anterior syndesmosis on external rotation. This test may also allow assessment of the deltoid ligament complex (see section "Deltoid ligament injury"). So, diagnosis is relatively straightforward but assessing the severity or extent of a syndesmotic injury is not.

Table 12.2 The West Point Ankle Grading System for ligamentous syndesmosis injuries (high ankle sprains)

West Point Ankle Grading System	Clinical features	MRI features	Treatment
Grade 1 (stable)	• Swelling anterior syndesmosis • Tenderness AITFL • Negative squeeze test • External rotation test negative • Deltoid ligament not tender	• AITFL sprain	• Non-weight-bearing 10 days • Boot 3 weeks • Syndesmosis taping from weeks 3–9
Grade 2A (stable)	• As for grade 1	• AITFL rupture + IOL injury	• Non-weight-bearing 10 days • Boot 3 weeks • Syndesmosis taping from weeks 3–9 • Arthroscopic assessment if doubt about instability
Grade 2B (dynamically unstable)	• Tenderness AITFT, extending >6 cm proximal to ankle joint • Deltoid ligament tenderness • Positive squeeze test and/or external rotation test	• AITFL, IOL rupture • PITFL rupture OR Posterior malleolus bone bruise or fracture • No diastasis	• Arthroscopic assessment and syndesmosis reconstruction if positive 'drive through' sign • If negative 'drive through' sign, simply debride anterior syndesmosis
Grade 3 (unstable)	• Extensive swelling • Tenderness AITFT, extending >6 cm proximal to ankle joint • Deltoid ligament tenderness/swelling • Positive squeeze test and/or external rotation test	• Frank diastasis at syndesmosis and talar shift • AITFL, IOL + PITFL rupture or posterior malleolus bone bruise or fracture	• Syndesmosis reconstruction +/− deltoid ligament reconstruction

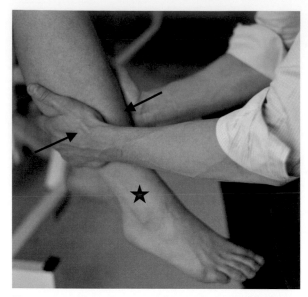

Figure 12.16 The squeeze test for syndesmosis instability. A positive test is pain felt in the anterior syndesmosis (*).

Investigations

Weight-bearing radiographs of both ankles allow comparison and may demonstrate a frank diastasis at the syndesmosis. Radiographs should be taken to rule out a Maisonneuve type injury if there is proximal fibula tenderness and also to exclude Tillaux-type or posterior malleolar avulsion fractures, which can be present in up to 50% of such injuries. The gold standard imaging is MRI, which is highly sensitive and specific for syndesmosis injury and should be performed early as sensitivity reduces with time (7). Early clinical examination (e.g., positive squeeze or external rotation tests) combined with MRI within 5–10 days of injury allows accurate differentiation of stable and unstable injuries (24). MRI features of instability include disruption of the posterior elements including, PITFL rupture, posterior malleolus bone bruise or posterior malleolus fracture (7). For chronic injuries, CT of both ankles is helpful. The gold standard assessment for patients with suspected syndesmosis instability is arthroscopic. If a 4.0 mm shaver can be 'driven through' the syndesmosis then reconstruction is warranted (7).

Management

Grade 1 and 2A injuries are stable and are managed non-operatively. The patient is mobilised non-weight-bearing for the first 10 days and kept in a boot for 3 weeks, followed by taping of the syndesmosis from weeks 3–9 (24).

A grade 2B injury is dynamically unstable and, if suspected, warrants an arthroscopic assessment. If proven to be unstable with a positive 'drive-through' sign, then syndesmosis reconstruction is necessary (Figure 12.18). If stable to probing then the anterior syndesmosis is simply debrided and reconstruction is not required. A grade 3 injury, with complete disruption of the syndesmosis and diastasis, requires reduction and stabilisation.

The method of syndesmosis fixation remains controversial and can be performed with suture buttons or screws. No optimal screw configuration has been established. Level 1 evidence has shown that a single suture button is superior to a single screw with lower rates of mal-reduction and better functional outcomes at 5 years, without the need for implant removal (25). However, this only applies to purely coronal plane instability. If there is either vertical plane instability (such as in the presence of a fractured and shortened fibula) or, there is sagittal plane instability (when all

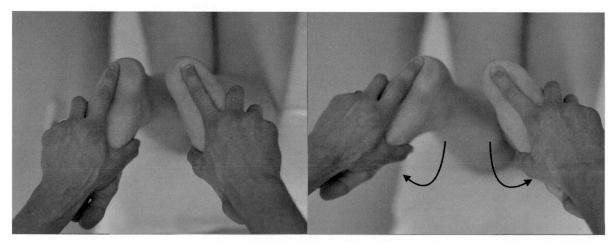

Figure 12.17 The external rotation test being applied with the patient positioned prone, which allows side-to-side comparison. This test can be used to test both the syndesmosis and also deltoid ligament (deep component).

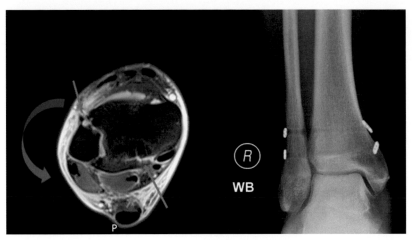

Figure 12.18 A 50-year-old patient with a complete syndesmosis injury following a skiing accident. The curved arrow indicates an external rotation mechanism. The straight arrows demonstrate rupture of the AITFL and a posterior malleolus fracture (to which the PITFL is attached). The syndesmosis proved to be unstable at arthroscopy (positive drive through sign) and was reconstructed using two suture buttons.

three components – AITFL, IOL and PITFL are injured), then a single suture button does not provide adequate stability. In fact, no combination of suture buttons can provide adequate vertical plane stability and should not be used in this situation. If there is sagittal plane instability then, if suture buttons are to be used in preference to a screw, two should be used in divergent fashion. Delayed surgical stabilisation (>6 months) is associated with significantly worse clinical function, and chronic injuries are difficult to manage, sometimes requiring reconstruction using tendon graft (7, 23).

Deltoid ligament injury

Deltoid ligament injuries frequently occur in association with ankle fracture dislocations or high grade syndesmosis injuries. Isolated deltoid ligament injuries are, in contrast, rare and account for only 3–4% of ankle sprains (8). Recovery from an acute deltoid ligament injury can be prolonged (from 4–6 months). Medial ankle pain can persist due to impingement or, in higher grade injuries, due to instability.

Clinical features

The typical mechanism of injury is high energy external rotation or abduction through the ankle. For rotational injuries, the foot can be either pronated or supinated as described by the Lauge-Hansen classification. There is medial swelling and palpation may help differentiate a deltoid ligament injury (tender tip of medial malleolus) from a spring ligament injury (tender between the sustentaculum tali and naviculum). Tenderness over the sustentaculum tali (bony prominence inferior to medial malleolus) may indicate an avulsion fracture. On standing, increased hindfoot valgus suggests

rupture of the deltoid ligament. Pes planus suggests rupture of the spring ligament. An inability to perform a single leg heel raise suggests instability or tibialis posterior tendinopathy. An external rotation stress test done prone (Figure 12.16) allows side-to-side comparison. Increased external rotation suggests a deep deltoid ligament rupture. Increased hindfoot valgus on a valgus stress test suggests injury to the superficial deltoid.

Investigations

If tolerated, weight-bearing foot and ankle radiographs should be obtained. An increased medial clear space on an AP weight-bearing projection indicates rupture of the posterior part of the deep deltoid, whilst valgus talar tilt indicates rupture of the superficial deltoid. A negative Meary's angle or uncovering of the talonavicular joint may indicate a spring ligament rupture. MRI is the gold standard imaging test and allows assessment of the deltoid ligament complex, spring ligament and tibialis posterior tendon. Where local expertise exists, ultrasound is also very good and has the advantage of being a dynamic imaging test as well.

Management

Treatment of an acute deltoid ligament injury varies depending upon the grade of injury and also upon the presence or otherwise of associated fractures or syndesmotic injury. For isolated deltoid ligament sprains without instability, weight-bearing in a boot for 6 weeks followed by ankle taping for a further 6 weeks is adequate. Physiotherapy work should focus on optimising tibialis posterior strength, calf strength and balance.

When associated with a fracture dislocation and increased talar tilt, the superficial deltoid is usually

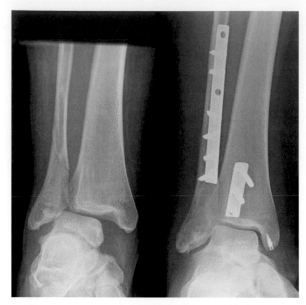

Figure 12.19 A patient with a Weber C ankle fracture dislocation, including a posterior malleolus fracture and complete disruption of the superficial deltoid ligament. As is common, the superficial deltoid ligament was found to be avulsed from the medial malleolus and reconstructed using a single suture anchor.

avulsed from the medial malleolus as a sleeve (6). Indications for reconstruction include an inability to reduce the talus due to entrapment of the deltoid ligament within the medial gutter or excessive talar tilt on intraoperative valgus stress testing after fracture fixation. Acute repair is technically straightforward, and the superficial deltoid can be reattached using one or two suture anchors (Figure 12.19). In the presence of a deep deltoid ligament rupture though, especially if it involves the posterior part (opening of the medial clear space on weight-bearing AP radiographs), repairing the superficial deltoid will make little difference. Unlike with the superficial deltoid ligament though, surgical access to the deep deltoid, especially to its posterior part, is more complex and, as such, controversy remains as to whether ankle fracture fixation should be routinely augmented with deltoid ligament repair. However, results of superficial deltoid ligament reconstruction can be excellent and in one study of elite athletes with Weber C ankle fractures, additional reconstruction of the superficial deltoid ligament resulted in better function (6).

Isolated deltoid ligament rupture leading to instability is relatively uncommon. This injury can be treated with immobilisation in plaster for 6 weeks, but considering the risk of long-term disability, surgical reconstruction is recommended, especially in athletes (8). Late deltoid ligament reconstruction is challenging and may require tendon graft, augmentation with suture tape and/or a medialising calcaneal osteotomy.

Injuries that occur to the distal insertion of the superficial deltoid also often involve the spring (calcaneonavicular) ligament. The superficial deltoid ligament insertion is broad and attaches to the spring ligament. Spring ligament injuries may also occur in isolation. Both injury patterns are rare and often occur during sport. This injury is very different to an acquired flatfoot due to tibialis posterior tendinopathy, and/or a degenerate tear or insufficiency of the spring ligament (the planovalgus foot is discussed in Chapter 8). An acute spring ligament sprain can be treated non-operatively, typically with a boot for 6–12 weeks, followed by a medial arch support orthotic. For partial or complete ruptures, with acquired pes planus and inability to perform a single-leg heel raise, then spring ligament reconstruction is necessary.

Take home messages

- The primary treatment for an acute LAS is RICE, followed by functional bracing and self-directed rehabilitation. 10 days of immobilisation in a boot or a cast may be warranted so as to manage pain, but longer periods of immobilisation are detrimental.
- Up to 40% of patients develop long-term disability following a LAS, due to secondary anterolateral soft tissue impingement, CLAI and/or OCL.
- Other injuries may present as a LAS and are easily missed including fractures, a high-ankle sprain (syndesmosis), peroneal traction tenosynovitis or, less commonly, injuries such as peroneal tendon dislocation and coalitions.
- For the surgical treatment of CLAI, the Broström-Gould lateral ligament reconstruction is considered the gold standard and achieves an anatomical repair, with low failure rates.
- Syndesmosis injuries are common in athletes and cause prolonged disability, especially if the diagnosis is delayed.
- Deltoid ligament injuries often occur in association with syndesmosis injuries and/or ankle fracture-dislocations.

Acknowledgement

The authors would like to thank Dr Kuljit Bhogal for the original artwork (surgical technique).

References

1. Waterman BR, Owens BD, Davey S, Zacchilli MA, Belmont PJ Jr. The epidemiology of ankle sprains in the United States. J Bone Joint Surg Am. 2010; 92(13):2279–2284.
2. Vuurberg G, Hoorntje A, Wink LM, et al. Diagnosis, treatment and prevention of ankle sprains: Update of an

evidence-based clinical guideline. Br J Sports Med. 2018; 52(15):956.

3. Verhagen RA, De Keizer G, Van Dijk CN. Long-term follow-up of inversion trauma of the ankle. Arch Orthop Trauma Surg. 1995; 114(2):92–96.

4. Doherty C, Bleakley C, Hertel J, Caulfield B, Ryan J, Delahunt E. Gait biomechanics in participants, six months after first-time lateral ankle sprain. Int J Sports Med. 2016; 37(7): 577–583.

5. Van Dijk CN, Vuurberg G. There is no such thing as a simple ankle sprain: Clinical commentary on the 2016 International Ankle Consortium position statement. Br J Sports Med. 2017; 51(6):485–486.

6. Hsu AR, Lareau CR, Anderson RB. Repair of acute superficial deltoid complex avulsion during ankle fracture fixation in National Football League Players. Foot Ankle Int. 2015; 36(11):1272–1278.

7. Randell M, Marsland D, Ballard E, Forster B, Lutz M. MRI for high ankle sprains with an unstable syndesmosis: Posterior malleolus bone oedema is common and time to scan matters. Knee Surg Sports Traumatol Arthrosc. 2019; 27(9): 2890–2897.

8. Lötscher P, Lang TH, Zwicky L, Hintermann B, Knupp M. Osteoligamentous injuries of the medial ankle joint. Eur J Trauma Emerg Surg. 2015; 41(6):615–621.

9. Van Dijk CN, Bossuyt PM, Marti RK. Medial ankle pain after lateral ligament rupture. J Bone Joint Surg Br. 1996; 78(4): 562–567.

10. Kobayashi T, Tanaka M, Shida M. Intrinsic risk factors of lateral ankle sprain: A systematic review and meta-analysis. Sports Health. 2016; 8(2):190–193.

11. Van Dijk CN, Lim LS, Bossuyt PM, Marti RK. Physical examination is sufficient for the diagnosis of sprained ankles. J Bone Joint Surg Br. 1996; 78(6):958 962.

12. van den Bekerom MP, Kerkhoffs GM, McCollum GA, Calder JD, van Dijk CN. Management of acute lateral ankle ligament injury in the athlete. Knee Surg Sports Traumatol Arthrosc. 2013; 21(6):1390–1395.

13. Struijs PA, Kerkhoffs GM. Ankle sprain. BMJ Clin Evid. 2010; 2010:1115.

14. Han LH, Zhang CY, Liu, Ting H, Jihong W. A meta-analysis of treatment methods for acute ankle sprain. Pakistan Journal of Medical Science 2012; 28(5):895–899.

15. Grice J, Marsland D, Smith G, Calder J. Efficacy of foot and ankle corticosteroid injections. Foot Ankle Int. 2017; 38(1): 8–13.

16. Gribble PA, Bleakley CM, Caulfield BM, et al. 2016 consensus statement of the International Ankle Consortium: Prevalence, impact and long-term consequences of lateral ankle sprains. Br J Sports Med. 2016; 50(24):1493–1495.

17. Krips R, Brandsson S, Swensson C, van Dijk CN, Karlsson J. Anatomical reconstruction and Evans tenodesis of the lateral ligaments of the ankle. Clinical and radiological findings after follow-up for 15 to 30 years. J Bone Joint Surg Br. 2002; 84(2):232–236.

18. So E, Preston N, Holmes T. Intermediate- to long-term longevity and incidence of revision of the modified Broström-Gould procedure for lateral ankle ligament repair: A systematic review. J Foot Ankle Surg. 2017; 56(5):1076–1080.

19. Mabit C, Tourné Y, Besse JL, et al. Chronic lateral ankle instability surgical repairs: The long term prospective. Orthop Traumatol Surg Res. 2010; 96(4):417–423.

20. Lee M, Kwon JW, Choi WJ, Lee JW. Comparison of outcomes for osteochondral lesions of the talus with and without chronic lateral ankle instability. Foot Ankle Int. 2015; 36(9):1050–1057.

21. Nery C, Raduan F, Del Buono A, Asaumi ID, Cohen M, Maffulli N. Arthroscopic-assisted Broström-Gould for chronic ankle instability: A long-term follow-up. Am J Sports Med. 2011; 39(11):2381–2388.

22. Valderrabano V, Horisberger M, Russell I, Dougall H, Hintermann B. Etiology of ankle osteoarthritis. Clin Orthop Relat Res. 2009; 467(7):1800–1806.

23. Kent S, Yeo G, Marsland D, Randell M, Forster B, Lutz M, Okano S. Delayed stabilisation of dynamically unstable syndesmotic injuries results in worse functional outcomes. Knee Surg Sports Traumatol Arthrosc. 2020; 28(10):3347 3353.

24. Calder JD, Bamford R, Petrie A, McCollum GA. Stable versus unstable grade II high ankle sprains: A prospective study predicting the need for surgical stabilization and time to return to sports. Arthroscopy. 2016; 32(4):634–642.

25. Ræder BW, Figved W, Madsen JE, Frihagen F, Jacobsen SB, Andersen MR. Better outcome for suture button compared with single syndesmotic screw for syndesmosis injury: Five-year results of a randomized controlled trial. Bone Joint J. 2020; 102-B(2):212–219.

Achilles disorders

Maneesh Bhatia, Nicholas Eastley, and Kartik Hariharan

Introduction

The Achilles tendon (AT) is a morphologically complex and functionally powerful lower limb tendon measuring an average of 15 cm in length. Patients with AT pathology usually present with tendon rupture (acute or chronic) or degeneration of the tendon, termed insertional or non-insertional tendinopathy depending on the site of the pathology. The latter tendon degeneration is a common cause of disability, and can affect a wide range of patients with hugely varied functional abilities and expectations.

Anatomy

The AT is the long lever arm in the plantarflexion mechanism of the ankle linking the gastrocsoleus muscle complex with the calcaneum (Figure 13.1). Distally before attaching to the posterior calcaneal tubercle, the AT's fibres undergo a change in orientation from a linear to twisted arrangement. This causes most of its deeper fibres to insert differentially (gastrocnemius portion laterally, soleus portion medially). The remaining superficial AT fibres pass plantar to the calcaneal tuberosity merging imperceptibly with the plantar fascia (1).

The retrocalcaneal bursa lies between the AT and posterior-superior calcaneum. Its function is to reduce friction between the AT and the calcaneum during ankle range of movement. Kager's fat pad is a pyramidal structure made of adipose tissue found between Flexor Hallucis Longus (FHL) anteriorly and the AT posteriorly. During plantarflexion Kager's pad is squeezed into the retrocalcaneal bursa posterolaterally, and is thought to provide a further mechanical advantage at the AT insertion (2).

A further subcutaneous calcaneal bursa lies between the posterior AT and the overlying skin, facilitating unimpeded and smooth movement of the skin over the tendon as the tendon is very subcutaneous in this region. The AT receives its blood supply from the posterior tibial (proximally and distally) and peroneal arteries (mid-portion). A significant proportion of this vascularity is via the AT paratenon which encases the AT posteriorly, laterally and medially, reducing friction between the tendon and its adjacent structures (1).

Function

Gastrocnemius is a fusiform muscle made principally of fast twitch type II fibres. The muscle acts across three joints, primarily facilitating ankle plantarflexion (with soleus) but also assisting in knee flexion and subtalar inversion. By transmitting forces from the triceps surae, the AT is key in each of the three gait rockers. During the first rocker, eccentric gastrocnemius contraction follows heel strike ensuring a controlled progression into the stance phase. Next, controlled soleus contraction facilitates the forward transfer of body weight over the ankle (second rocker), before concentric gastrocnemius contraction and eccentric Tibialis Anterior contraction facilitates toe off during the third rocker (when AT forces may reach 12.5 times a patient's body weight).

Achilles tendinopathy

Achilles tendinopathy is a common cause of heel pain and disability and is categorised into two types based on its location – insertional Achilles tendinopathy (IAT) or non-insertional Achilles tendinopathy (NIAT).

Aetiology

The anatomy of the AT is so fashioned that different regions of the tendon are subject to different forces during mobilisation. The AT paratenon is deficient anteriorly. This exposes the tendon's deeper fibres to transverse and tangential compressive forces from impingement by the posterior part of the calcaneum in dorsiflexion, particularly in certain morphologic variations in the bony anatomy of the calcaneum. In contrast, the tendon's superficial fibres are subjected to longitudinal tensile forces created by the contracting triceps surae in active plantarflexion during the toe off phase of gait.

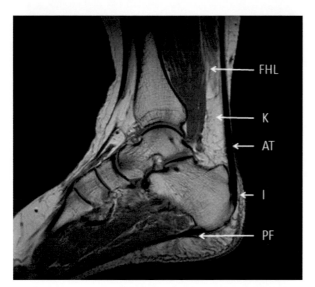

Figure 13.1 Normal Achilles tendon. A T1-weighted sagittal magnetic resonance imaging (MRI) scan showing a normal Achilles tendon and adjacent anatomy. (Abbreviations: AT, Achilles tendon; FHL, FHL muscle; I, Achilles tendon insertion; K, Kager's fat pad; PF, Plantar fascia.)

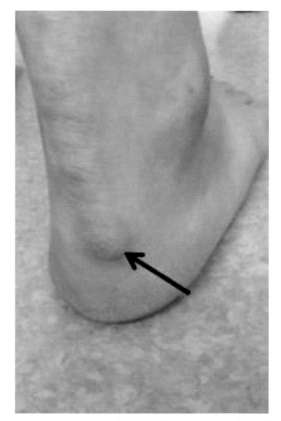

Figure 13.2 A clinical photograph of insertional Achilles tendinopathy. The characteristic swelling on the postero-lateral heel is highlighted (black arrow).

Thus a combination of these compressive and tensile forces predisposes the tendon to repetitive microtrauma and eventually degenerative change within the substance of AT and also just proximal to its insertion, giving rise to the insertional and non-insertional varieties of tendinopathy. This process has also been shown to be accelerated by mechanical overloading, altered ankle biomechanics, abnormal heel strike, preexisting malalignment of the hindfoot, enthesophytes, a posterior-superior calcaneal prominence (termed as Haglund's deformity) (3–6) and in inflammatory diseases such as rheumatoid arthritis. A Haglund's deformity may also compress the retrocalcaneal bursa in terminal ankle dorsiflexion, triggering retrocalcaneal bursitis (a pathology commonly seen alongside IAT).

To identify other risk factors for Achilles tendinopathy a systematic review was performed in 2018 (7). Nine risk factors were successfully identified including previous lower limb tendinopathy or fractures, Quinolone antibiotics, moderate alcohol use, training during cold weather, ankle plantarflexion weakness, several gait abnormalities and two factors specific to heart transplant patients.

Insertional Achilles tendinopathy

Presentation

Patients with IAT classically present with heel pain worse when first rising after rest and with weight-bearing. They commonly complain of a swelling in the region of the AT's insertion, which often cause significant problems with footwear. Clinical examination may confirm localised swelling, erythema, warmth and tenderness at the AT's calcaneal insertion (Figure 13.2). Sometimes intratendinous calcification at the tendon's insertion can also be palpated as a hard lump.

Histopathology

In IAT the AT undergoes several histopathological changes. These include replacement of type I collagen by type III collagen, disorganisation of collagen fibres, fatty tendon infiltration, increased tendon vascularity and an increase in overall tendon thickness (4).

Radiological investigations

A plain lateral radiograph is usually the first imaging modality performed (Figure 13.3). In addition, an ultrasound (US) or magnetic resonance image (MRI) scan is performed in most cases. MRI is particularly useful and can provide an important assessment of other potential causes of a patient's symptoms (such as retrocalcaneal bursitis or intraosseous pathologies) and quantifying the extent of any tendinopathy present (Figure 13.4). US performed by an experienced radiologist offers excellent

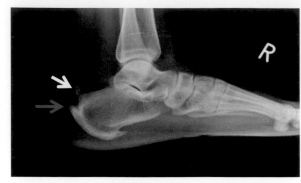

Figure 13.3 A lateral weight-bearing radiograph of insertional Achilles tendinopathy. Intratendinous Achilles tendon calcification (white arrow) and a traction spur (blue arrow) are highlighted.

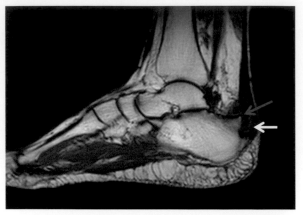

Figure 13.4 Insertional Achilles tendinopathy with Haglund's lesion and retrocalcaneal bursitis: A T1-weighted sagittal MRI of the hindfoot showing a thickened Achilles tendon insertion (white arrow) and Haglund's lesion with surrounding inflammation of the retrocalcaneal bursa (blue arrow).

visualisation of the structures around the insertion of AT, and a good means to assess tenosynovitis and vascularity – both indicators of the activity of the degenerative process. It is also especially useful for US guided therapeutic intervention.

Management

Conservative management

Conservative management is the first line treatment for IAT. This includes activity modification, shoe adjustments (to include shock-absorbing insoles and adequate space to prevent direct AT compression), ice packs, analgesia (including topical or oral non-steroidal anti-inflammatory drugs [NSAIDs]) and 1–2 cm heel lifts (to reduce tensile and compressive strain). Orthoses should also be used to correct suboptimal biomechanical alignment. These may include medial arch supports for patients with flatfeet or lateral heel wedges for those that bear weight through the lateral border of their feet. Occasionally a walking aid such as a pneumatic walking boot with heel wedges, or a dynamic hinged boot fixed in mild plantarflexion may be required to relieve pain.

Physiotherapy

Eccentric stretching of the AT (Figure 13.5) forms the mainstay of physiotherapy for IAT, with various

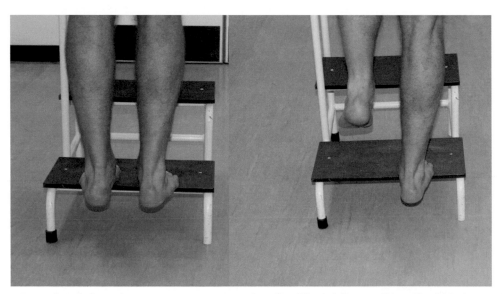

Figure 13.5 Examples of physiotherapy exercises commonly utilised for Achilles tendinopathy. (a) It shows a bilateral seated heel drop, (b) it shows single heel drop. Both exercises are repeated with knee straight and bent.

regimens shown to reduce pain and improve function (8). Although physiotherapy may take many months to work (particularly in the presence of other comorbidities), successful treatment may allow patients to avoid the need for surgery. Pain is often a barrier to compliance. This makes it important to establish an exercise regime that does not aggravate symptoms where possible, or gain control of pain by pharmacological and/or other means before embarking on treatment.

Image guided corticosteroid injection for retrocalcaneal bursitis

The use of direct AT corticosteroid injections for Achilles tendinopathy is no longer recommended. This is based on their limited long-term effect, and concerns over accelerated tendon degeneration and rupture (9). In contrast corticosteroid injections may be considered to treat retrocalcaneal bursitis (which often accompanies IAT) where they appear to result in significant improvements in pain (10). Unfortunately a small number of AT ruptures have been reported following retrocalcaneal bursal injections, which may be explained by small anatomic connections between the retrocalcaneal bursa and AT (11). Considering these connections, in order to minimise bursal damage and corticosteroid dispersal we strongly recommend that any retrocalcaneal bursal injection is performed only under US guidance.

Extracorporeal shock wave therapy (ESWT)

During ESWT pressure waves or transient pressure oscillations are passed through the skin to the AT. These waves stimulate several biological changes in the AT including the breakdown of scar tissue, a reduction in inflammation, increased production of collagen and glycosaminoglycans as well as activation of tissue healing pathways by increasing expression of growth factors (12). ESWT also directly alters pain transmission by triggering changes in the peripheral and central nervous system (13). Multiple studies have shown that ESWT reduces symptoms in IAT and NIAT, and furthermore that a combination of ESWT and eccentric Achilles stretching exercises is more effective than eccentric stretching alone (14). ESWT should be offered to all patients undergoing non-operative treatment where it is available. Patients need to be counselled as to the nature and function of ESWT to meet their expectations and to prepare them for their treatment. The duration and frequency of the regime (usually 3–4 sessions), the risk of symptoms worsening (leading to discontinued treatment in up to 20%) (15) and the small risk of tendon rupture should be highlighted.

Operative management

Surgery is considered in cases refractory to a trial of conservative treatment. Several surgical options have been described for IAT, depending on the degree of AT pathology. Preoperative MRI can help predict this, and has been shown to correlate excellently with intraoperative findings (16).

Open resection of retrocalcaneal bursa, Haglund's deformity and AT debridement

Open excision of the retrocalcaneal bursa, AT debridement plus excision of Haglund's deformity is the most commonly performed procedure for recalcitrant IAT. This is usually performed through a posterolateral approach (Figure 13.6). However, in cases with significant intratendinous calcification or large enthesophytes, a midline AT splitting approach or AT detachment from its insertion may be advantageous (Figure 13.7). Based on biomechanical studies it is generally accepted that 50% of AT can be debrided without

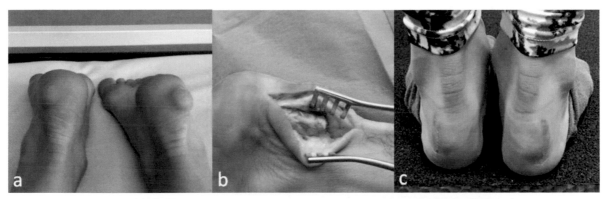

Figure 13.6 Clinical photographs of bilateral insertional Achilles tendinopathy with Haglund's deformity. (a) It shows the classical posterolateral swellings. (b) It is an intraoperative photograph showing a Haglund's deformity exposed via a posterolateral approach. (c) It shows the expected postoperative scarring.

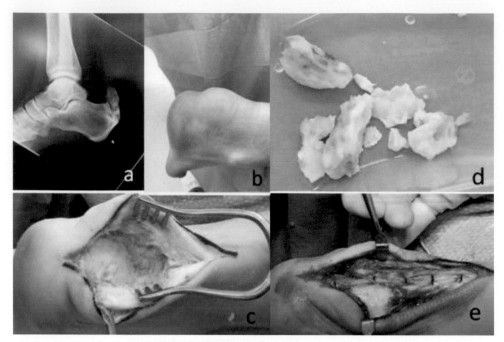

Figure 13.7 Example of insertional Achilles tendinopathy with large central enthesophytes. (a) X-ray shows large enthesophytes. (b) It shows the central swelling at insertion of Achilles. (c) It is an intraoperative photograph shows posterior midline approach. (d) It shows the excised enthesophytes. (e) It is following reattachment and repair of Achilles tendon.

seriously compromising overall insertion strength (17). In most cases, suture anchors are used to re-attach the AT. In the last few years, the use of more robust anchoring devices has strengthened the case for the surgical management of IAT, although to our knowledge no biomechanical or clinical studies have compared these modalities of fixation.

Endoscopic resection of retrocalcaneal bursa and Haglund's deformity

To reduce the risk of soft tissue break down, the retrocalcaneal bursa and Haglund's deformity can be excised endoscopically. This approach has a reduced complication rate compared to open surgery, including a reduced

incidence of postoperative altered sensation (6). Unfortunately, endoscopic surgery does not allow for the debridement and repair of a degenerate AT thereby limiting its use in the management of IAT. Therefore, endoscopic surgery is reserved for those patients who have a reasonably normal distal tendon.

Zadek's dorsal closing wedge osteotomy

This technique aims to decrease the power of the lever arm of the AT by reducing the axial length of the dorsal calcaneum. This is achieved by excising a dorsally based wedge of the calcaneal body posterior to the posterior facet of subtalar joint (Figure 13.8). This in turn

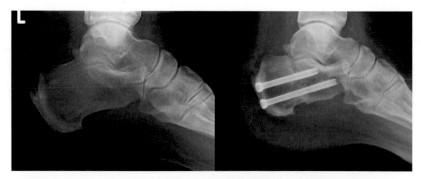

Figure 13.8 An example of IAT treated with Zadek's calcaneal osteotomy.

reduces the pull of the AT on its calcaneal insertion, which has been shown to help symptoms in recalcitrant patients. The ability to perform this procedure by minimally invasive percutaneous techniques has added to its attraction, and avoids the wound problems associated with a posterior heel incision. A similar effect can be achieved using a proximal medial gastrocnemius recession, which aims to decrease the power of the gastrocsoleus lever arm.

Non-insertional Achilles tendinopathy (mid-portion Achilles tendinopathy)

Aetiology

NIAT is more common than IAT with a reported incidence of 37/100000 (18). This is often characterised as an 'overuse condition', and typically develops after an increase in the frequency, duration or intensity of weight-bearing exercise. It should be noted that in elderly patients, a seemingly small increase in activity may be enough to trigger symptoms. Like IAT, NIAT is characterised by the cumulative microtrauma and degenerative changes within the AT. However, unlike IAT, these typically occur 2–6 cm proximal to the AT's insertion, which is a recognised vascular watershed in the tendon. In addition to the general risk factors for Achilles tendinopathy outlined earlier, several other NIAT specific factors have been identified. These include foot malalignment (which increases the strain on the AT), a pre-existing injury elsewhere in the kinetic chain (leading to AT overload), increasing age (resulting in a reduction in AT elasticity and accumulation of degenerative changes), obesity, diabetes mellitus, hypertension and steroid use (19). Another potential trigger for NIAT are local compressive forces created by a hypertrophied or overactive Plantaris tendon. This is supported by the posteromedial nature of most patients' symptoms and the association of similar forces with the development of IAT.

Presentation

Patients with NIAT typically present with pain which worsens during mobilisation and is particularly symptomatic after a period of rest, such as on waking in the morning. On examination, swelling and tenderness is found over the posteromedial AT 2–6 cm proximal to its calcaneal insertion (Figure 13.9) and often presents as a fusiform swelling of the tendon in this region. The swelling either moves or remains stationary during ankle movements. This forms the basis of the 'painful arc sign', which describes a tender swelling of the AT reciprocally moving with ankle movements, indicating tendinopathy rather than paratendinopathy. Occasionally, NIAT

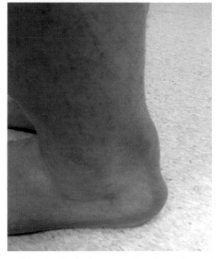

Figure 13.9 Clinical photograph of non-insertional Achilles tendinopathy. Swelling can be seen posteriorly over Achilles tendon.

presents acutely following a partial or complete rupture of the AT, on a background of chronic degenerative changes.

Role of imaging

MRI and US are the two most useful radiological modalities for NIAT, and have similar diagnostic sensitivities (18). Radiological appearances of the AT are similar to those seen in IAT, although changes are more proximal in location (Figure 13.10). The severity of imaging changes generally correlate well with patients'

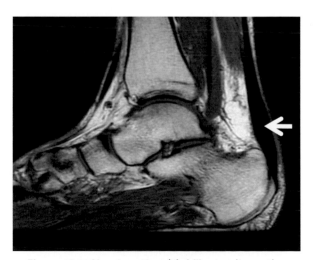

Figure 13.10 Non-insertional Achilles tendinopathy. A T1-weighted sagittal MRI of the hindfoot showing diffuse fusiform thickening of the mid-portion of the Achilles tendon (white arrow).

symptoms, although it should be noted that degenerative changes may be identified on imaging in asymptomatic patients.

Management

Non-operative management

The majority of NIAT treatment is non-operative, with surgery only reserved for refractory cases. All modifiable triggers (i.e., quinolone antibiotics) should be addressed, and any excessive training regimes adjusted (including periods of rest as required). Footwear should also be modified, and any foot and ankle malalignment addressed using orthotics such as heel raises. Analgesia (including NSAIDs) should be initiated as required.

Physiotherapy

Most patients who present with NIAT will recover following appropriate physiotherapy and exercise/activity modulation (see Figure 14). There is ongoing debate as to whether eccentric exercises provide the most effective exercise regimen and systematic reviews have failed to conclude the most superior training program. There is however evidence confirming that other than short periods of rest for pain control, protracted immobilisation worsens NIAT, thus highlighting the importance of early functional treatment. To maximise compliance patients should be warned that exercises may be painful, treatment is protracted, and that surgical intervention may be required if conservative measures fail to resolve the condition.

Extracorporeal shock wave therapy

ESWT should also be considered in NIAT prior to any surgical treatment. The current literature suggests that ESWT is more successful for the management of NIAT compared to IAT, with success rates of 78–87% reported after 6–12 months follow up. These high rates combined with the relatively low complication profile of ESWT make it an attractive option to offer patients prior to embarking on more invasive treatment modalities.

Ultrasound guided paratenon stripping

As neovascularisation occurs in NIAT, new nerve fibres thought to play a central role in pain grow from the paratenon into the AT. To target these, high volumes of saline can be injected into the AT's paratenon under US guidance (Figure 13.11). This effectively strips the nerve fibres from the AT, whilst simultaneously breaking down any adhesions present reducing friction. Paratenon stripping in this way has been shown to result in a sustained improvement in patients' pain and function (20). Clinical improvement can take up to 2 months, and patients should be made aware that symptoms may worsen following treatment.

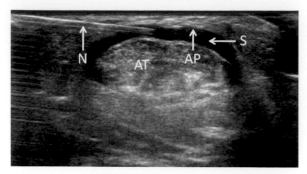

Figure 13.11 An axial ultrasound examination during high volume saline injection for non-insertional Achilles tendinopathy. (Abbreviations: AT, Achilles tendon; AP, Achilles paratenon; N, Needle; S, Injected saline.)

Platelet-rich plasma (PRP)

PRP is created by spinning a patient's whole blood using centrifugation to separate its constituents based on their specific gravities. This allows plasma with a high concentration of platelets to be isolated, which are known to release a variety of growth factors involved in injured tissue repair. The injection of autologous PRP around an AT with NIAT has attracted considerable attention in recent years. Disappointingly, the current body of evidence investigating the efficacy of this approach is inconclusive. A meta-analysis performed in 2018 tried to evaluate this work in more detail (21). A lack of conclusive benefit led the authors to conclude that the routine use of PRP injection for chronic Achilles tendinopathy cannot be recommended at present.

Operative management

Minimally invasive procedures

Various minimally invasive procedures have been described to treat NIAT including mechanical stripping of the paratenon and percutaneous longitudinal AT tenotomies. These have shown promising results and may be used as an intermediate therapy before surgical treatment is considered. A systematic review in 2016 concluded that, although the success rates of minimally invasive and open treatments are comparable, open procedures have a tendency for higher complication rates (22). Considering this, minimally invasive surgery seems most suitable for those at particular risk of wound healing problems, for example, patients with peripheral vascular disease, peripheral neuropathy or diabetes mellitus.

Open AT debridement +/− Augmentation

Despite conservative treatment, around a third of patients' symptoms will persevere necessitating open surgery. This involves open excision of diseased AT,

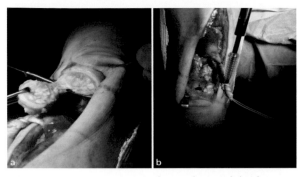

Figure 13.12 Intraoperative photos during debridement and Flexor Hallucis Longus transfer for a severe case of non-insertional Achilles tendinopathy. (a) It shows the Achilles tendon debrided fully confirming almost 100% involvement. (b) It shows calcaneal biotenodesis screw fixation of the transferred FHL tendon being performed.

combined with FHL augmentation in severe tendinopathy requiring excision of more than 50% of tendon (Figure 13.12). Although time to recovery may be prolonged, this procedure is successful in returning 80% of patients to meaningful function. During surgery, any diseased paratenon should also be removed, and the remaining healthy AT tubularised to minimise postoperative adhesions. Although the risks of complications are lower than IAT, they may still be as high as 11% (23).

Plantaris excision

To eliminate its local compressive effects on the AT several groups have advocated the surgical division of the Plantaris tendon. This can be performed during open or endoscopic surgery and has shown promising results with improved pain and function reported (24).

Gastrocnemius recession

Gastrocnemius recession has been proposed as a treatment for Achilles tendinopathy associated with gastrocnemius tightness (4). This tightness can be identified clinically using the Silfverskiöld test (Chapter 1). There are two ways of releasing the Gastrocnemius. The classical operation is the Strayer procedure where the release of Gastrocnemius is done in the mid-calf. The other surgery which has gained popularity recently is proximal medial Gastrocnemius recession. Although some evidence exists for the use of isolated gastrocnemius release for both IAT and NIAT a paucity of high quality data precludes any statements on its routine use.

Take home messages

- Most patients with Achilles tendinopathy can be managed conservatively.
- Non-surgical measures include activity and foot wear modification, physiotherapy, ESWT, US guided retrocalcaneal bursal corticosteroid injection (IAT), US guided paratenon stripping or PRP injection (NIAT).
- Surgical treatment of IAT involves excision of retrocalcaneal bursa and Haglund's deformity.
- Surgical treatment of NIAT involves stripping of paratenon and debridement of Achilles.
- If tendinopathy is severe, FHL tendon transfer to the calcaneal footprint of the AT can be performed to augment the strength of repair.

Acknowledgement

The authors would like to acknowledge Annette Jones for her input regarding the rehabilitation section.

References

1. Benjamin M, Theobald P, Suzuki D, Toumi H. The anatomy of the Achilles tendon. The Achilles tendon. 2007, pp 5–16.
2. Canoso JJ, Liu N, Traill MR, Runge VM. Physiology of the retrocalcaneal bursa. Ann Rheum Dis. 1988; 47(11):910–2.
3. Chimenti RL, Flemister AS, Tome J, McMahon JM, Houck JR. Patients with insertional Achilles tendinopathy exhibit differences in ankle biomechanics as opposed to strength and range of motion. J Orthop Sports Phys Ther. 2016; 46(12):1051–60.
4. Chimenti RL, Cychosz CC, Hall MM, Phisitkul P. Current concepts review update: Insertional Achilles tendinopathy. Foot Ankle Int. 2017; 38(10):1160–9.
5. Chimenti RL, Chimenti PC, Buckley MR, Houck JR, Flemister AS. Utility of ultrasound for imaging osteophytes in patients with insertional Achilles tendinopathy. Arch Phys Med Rehabil. 2016; 97(7):1206–9.
6. Leitze Z, Sella EJ, Aversa JM. Endoscopic decompression of the retrocalcaneal space. J Bone Jt Surg - Ser A. 2003; 85(8):1488–96.
7. Van Der Vlist AC, Breda SJ, Oei EHG, Verhaar JAN, De Vos RJ. Clinical risk factors for Achilles tendinopathy: A systematic review. Br J Sports Med. 2019; 53(21):1352–61.
8. Alfredson H, Pietilä T, Jonsson P, Lorentzon R. Heavy-load eccentric calf muscle training for the treatment of chronic Achilles tendinosis. Am J Sports Med. 1998; 26(3):360–6.
9. Coombes BK, Bisset L, Vicenzino B. Efficacy and safety of corticosteroid injections and other injections for management of tendinopathy: A systematic review of randomised controlled trials. Lancet. 2010; 376(9754):1751–67.
10. Goldberg-Stein S, Berko N, Thornhill B, Elsinger E, Walter E, Catanese D, Popowitz D. Fluoroscopically guided retrocalcaneal bursa steroid injection: Description of the technique and pilot study of short-term patient outcomes. Skeletal Radiol. 2016; 45(8):1107–12.
11. Turmo-Garuz A, Rodas G, Balius R, Til L, Miguel-Perez M, Pedret C, Del Buono A, Maffulli N. Can local corticosteroid injection in the retrocalcaneal bursa lead to rupture of the Achilles tendon and the medial head of the gastrocnemius muscle? Musculoskelet Surg. 2014; 98(2):121–6.
12. Wang CJ, Ko JY, Kuo YR, Yang YJ. Molecular changes in diabetic foot ulcers. Diabetes Res Clin Pract. 2011; 94(1):105–10.
13. Rompe JD, Furia JP, Maffulli N. Mid-portion Achilles tendinopathy – Current options for treatment. Disabil Rehabil. 2008; 30(20–22):1666–76.

14. Stania M, Juras G, Chmielewska D, Polak A, Kucio C, Król P. Extracorporeal shock wave therapy for Achilles tendinopathy. Biomed Res Int. 2019; 26:3086910.

15. Wei M, Liu Y, Li Z, Wang Z. Comparison of clinical efficacy among endoscopy-assisted radio-frequency ablation, extracorporeal shockwaves, and eccentric exercises in treatment of insertional achilles tendinosis. J Am Podiatr Med Assoc. 2017; 107(1):11–6.

16. Schepsis AA, Wagner C, Leach RE. Surgical management of Achilles tendon overuse injuries: A long-term follow-up study. Am J Sports Med. 1994; 22(5):611–9.

17. DeOrio M, Easley M. Surgical strategies: Insertional Achilles tendinopathy. Foot Ankle Int. 2008; 29(5):542–50.

18. Pearce CJ, Tan A. Non-insertional Achilles tendinopathy. EFORT Open Rev. 2016; 1(11):383–90.

19. van Sterkenburg MN, van Dijk CN. Mid-portion Achilles tendinopathy: Why painful? An evidence-based philosophy. Knee Surg Sport Traumatol Arthrosc. 2011; 20(8):1653–4.

20. Maffulli N, Spiezia F, Longo UG, Denaro V, Maffulli GD. High volume image guided injections for the management of chronic tendinopathy of the main body of the Achilles tendon. Phys Ther Sport. 2013; 14(3):163–7.

21. Liu CJ, Yu KL, Bai JB, Tian DH, Liu GL. Platelet-rich plasma injection for the treatment of chronic Achilles tendinopathy: A meta-analysis. Medicine (Baltimore). 2019; 98(16): e15278.

22. Lohrer H, David S, Nauck T. Surgical treatment for Achilles tendinopathy – A systematic review. BMC Musculoskelet Disord. 2016; 10(17):207.

23. Paavola M, Orava S, Leppilahti J, Kannus P, Järvinen M. Chronic Achilles tendon overuse injury: Complications after surgical treatment – An analysis of 432 consecutive patients. Am J Sports Med. 2000; 28(1):77–82.

24. Calder JDF, Freeman R, Pollock N. Plantaris excision in the treatment of non-insertional Achilles tendinopathy in elite athletes. Br J Sports Med. 2015; 49(23):1532–4.

14 Achilles tendon rupture

Manuel Monteagudo and Pilar Martínez de Albornoz

Introduction

The human musculoskeletal system remains poorly adapted to bipedalism. We are demanding more and more from the Achilles tendon as we are challenged by sports at an older age. Additionally, the obesity rate has increased, and more people are engaging in high-impact activities. Collagen composition and mechanical properties of the tendon change with age, making the Achilles more prone to rupture. The poor vascular supply at the narrowest portion of the tendon also predisposes it to rupture. The incidence of Achilles tendon rupture has been steadily increasing over the last two decades, more commonly in men than women.

There is no clear consensus as to the superiority of any treatment strategy for acute Achilles tendon ruptures. Early mobilisation techniques and early weight-bearing have revolutionised both surgical and non-surgical management. The decision for treatment should be individualised.

Some acute ruptures are initially neglected causing severe impairment with loss of calf power and a limping gait. Although the management of acute ruptures is controversial, there is not much debate in relation to the indications for surgery for chronic ruptures. There are many reconstructive strategies for chronic Achilles ruptures depending on different factors such as the gap size, functional demands of the patient, the quality of existing tissue, and surgeons' experience with each technique.

This chapter aims to provide the reader with a perspective on the causes and consequences of acute and chronic Achilles tendon ruptures and the various treatments available. The structure we present might serve as a guide to personalise treatment choice for each patient in view of current knowledge and the latest evidence.

Understanding Achilles ruptures

The Achilles tendon works under considerable stress in all phases of gait. This is because evolution placed the foot in a biomechanically disadvantaged position due to the leveraged forces placed upon it by ground reaction forces. The cause of rupture is multifactorial. The potential combination of different mechanisms may explain most acute ruptures. Coalescent tendinous fibres of the gastrocnemius originating from the distal femur, and of the soleus originating from the proximal tibia, form the tendon that twists around 90° internally upon descending towards its calcaneal insertion. The twisting of the tendon allows for the accumulation and release of energy when walking or running. The midsection receives a relatively poor blood supply, which might make it more vulnerable to degeneration and rupture. The blood supply decreases with increasing age and might be another factor that would facilitate rupture when exposed to minor trauma. A torsional ischaemic effect, with the transient vasoconstriction of the intratendinous vessels may cause hyperthermia that damages tenocytes. The Achilles tendon may be susceptible to the effects of this temperature increase in its relatively avascular area, where most ruptures occur.

Some drugs have been associated with Achilles tendinopathy and rupture: corticosteroids, quinolone antibiotics, aromatase inhibitors, and statins (as HMG-CoA-reductase inhibitors). These agents cause cellular and molecular changes that modify the architecture of the tendon thereby altering its mechanical properties and increasing fragility.

Some mechanical factors – overpronation on heel-strike, tight gastrocnemius, training mistakes, malfunction, or suppression of the proprioceptive component of the muscle-tendon unit – may also predispose to rupture. Malfunction of the proprioceptive component of the gastrocnemius-soleus-Achilles-calcaneal-plantar fascia system may be responsible for the higher incidence of ruptures in athletes who resume training after a period of rest (1).

The convergence of this apparently multifactorial aetiology in the "weekend warrior" is probably what accounts for most acute ruptures. The Achilles-weekend-warrior is usually a sedentary worker who participates in strenuous sports and activities on his/her

Table 14.1 Physical examination in Achilles ruptures (3)

Test	Description	Sensitivity	Specificity
Palpation	Touch gap between 3 and 8 cm above calcaneal insertion	0.73	0.89
Calf squeeze (Simmonds, Thompson)	Patient prone with both feet hanging from examination table. With intact Achilles the foot plantarflexes with calf squeeze. When ruptured the foot will show no passive (or minimal) plantarflexion. Comparison with contralateral is advised.	0.96	0.93
Knee flexion (Matles)	Patient prone is asked to flex both knees to 90°. When there is a ruptured Achilles, the foot will fall intro neutral or slight dorsiflexion.	0.88	0.85
Needle (O'Brien)	Patient prone with both feet hanging from examination table. 25-gauge needle inserted medial to the midline 10 cm proximal to the calcaneal insertion. Foot is passively dorsi/plantarflexed. Needle movement in the opposite direction of the foot indicates the tendon is intact. No movement means rupture.	-	-
Sphygmomanometer (Copeland)	Patient prone with both feet hanging the examination table. The ankle is passively plantarflex and a sphygmo cuff placed halfway up the calf and inflated to 100 mmHg. When passively dorsiflexing the ankle, no pressure rise when Achilles is ruptured. When intact, pressure rise around 40–60 mmHg.	0.78	-

(usually his) days off. These bursts of activity and the inconsistency in these efforts put the participant at risk for an acute rupture. There is an increasing incidence of acute rupture in the 49–60-year age group (2).

Diagnosis

The diagnosis of an acute Achilles rupture is clinical. Patients usually describe having heard a popping sound in the back of the leg/ankle and the feeling of having been kicked in the back of the ankle. Most patients also describe falling to the ground and turning around to check who hit them only to find there is nobody close. The different physical tests to aid in the diagnosis of a torn Achilles are listed in Table 14.1, with their sensitivity and specificity where available (3).

Up to 25% of Achilles acute ruptures may be initially missed by the first evaluating physician (4). The false negatives might be due to the presence of some active plantarflexion from the preserved action of the long toe flexors, the peroneals and the tibialis posterior tendon, but this plantarflexion is always insufficient (both in acute and chronic ruptures) to perform a single heel rise test. To reduce false negative cases, the American Academy of Orthopaedic Surgeons advised establishing the diagnosis by two or more physical examination tests (Table 14.2) (5).

Ultrasonography may be used if any diagnostic doubt exists after physical examination and may also be of aid in checking whether or not there is apposition of the tendon stumps. In turn, this may contribute to a decision as to whether or not nonoperative management

is an option. Magnetic resonance imaging (MRI) reveals the disruption of the tendon, helps to evaluate the size of the distal stump in chronic ruptures, and the presence of fatty atrophy of the gastrocsoleus complex and/or flexor hallucis longus muscle (Figure 14.1).

Treatment of acute Achilles ruptures

The goal of management of an acute Achilles rupture is the restoration of tendon length, tension, and function with as few complications as possible and the quickest possible return to work and sport. The optimal initial treatment of an acute rupture has been debated for the last four decades.

In the past, conservative treatment was compared to open surgical treatment in terms of complications and re-rupture rates. Conservative treatment included 6–8 weeks of cast immobilisation with fewer complications

Table 14.2 Recommendation of tests for the diagnosis of Achilles ruptures from the American Academy of Orthopaedic Surgeons (5)

Clinical Thompson test (i.e., Simmonds squeeze test)

Decreased ankle plantarflexion strength

Presence of a palpable gap (defect, loss of contour)

Increased passive ankle dorsiflexion with gentle manipulation

Two or more are needed to establish diagnosis of acute Achilles rupture

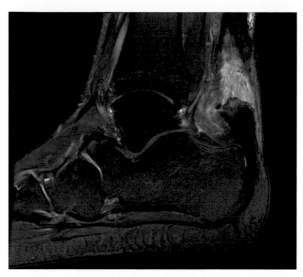

Figure 14.1 Magnetic resonance imaging in a case of chronic rupture revealing a disruption of the signal within the tendon substance.

than surgery but a higher re-rupture rate compared with operative repair (12.6% vs 3.5%) (6). Surgery evolved from open to percutaneous repair but at the cost of sural nerve complications. Later, mini-open repair allowed for a lower nerve injury rate, maintenance of a low re-rupture rate and with fewer wound complications than reported with open surgery. Conservative, percutaneous, and mini-open repairs were soon followed by functional rehabilitation. For tendon healing, early functional rehabilitation is more important than the type of surgery itself. The combination of non-surgical treatment and functional rehabilitation demonstrated similar outcomes to surgically treated patients with even greater patient satisfaction (7). In the last two decades, as a result of these findings, some surgeons modified their practice to treating acute ruptures non-surgically and, consequently, surgery has declined by up to 55% in some countries (8). A recently published randomised controlled trial with minimum follow up of 13 years has reported that surgical treatment is not superior in terms of long-term patient reported outcome when compared to nonoperative treatment (9).

Non-surgical

The rationale for non-surgical management includes the avoidance of wound and sural nerve complications that are associated with surgery. Non-surgical treatment has evolved from 4–9 weeks of cast immobilisation towards the use of early functional rehabilitation with functional bracing for early motion and protected early weight-bearing. Swansea (SMART) and Leicester (LAMP) in the UK have reported re-rupture rates of 1.1% and 2%, respectively, following nonoperative functional

treatment (27, 28). Several studies show that there is no significant difference in the clinically important parameters for patients who underwent surgical or non-surgical treatments provided the accelerated rehabilitation protocol is indicated and followed correctly (7, 9, 10). Rehabilitation is an integral part of management, regardless of the initial decision of treatment. Several studies and meta-analyses have demonstrated that the combination of initial non-surgical treatment followed by functional rehabilitation allows for improved healed tendon strength, better range of motion, and patients being more satisfied when compared with surgically treated patients (11–13). Complications were also lower in non-surgical groups.

Successful non-surgical management depends on similar principles to surgery; namely, the complete apposition of tendon stumps to restore length and appropriate tension of the Achilles. Delayed presentation may prevent the correct apposition of the stumps because of the presence of a well-organised hematoma. The ideal timing for the initiation of non-surgical treatment is controversial. Some authors defend non-surgical management if the patient is diagnosed within 48 hours from injury with minimal weight-bearing during that period (14). Others allow up to 72 hours and have reported a clinically insignificant re-rupture rate with non-surgical management with a delayed presentation at 2 weeks (10). Patient compliance is an important issue in non-surgical management. The patient must be managed with immobilisation with an equinus cast or walker boot with heel wedges, and comply with the functional rehabilitation protocols (Figure 14.2). The exclusion criteria for nonoperative treatment would be open ruptures, any physical or mental impairment that would affect patient compliance, avulsion from the calcaneum, diabetes, immunosuppressive therapies, or a tendon that had not been managed with the ankle in an equinus position (plantarflexed) in a cast within the first 48 hours from injury (14).

Functional rehabilitation following initial conservative treatment

The benefits of early motion and early protected weight-bearing have been well documented in animal models (15). Mechanical loading of a healing Achilles tendon induces the stimulation of fibroblasts which produces a stronger tendon repair. Protocols for functional rehabilitation involve immobilisation in a plaster cast with maximum passive plantarflexion and non–weight-bearing for the initial 2 weeks (14). The patient is then placed in a walking boot with around 40° heel wedges and protected weight-bearing with crutches is allowed. Functional treatment should ideally be supervised by a physiotherapist and an orthopaedic surgeon so as to improve patient compliance, which is the key to a

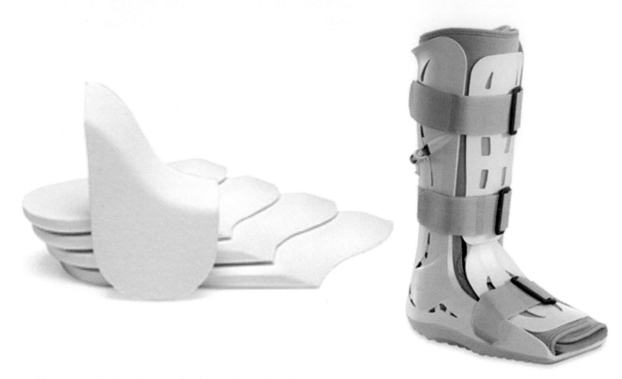

Figure 14.2 Heel wedges and orthopaedic walker boot are used in non-surgical and surgical treatment of acute Achilles tendon ruptures.

good outcome. From the 3rd to the 6th week patients are advised to progress with weight-bearing and a heel wedge is removed every week from the 3rd week. Commercially available specialist hinged boots are now available, which allow the physiotherapist/surgeon to adjust and lock the ankle at varying (reducing) angles, as required. A detailed protocol of functional rehabilitation following non-surgical and surgical treatments is outlined in Table 14.3. Patients are advised to match the height of the boot on the uninjured side to reduce stress on other joints. Appropriate thromboprophylaxis should be prescribed for the first 4 weeks to avoid deep venous thrombosis. It is very important to avoid dorsiflexion beyond 90° during the first 4 months and that the patient understands that the Achilles will still be vulnerable within those first 4 months and that any sudden loading may end up in a re-rupture. From the 10th to the 16th week post rupture, the two most important complications – elongation and re-rupture – may be more common because of the patient returning to previous daily activities out of the boot.

Surgical

Surgical management of acute ruptures has historically resulted in low re-rupture rates and low incidence of lengthening of the tendon. Wound-related complications were inherent to open surgery. The development of percutaneous techniques popularised by Ma and Griffith in 1977 decreased wound-related problems but at the expense of sural nerve injury (16). Mini-open techniques seemed to reduce the rate of both skin and sural nerve injury very close to the incidence reported for non-surgical treatment. The use of local anaesthesia and sedation allows protection of the sural nerve while suturing the tendon, and permits intraoperative tension testing, as the patient can actively plantarflex the foot when asked to do so after provisional tying of the suture. A step-by-step mini-open technique is shown in Figure 14.3.

Different studies comparing non-surgical treatment with open surgery have shown a small but statistically significant higher plantarflexion strength and a higher rate of resuming sports after surgical repair (7, 17). Earlier return to work by around 3 weeks in operated patients has been demonstrated (17). The introduction of functional rehabilitation also showed a trend towards better functional results in surgical groups, especially in jumping and hopping, but also in heel-rise work, heel-rise height, and concentric power at 6 months from surgery with respect to non-surgical groups (9).

A critical analysis of the existing randomised controlled trials does not demonstrate a statistically significant difference in re-rupture rates. However, all of them showed fewer re-ruptures after surgery and with a comparable rate of other complications. In this context,

Table 14.3 Sample functional rehabilitation plan after non-surgical and surgical treatment of an acute Achilles tendon rupture (Author's protocols)

	Non-surgical	Surgical
Week 1 Week 2 Week 3	Walker boot with four heel wedges all the time, including night sleep Crutches and put some weight through foot when you walk Do not stretch your calf muscle	Walker boot with four heel wedges all the time, including night sleep. Weight-bearing as tolerated with crutches Remove one wedge (bottom of the stack) + boot at all times, last week of heparin. Progress with weight-bearing. Remove one wedge. Progress with weight-bearing without crutches
Week 4	Remove one wedge (bottom of the stack) + boot at all times, last week of heparin. Progress with weight-bearing with the aid of crutches. Do not stretch your calf muscle	Remove one wedge. Progress with weight-bearing without crutches. Do not stretch your calf muscle
Week 5	Remove one wedge and progress with weight-bearing as tolerated with the aid of crutches. Do not stretch your calf muscle	Remove last wedge and progress with weight-bearing abandoning crutches Keep boot and orthopaedic clinic visit
Week 6	Remove one wedge and progress with weight-bearing as tolerated with the aid of crutches. Do not stretch your calf muscle. Orthopaedic clinic visit	Wean out of boot. This may take 7–10 days. Try short distances indoors and outdoors wearing sport shoes. You do not need to wear the boot at night
Week 7	Remove last wedge and progress with weight-bearing abandoning crutches. Do not stretch your calf muscle	Physiotherapy appointment. Do not start exercises until guided by your physiotherapist
Week 8	Wean out of boot. This may take 7–10 days. Try short distances indoors and outdoors wearing sport shoes. You do not need to wear the boot at night Physiotherapy appointment. Do not start exercises until guided by your physiotherapist	Add stationary bicycle, walking on treadmill as tolerated. Physiotherapy 1–2 times/wk. Orthopaedic clinic visit **Ensure patient understands that tendon is still very vulnerable and any sudden loading (step up stairs, trip) may result in rerupture**
Weeks 8–12	Progress to ROM, strength, proprioception exercises. Add stationary bicycle, walking on treadmill as tolerated. Physiotherapy 1–2 times/wk. Orthopaedic clinic visit **Ensure patient understands that tendon is still very vulnerable and any sudden loading (step up stairs, trip) may result in re-rupture**	Retrain strength, power, endurance. Work on proprioception exercises Avoid lunges, squats. **Excessive stretch on the tendon may result in elongation and permanent loss of calf power**
Weeks 12–16	Retrain strength, power, endurance. Work on proprioception exercises. Avoid lunges, squats. **Excessive stretch on the tendon may result in elongation and permanent loss of calf power**	Increase dynamic weight-bearing exercises (jogging, weight training, eccentric loading)
Months 4–6	Increase dynamic weight-bearing exercises (jogging, weight training, eccentric loading)	Return to normal sporting activities without contact or sprinting, cutting, jumping that should be resumed at around 6 months and after regaining 80–90% strength with respect to the contralateral calf
Months 6–9	Return to normal sporting activities without contact or sprinting, cutting, jumping that should be resumed at around 9 months and after regaining 80–90% strength with respect to the contralateral calf	Sport-specific training Plyometric training

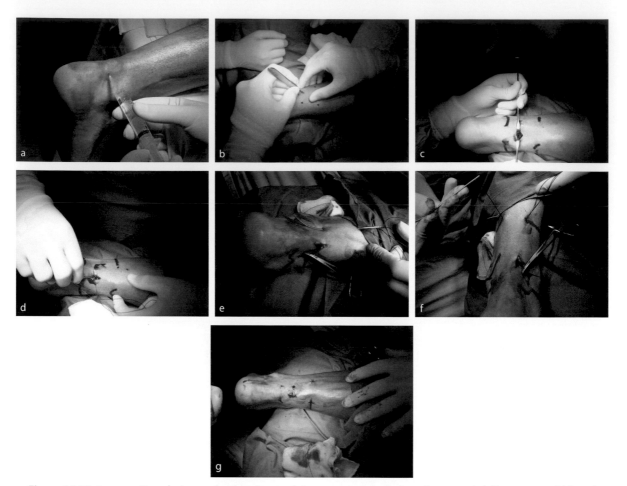

Figure 14.3 Intraoperative photographs showing a mini-open repair technique for acute Achilles rupture. (a) Local anaesthesia is very effective and safe to avoid sural nerve injury. (b) Five stab incisions are made around 6–8 cm proximal and distal to the rupture site. (c) A mini-open incision is made in the medial side of the gap. (d) The suture is inserted through the mini-open incision with the help of a long-curved needle. (e) A modified Kessler technique is used through the incisions. (f) After freeing the subcutaneous tissue underneath the incisions, sutures are tightened and tied at the mini-open incision. (g) Skin closure after checking symmetry of the suture and continuity of the tendon.

some surgeons still believe that surgical restoration of tendon length will allow their patients to improve functional outcome (18).

Percutaneous, mini-open, and open repair strength has been tested in cadavers showing open surgery is almost twice as resistant when testing ankle dorsiflexion and pull-out strength as compared to percutaneous conventional Kessler repair (19). Absorbable sutures that hold the tendon properly, and allow healing for a period of around 3 months after the repair, are preferable to nonabsorbable sutures, which increase the risk of delayed granuloma formation and infection. The use of new devices with more sutures running parallel and creating a box-type configuration also demonstrated more resistance to elongation and re-rupture in cadaver studies. However, these results may not be

clinically relevant during the early postoperative period with protected weight-bearing and wedges preventing stress in the repaired tendon. These new devices for acute Achilles repair have been developed over the last few years to protect the sural nerve and to keep the re-ruptures rate low. Most of these instruments yield similarly functional good results (19). A summary of the devices available is shown in Table 14.4.

Functional rehabilitation following initial surgical treatment

In active young patients and recreational or professional athletes, the bias continues to be towards surgical management. Functional rehabilitation after surgical repair has shortened return to work and sports. In athletes,

Table 14.4 Devices for mini-open repair of acute Achilles tendon ruptures

Device	Company	Description	First publication
Tenolig	FH Orthopaedics, Chicago, Illinois, U.S.A.	Single-use sutures with preloaded needles into which small harpoons are embedded. Sutures are tightened to approximate tendon stumps and are locked with polyethylene discs against the skin	1992
Achillon	Integra Lifesciences, Plainsboro, New Jersey, U.S.A.	Single-use device that assists in the passage of sutures through the tendon creating three box configurations and protecting sural nerve by placing the tendon in a different plane from the nerve	2002
Dresden	Intercus, Bad Blankenburg, Germany	Reusable custom-made suture retrievers with palpable holes through the skin for the insertion of sutures at distal tendon stump and pulled from the proximal wound to create a Kessler repair	2006
PARS (Percutaneous Achilles Repair System)	Arthrex, Naples, Florida, U.S.A.	Reusable anatomically designed jig that provides capture of proximal and distal stumps of the ruptured tendon and allows for locked suture fixation	2010

surgery has been traditionally favoured because, as the recovery time is long, a re-rupture and/or elongation would be devastating and likely lead to the end of the sporting career. Functional rehabilitation after operative repair is not too different from that after nonoperative management, except for a quicker progression from week 12 that allows for dynamic weight-bearing exercise (water-running/aqua-jogging) at around 14 weeks and returning to normal sporting activities including sprinting, cutting, jumping, etc., at around 6 months from surgery. A protocol of functional rehabilitation after surgical repair is shown in Table 14.3.

Treatment of chronic Achilles ruptures

Improved education has reduced the rate of chronic ruptures because most are diagnosed and managed acutely. Patients with a chronic rupture present with weakness of push-off but are rarely in pain. There is consensus on chronic ruptures needing surgical treatment.

Non-surgical

Nonoperative management is only indicated in low-demand patients or in those who cannot tolerate surgery. In those cases, a carbon composite ankle-foot orthosis may allow for keeping the foot up during swing phase, a soft heel strike, and stability in stance and a better toe-off.

Surgical

Although several reconstructive strategies exist for chronic ruptures, most reported outcomes are limited to case reports and case series, so there is no clear gold standard technique for all chronic cases. Although the Myerson classification, which considers the size of the defect, is useful when determining the type of surgery, other factors such as patient age, activity level, comorbidities, the quality of soft the tissue envelope, and surgeon's comfort with each technique, should all be considered (20). Surgery is challenging because it requires a large incision in an anatomic region with a high rate of skin/wound complications. Most techniques have been studied with homogeneous good results with almost no re-rupture and most patients returning to pre-injury levels of activity. Regardless of the technique and type of repair planned, a preoperative MRI of the whole calf, so as to rule out denervation (and fatty atrophy) of the gastrocsoleus complex or the flexor hallucis longus (FHL) muscle, is mandatory. If MRI of the whole calf shows extensive muscle atrophy, turndown flap or V-Y advancement will not restore enough function and the use of an alternative tendon transfer such as FHL will be needed.

After tourniquet application to the thigh, the patient is usually operated on in the prone position and the ruptured tendon is approached through a medial incision parallel to the medial border of the Achilles tendon. The sural nerve and saphenous vein should be identified and protected during the initial steps of the procedure. In all techniques, non-elastic thickened tissue should be excised and the adhesions between the tendon and sheath released so that the whole complex slides distally to allow for the tendon stumps to approximate and be in contact, with the foot in approximately 30–40° of plantarflexion.

- ***Primary end-to-end repair*** without augmentation may be considered if there is less than 2–3 cm of retraction after debridement of scar tissue. This usually corresponds to cases that present less than 3–4 months following rupture. A modified Krackow suture technique, with a heavy absorbable suture, may be used for the tendon, and the paratenon is repaired as a separate layer (Figure 14.4).

- *Turndown flap* technique is used for the reconstruction of moderate-sized defects and as reinforcement of primary repairs with small defects after suture. Since the introduction of the technique by Christensen in 1956, several variations have been developed involving a distally based flap or two adjacent flaps to span or reinforce the gap in the Achilles (21). The end-to-end repair is reinforced with a 10–12-cm-long and 2–3-cm-wide strip of gastrocsoleus fascia that is twisted 180° on its distal pedicle so that its smooth surface underlies the tendon sheath and the subcutaneous tissues (Figure 14.5).

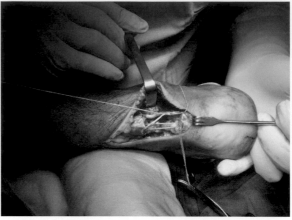

Figure 14.4 Intraoperative photograph showing an end-to-end repair in a neglected rupture 3 months after injury.

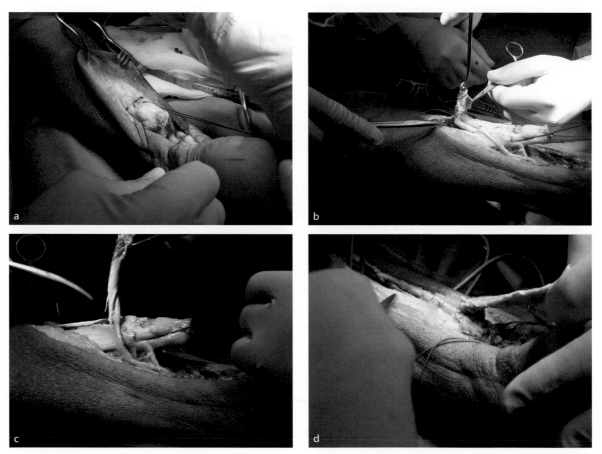

Figure 14.5 Intraoperative photographs showing a turndown flap repair technique for a chronic Achilles rupture. (a) Fibrotic non-healthy scar tissue has been removed and the proximal stump is secured with a modified Krackow technique. (b) A distally based flap with a 2-cm cuff left attached, measuring around 4 cm in width and around 12 cm in length is made. (c) The flap is then mobilised and turned down through the remaining tendon. The gastrocnemius has been released to allow for the maximum distal excursion of the proximal stump. (d) The turndown flap is able to cover the sutured tendon and is then sutured to augment the repair.

- ***V-Y tendon advancement*** was first described in 1975 by Abraham and Pankovich to salvage neglected ruptures of the Achilles with moderate-big-sized defects (5–10 cm after debridement of scar tissue) (22). An inverted V incision is made within the myotendinous portion of the gastrocsoleus with the apex of the V sited midline, as proximal as possible over the gastrocnemius fascia. With forced plantarflexion of the foot, the gap is measured and the size of the gap is transferred to the lateral and medial borders of the proximal stump to draw the limbs of the V so that they converge proximally. The limbs should be at least twice the length of the measured true gap. The V is then carefully incised through the fascia only, leaving the underlying muscle intact. A heavy absorbable suture is then placed into the ends of the ruptured tendon using a locking Krakow technique and longitudinal traction applied to the proximal tendon stump, while gently dissecting the muscle fibres longitudinally, to allow the myotendinous junction to slide distally. This manoeuvre should be done with great care so as not to detach the tendon from the underlying muscle, which could cause devascularisation of the tendon. The V-shaped incision is then repaired creating an inverted Y (Figure 14.6).

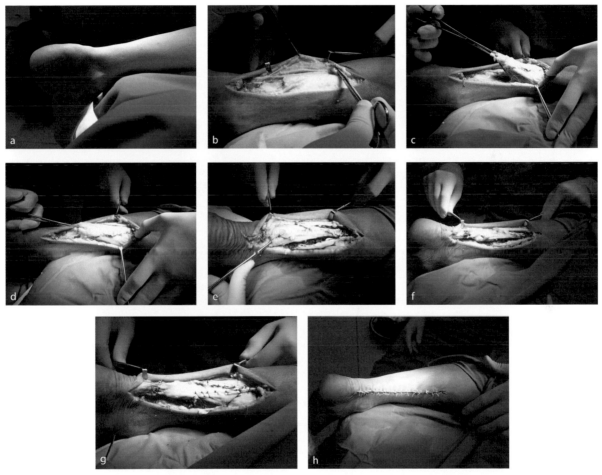

Figure 14.6 Intraoperative photographs showing a V-Y tendon advancement technique for a chronic Achilles rupture. (a) Neglected Achilles ruptures 8 months after injury. Note the gap and calf atrophy. (b) After debridement of all scar tissue at the rupture site, the sural nerve is identified and protected. (c) Gastrocsoleous complex is released. (d) An inverted V incision is made with the apex of the V placed midline as proximal as possible over the gastrocnemius fascia. With forced plantarflexion of the foot the gap is measured, and the size of the gap transferred to the borders of the proximal stump to draw the limbs of the V. (e) The V is then carefully incised through the fascia only, leaving the underlying muscle intact. The dissection of the muscle fibres longitudinally should be done with great care not to detach the tendon from the underlying muscle. (f) Tendon stumps are sutured with the foot in maximum plantarflexion. (g) The V-shaped incision is then repaired creating an inverted Y. (h) Final clinical picture following wound closure.

- *Flexor hallucis longus transfer* was first described by Mann and Collins in 1991 to manage large defects in a chronic rupture (23). FHL transfer may be used alone or in combination with V-Y advancement or turndown. FHL is biomechanically a strong tendon and the phase of action is in line of pull with the Achilles. Besides, its rich vascularity allows for a more elastic repair after being transferred. It was traditionally harvested in the master knot of Henry using two separate incisions to obtain a longer length of tendon for a tunnelled tenodesis through the calcaneus. With the development of interference screws, there is no need for a long tendon end and harvesting may be done either using a single incision, minimal invasive technique or endoscopically under the sustentaculum tali via posterior ankle arthroscopy. There is apparently no significant difference in terms of strength, peak stress, and failure between bone tunnel fixation and interference screw fixation of the FHL (20). There is a higher risk of infection and wound complications associated with the open FHL transfer compared to the endoscopic approach (21).
- *Other techniques* may also allow for the repair of chronic ruptures. Peroneus brevis transfer, autograft reconstruction using quadriceps, hamstring tendon allograft (when FHL or peroneus brevis cannot be transferred), and synthetic graft techniques have also been described for chronic ruptures when large defects are present.

Functional rehabilitation in chronic ruptures

The large incision may compromise early movement and weight-bearing. As soon as the wound is healed, functional rehabilitation in chronic ruptures follows almost the same steps as the protocol presented in Table 14.3 for nonoperative management of acute ruptures.

Complications and management

Complications after non-surgical management of an acute or chronic Achilles rupture include deep venous thrombosis, re-rupture, and tendon elongation/calf muscle weakness. In addition open surgery may (rarely) cause hypertrophic painful scars, infection, sural nerve injury, and wound breakdown. The more common complications cited in the literature are re-rupture, deep venous thrombosis, and deep infection. In a recent meta-analysis that included twenty-nine randomised controlled trials with 2060 patients with an acute rupture of the Achilles, the mean incidence of overall major complications from all managements was 9.13% (24). The mean incidence rates from all managements of re-rupture, deep venous thrombosis, and deep infection

were 5%, 2.67%, and 1.50%, respectively. Sural nerve injury is not among the most common complications as around half of cases were managed without surgery and minimal invasive surgery has lowered the incidence of sural nerve problems. In terms of relative risk, nonoperative treatment combined with early immobilisation was associated with a higher risk of major complications. According to the area under the cumulative ranking curve, minimally invasive surgery with accelerated rehabilitation had the highest possibility (79.7%) of being the best management with regard to minimising major complications (24).

Deep infection is usually followed by wound dehiscence and should be addressed with intravenous antibiotics and aggressive early treatment with debridement and a negative-pressure wound device. It is important to consult plastic surgery early in this process as most cases end up needing a flap for coverage of the defect (Figure 14.7).

Tendon elongation is more common with non-surgical management if the protocol is not administered

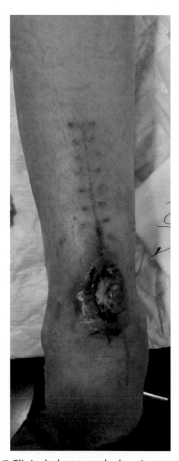

Figure 14.7 Clinical photograph showing wound breakdown and infection 4 weeks after open repair of an acute Achilles tendon rupture.

properly or in patients who are noncompliant. It is more likely to occur during the 10th to the 16th weeks as patients start walking and gain confidence. Achilles tendon shortening surgery may be indicated in severe cases although it is not easy to define the amount of non-elastic tissue requiring resection so as to achieve adequate tension of the remaining tendon.

Outcome

Most low-demand patients resume work and amateur sports uneventfully. The effect of an acute Achilles rupture on professional athletes in various sports has been studied (25). In the National Football League (NFL) around 70% of players were able to return to sport but it took around 1 year to return to pre-injury performance level and those that returned had shorter postoperative careers than matched controls. In the National Basketball Association (NBA), only 61% of players were able to return to competition after rupture and those that did return showed a significant decrease in performance and playing time. Performance normalised by 2 years after injury. So, an acute Achilles rupture is a change-of-career (and potentially end-of-career) injury for a professional athlete.

Take home messages

- Achilles tendon rupture incidence has increased significantly in the last few decades, mainly in sports with repetitive jumping and sprinting.
- The diagnosis is clinical, and single-leg heel rise is impossible with a ruptured tendon.
- Nonoperative management with functional early movement and protected weight-bearing is a suitable treatment for most patients, but requires physician/physiotherapist supervision and patient compliance and diligence for a good outcome.
- Minimally invasive techniques have lowered historical complication rates of open surgery to negligible.
- Chronic rupture requires surgery and the type of repair depends on many factors, including the size of the gap and the surgeon's comfort with the technique. Surgery for chronic ruptures is associated with higher wound complications. The rehabilitation guideline is similar to that of an acute rupture.

References

1. Myer GD, Faigenbaum AD, Cherny CE, Heidt RS Jr, Hewett TE. Did the NFL lockout expose the Achilles heel of competitive sports? J Orthop Sports Phys Ther. 2011; 41(10):702–5.
2. Huttunen TT, Kannus P, Rolf C, Felländer-Tsai L, Mattila VM. Acute Achilles tendon ruptures: Incidence of injury and surgery in Sweden between 2001 and 2012. Am J Sports Med. 2014; 42(10):2419–23.
3. Maffulli N. The clinical diagnosis of subcutaneous tear of the Achilles tendon: A prospective study in 174 patients. Am J Sports Med. 1998; 26(2):266–70.
4. Nillius SA, Nilsson BE, Westlin NE. The incidence of Achilles tendon rupture. Acta Orthop Scand. 1976; 47(1):118–21.
5. Chiodo CP, Glazebrook M, Bluman EM, et al. Diagnosis and treatment of acute Achilles tendon rupture. J Am Acad Orthop Surg. 2010; 18(8):503–10.
6. Khan RJ, Fick D, Keogh A, Crawford J, Brammar T, Parker M. Treatment of acute Achilles tendon ruptures. A meta-analysis of randomized, controlled trials. J Bone Joint Surg Am. 2005; 87(10):2202–10.
7. Willits K, Amendola A, Bryant D, Mohtadi NG, Giffin JR, Fowler P, Jear CO, Kirkly A. Operative versus nonoperative treatment of acute Achilles tendon ruptures: A multicenter randomized trial using accelerated functional rehabilitation. J Bone Joint Surg Am. 2010; 92(17):2767–75.
8. Mattila VM, Huttunen TT, Haapasalo H, Sillanpää P, Malmivaara A, Pihlajamäki H. Declining incidence of surgery for Achilles tendon rupture follows publication of major RCTs: Evidence-influenced change evident using the Finnish registry study. Br J Sports Med. 2015; 49(16):1084–6.
9. Nilsson-Helander K, Silbernagel KG, Thomeé R, Faxén E, Olsson N, Eriksson BI, Karlsson J. Acute Achilles tendon rupture: A randomized, controlled study comparing surgical and nonsurgical treatments using validated outcome measures. Am J Sports Med. 2010; 38(11):2186–93.
10. Wallace RG, Heyes GJ, Michael AL. The non-operative functional management of patients with a rupture of the tendo Achillis leads to low rates of re-rupture. J Bone Joint Surg Br. 2011; 93(10):1362–6.
11. Aufwerber S, Heijne A, Edman G, Silbernagel KG, Ackermann PW. Does early functional mobilization affect long-term outcomes after an Achilles tendon rupture? A randomized clinical trial. Orthop J Sports Med. 2020; 8(3):2325967120906522.
12. Manent A, López L, Coromina H, Santamaría A, Domínguez A, Llorens N, Sales M, Videla S. Acute Achilles tendon ruptures: Efficacy of conservative and surgical (percutaneous, open) treatment – A randomized, controlled, clinical trial. J Foot Ankle Surg. 2019; 58(6):1229–34.
13. Young SW, Patel A, Zhu M, van Dijck S, McNair P, Bevan WP, Tomlinson M. Weight-Bearing in the nonoperative treatment of acute Achilles tendon ruptures: A randomized controlled trial. J Bone Joint Surg Am. 2014; 96(13):1073–9.
14. Glazebrook M, Rubinger D. Functional rehabilitation for non-surgical treatment of acute Achilles tendon rupture. Foot Ankle Clin. 2019; 24(3):387–98.
15. Hammerman M, Aspenberg P, Eliasson P. Microtrauma stimulates rat Achilles tendon healing via an early gene expression pattern similar to mechanical loading. J Appl Physiol (1985). 2014; 116(1):54–60.
16. Ma GW, Griffith TG. Percutaneous repair of acute closed ruptured Achilles tendon: A new technique. Clin Orthop Relat Res. 1977; 128:247–55.
17. Cetti R, Christensen SE, Ejsted R, Jensen NM, Jorgensen U. Operative versus nonoperative treatment of Achilles tendon rupture. A prospective randomized study and review of the literature. Am J Sports Med. 1993; 21(6):791–9.
18. Kadakia AR, Dekker RGII, Ho BS. Acute Achilles tendon ruptures: An update on treatment. J Am Acad Orthop Surg. 2017; 25(1):23–31.

19. Patel MS, Kadakia AR. Minimally invasive treatments of acute Achilles tendon ruptures. Foot Ankle Clin. 2019; 24(3):399–424.

20. Chen C, Hunt KJ. Open reconstructive strategies for chronic Achilles tendon ruptures. Foot Ankle Clin. 2019; 24(3):425–37.

21. Christensen I. Rupture of the Achilles tendon; analysis of 57 cases. Acta Chir Scand. 1953; 106(1):50–60.

22. Abraham E, Pankovich AM. Neglected rupture of the Achilles tendon. Treatment by V-Y tendinous flap. J Bone Joint Surg Am. 1975; 57(2):253–5.

23. Mann RA, Holmes GB Jr, Seale KS, Collins DN. Chronic rupture of the Achilles tendon: A new technique of repair. J Bone Joint Surg Am. 1991; 73(2):214–9.

24. Wu Y, Mu Y, Yin L, Wang Z, Liu W, Wan H. Complications in the management of acute Achilles tendon rupture: A systematic review and network meta-analysis of 2060 patients. Am J Sports Med. 2019; 47(9):2251–60.

25. Caldwell JE, Vosseller JT. Maximizing return to sports after Achilles tendon rupture in athletes. Foot Ankle Clin. 2019; 24(3):439–45.

26. Maempel JF, Clement ND, Wickramasinghe NR, Duckworth AD, Keating JF. Operative repair of acute Achilles tendon rupture does not give superior patient-reported outcomes to nonoperative management. Bone Joint J. 2020; 102-B(7):933–40. doi:10.1302/0301-620X.102B7.BJJ-2019-0783.R3

27. Hutchison AM, Topliss C, Beard D, Evans RM, Williams P. The treatment of a rupture of the Achilles tendon using a dedicated management programme. Bone Joint J. 2015; 97-B(4):510–5. doi:10.1302/0301-620X.97B4.35314

28. Aujla RS, Patel S, Jones A, Bhatia M. Non-operative functional treatment for acute Achilles tendon ruptures: The Leicester Achilles Management Protocol (LAMP). Injury. 2019; 50(4):995–9. doi:10.1016/j.injury.2019.03.007

15 Ankle fractures

Oliver Chan and Anthony Sakellariou

Introduction

Ankle fractures are common. In the United Kingdom, ankle fractures accounted for over 17,000 admissions in 2016-2017 (1). The management of these injuries has evolved over the past decade as our appreciation of ankle biomechanics has improved. As such, it has become apparent that the key factors in achieving a good outcome after such injuries are to follow the principle of restoring stability and alignment of the fractured ankle regardless of whether such injuries are treated non-operative or surgically (2). Malunion of unstable ankle fractures is associated with altered biomechanics such as increased contact stresses (3).

Applied anatomy/classification

The ankle joint consists of three bones (tibia, fibula and talus) and three ligament complexes (Figure 15.1):

1. The lateral ligament complex is the collective name for the three ligaments connecting the fibula to the hindfoot – the anterior (ATFL) and posterior (PTFL) talofibular ligaments and the calcaneofibular ligament (CFL).
2. The syndesmosis itself is a strong three-ligament structure. Formed by the anterior inferior tibiofibular ligament (AITFL), interosseous ligament and the posterior inferior tibiofibular ligament (PITFL). The syndesmosis provides strength to the distal tibiofibular joint by preventing diastasis whilst also allowing micro-motion in gait. During ankle motion, the fibula is allowed to translate in the anterior/posterior plane and rotate at the same time. This movement is guided by the syndesmotic ligaments when they are intact, in the right position and at the right length and tension (4).
3. The deltoid ligament consists of superficial and deep components, the second of which can be further subdivided into anterior and posterior talo-tibial ligaments (ATTL and PTTL). The significance of the PTTL is that of a key stabiliser of the ankle whilst bearing weight. This ligament is tightest when the foot is in the plantigrade position.

Models of the ankle relating to stability

The 'ring' model

The ankle joint can be thought of as a "ring" structure (three bones connected to three ligament complexes) (Figure 15.2), which holds the talus securely in anatomical alignment beneath the tibial plafond when bearing weight. If this "ring" is broken at one site only, it will remain stable. Two or more disruptions to the ring structure, whether bony or ligamentous, can result in instability and movement of these bones relative to one another.

The column model

It is possible to divide the ankle into two columns: lateral and medial. The lateral column consists of the fibula, the syndesmosis and lateral ligament complex. It had previously been thought that lateral column integrity was key to ankle fracture stability. However, over the last 20 years, it has been recognised that it is the medial column (medial malleolus and deltoid ligament) that is more significant (5), and that stability of a lateral malleolus fracture is important only if medial stability is compromised.

Classification systems

The two most commonly known systems in clinical practice are the Danis-Weber and Lauge-Hansen classifications.

Danis-Weber classification

Based upon the theory that the lateral column was the most important in assessing ankle stability, the Danis-Weber classification was devised to describe ankle fractures in relation to the distal fibula.

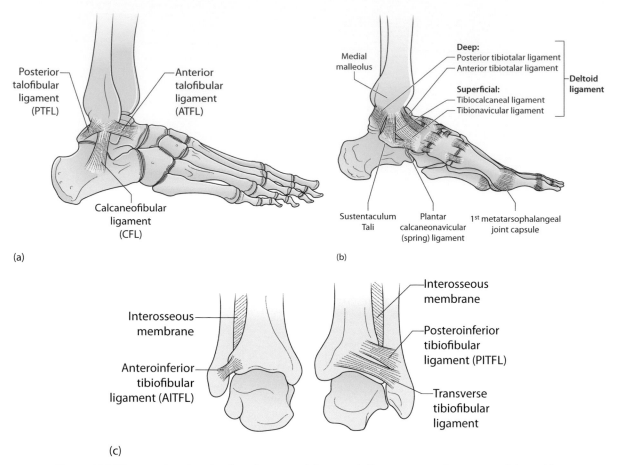

(a)

(b)

(c)

Figure 15.1 Diagram showing the three bones and three main ligament complexes around the ankle.

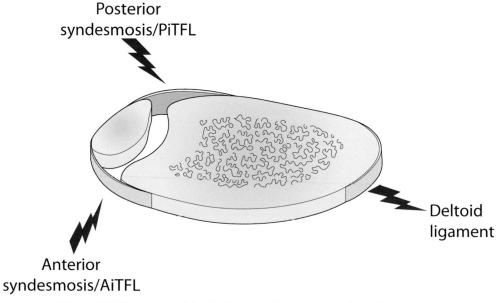

Figure 15.2 The ring model with the three ligament complexes highlighted.

Table 15.1 Different stages of the Lauge-Hansen classification system

Level of fibula fracture	Lauge-Hansen stages
Infra-syndesmotic	**Supination adduction (SAD)**
	1. Transverse fracture of the lateral malleolus 2. Vertical fracture of the medial malleolus
Trans-syndesmotic	**Supination external rotation (SER)**
	1. Injury to AITFL 2. Short oblique fracture of the lateral malleolus 3. Injury to PITFL or posterior malleolus fracture 4. Deltoid ligament injury or medial malleolus fracture
Supra-syndesmotic	**Pronation external rotation (PER)**
	1. Deltoid ligament injury or medial malleolus fracture 2. Injury to AITFL 3. Spiral fracture of the fibula (or Maisonneuve) 4. Injury to PITFL or posterior malleolus fracture
	Pronation abduction (PAB)
	1. Deltoid ligament injury or medial malleolus fracture 2. Injury to AITFL 3. Transverse or comminuted fracture of the fibula

Type A – a transverse fracture of the distal fibula beneath the tibiofibular syndesmosis.

Type B – an oblique sagittal plane fracture of the distal fibula at the level of the tibiofibular syndesmosis.

Type C – a fracture of the fibula above the level of the tibiofibular syndesmosis. This is often indicative of a more severe injury due to the forces extending through the syndesmotic ligaments. The fracture pattern of the fibula is often comminuted.

This simple descriptive classification is widely used in medical practice and well understood. The main weakness of this system is that it does not describe injuries to the tibial (medial and posterior malleoli) or ligamentous components, and therefore does not lend any weight to the assessment of stability.

Lauge-Hansen classification

This classification system is based upon the mechanism of injury of which there are four basic types: supination external rotation (SER), supination adduction (SA), pronation external rotation (PER) and pronation abduction (PA) (Table 15.1 and Figures 15.3 and 15.4). The first word in the classification system describes the position of the foot at the time of injury and the second the direction of force applied across the talus at this time (6).

The classification system is then subdivided into a number of 'stages' which represent the bony/ligamentous structures injured, and which fail in a predictable sequence, beginning at the malleolus or ligament most under tension at the time of injury. This is best illustrated by comparing an isolated fibula fracture at the

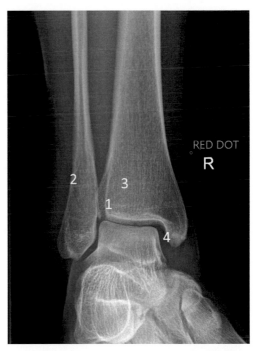

Figure 15.3 Radiograph demonstrating the progression of the supination external rotation (SER) ankle injury. An injury to the anterior syndesmosis occurs first (1). The external rotation force causes injury to progress in a clockwise fashion. A fibula fracture occurs next (2), followed by a posterior malleolus/posterior syndesmosis injury (3). Lastly, the deltoid ligament/medial malleolus is injured (4).

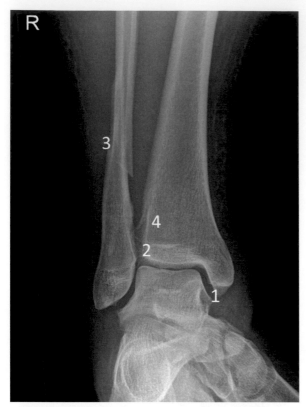

Figure 15.4 Radiograph demonstrating the progression of the pronation external rotation (PER) ankle injury. The deltoid ligament/medial malleolus (1) is first to be injured. The anterior syndesmosis (2) is then injured followed by high fibula fracture (3). If the external rotation force progresses, the posterior syndesmosis or posterior malleolus (4) is injured last.

of the distal fibula (SER-2), posterior syndesmotic ligament tear (PITFL) or posterior malleolus fracture (SER-3) and, finally, a medial malleolus fracture or deltoid ligament rupture (SER-4).

The Lauge-Hansen classification system allows a better understanding of the mechanism of injury and can be used to predict hidden injuries which may not be easily appreciable on initial non–weight-bearing radiographs of the ankle. More importantly, this system can aid management as stability can be inferred based on the classification grading. More recently the SER Type 4 injury (Lauge-Hansen classification) has been modified to 4a (PTTL portion of the deltoid ligament intact, thereby conferring stability whilst bearing weight, despite talar shift on NWB radiographs) and 4b (PTTL portion ruptured, no stability, with talar shift on both NWB and WB radiographs) (7).

CT-based classification systems

Fractures involving the posterior malleolus have been classified by two systems based on CT scan findings. Haraguchi et al (8) described three types of posterior malleolus fracture based on the axial reconstructions of the CT scan (Figure 15.5). With a Type 1, there is a single posterolateral fragment. A Type 2 includes extension of the fracture to the posteromedial side of the distal tibia and Type 3 fractures represent a thin shell of bone. This system is useful as Type 3 fractures may be too small to fix and the presence of a Type 2 fracture may dictate a posteromedial approach.

Bartoníček et al (9) classified posterior malleolus fractures based on more advanced CT scan reconstructions. The system (Type 1: Extraincisural, Type 2: Posterolateral, Type 3: Posteromedial, Type 4: Large posterolateral, Type 5: Irregular osteoporotic) places emphasis on recognising fractures that extend into the incisura, a fact that dictates the need for fixation and which may also influence choice of incision and approach. In 2017, Bartoníček et al. (10) and Mason et al (11), independently, refined this classification.

level of the syndesmosis (Danis-Weber Type-B), which corresponds to an SER-2 type injury, with a bi-malleolar SER-4 type ankle fracture. These two injuries share the same SER mechanism of injury, which starts with injury to the AITFL (SER-1), progression to an oblique fracture

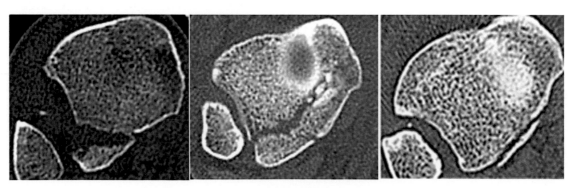

Figure 15.5 CT scan axial views of the ankle demonstrating different posterior malleolus fracture configurations as described by the Haraguchi classification system. Left: Type 1, Middle: Type 2, Right: Type 3.

Overall stability

Regardless of which classification system is used to categorise ankle fractures, it is most important that the surgeon identifies all bony and ligamentous components of the injury and understands the implications of these in relation to the stability of the ankle joint. The current view is that bi- and tri-malleolar ankle fractures are most likely unstable, as the ankle 'ring' has broken in at least two places. Unstable injuries are most commonly those resulting from PER and SER.

Diagnosis

Clinical assessment

The presentation of patients with ankle fractures is usually associated with a history of trauma followed by an inability to bear weight. Where possible, a history of the injury circumstances and mechanism are essential alongside an understanding of patients' past medical and social history. Co-morbidities such as diabetes mellitus as well as smoking status should be documented as they are prognostic factors for healing of bone and soft tissues and may affect the choice of management (12, 13).

Examination of the affected limb should be performed, looking for gross deformity, skin integrity and for assessment of the soft tissues. Neurological status and vascular perfusion should be assessed. Tenderness over the proximal fibula should be tested for because, when present, it may indicate a Maisonneuve injury type – a Weber C/PER variant with probable disruption of the whole length of the interosseous membrane. Clinical signs over the deltoid ligament (tenderness, swelling and bruising) are not, as previously thought, reliable predictors of instability. These signs can be present as a result of injury to the superficial deltoid ligament with the underlying deep deltoid structures remaining intact and conferring stability to the talus (5).

Investigations

Anteroposterior and lateral (non–weight-bearing) ankle radiographs are the initial imaging modalities obtained with most ease in an emergency department. It should be emphasised at this point that these images are rarely sufficient in isolation to comprehensively assess all the different components of ankle injuries. Mortise views can be useful if there is doubt on the initial views and additional views of the proximal fibula (whole length tibia/fibula views or knee radiographs) should be sought if a Maisonneuve injury is suspected.

Assessment of ankle fracture stability

The role of dynamic stress radiographs in ankle fractures is primarily indicated in isolated trans-syndesmotic lateral malleolus fractures (Weber B, SER-2) to assess competence of the deep deltoid ligament and to differentiate between SER-2 and SER-4 injuries, and therefore the type of management. This is performed with a mortise view of the ankle joint taken with the patient partially bearing weight (at least 50% body weight) through a plantigrade (heel must be planted on the ground) foot (14). This projection can often be difficult to achieve in acute ankle fractures as patients are reluctant to tolerate any weight through the ankle. Therefore, in an emergency setting where there is suspicion of deltoid injury (tenderness, ecchymosis, etc.), patients should be treated initially in a plaster of Paris back slab – non–weight-bearing, and reviewed with subsequent weight-bearing views (back-slab off) 5–10 days post injury (5, 15). There is significant injury to the deep deltoid ligament when there is widening of the medial clear space (MCS) >4 mm (3) as seen on the weight-bearing view (Figure 15.6).

Other stress tests have been described. These include the manual stress test radiograph which involves gentle abduction of the ankle to assess for opening on the medial side and gravity stress radiographs where the patient lies with the injured side down and with the foot

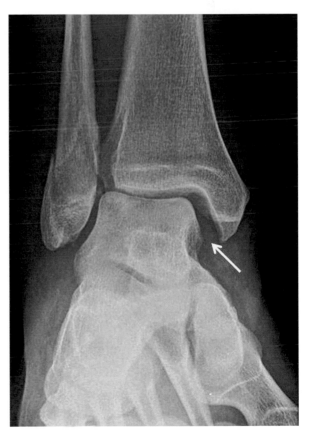

Figure 15.6 Weight-bearing AP radiograph demonstrating talar shift with a medial clear space >4 mm (represented by the white arrow).

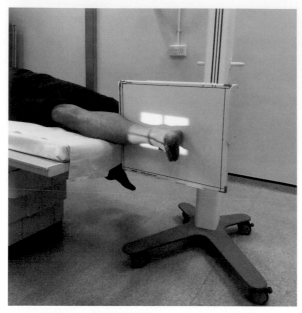

Figure 15.7 The position of the patient's limb during acquisition of gravity-stress radiographs. The lateral aspect of the ankle faces the floor so that gravity affects an external rotation force to the ankle thereby stressing the medial ligaments (deltoid).

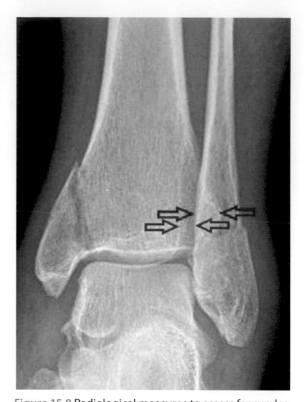

Figure 15.8 Radiological measures to assess for syndesmotic stability. Red arrows demonstrate the degree of tibio-fibular overlap (TFO) which is measured at the point of maximal overlap. Less than 1 mm on the mortise view or less than 6 mm on an AP are believed to be abnormal.

Blue arrows demonstrate the tibio-fibular clear space (TFCS). This is measured 1 cm proximal to the joint and should be compared to the unaffected contralateral limb.

hanging over the end of the x-ray table (Figure 15.7). The aim is to stress the medial ligaments with the effect of gravity.

However, both of these techniques tend to overestimate fracture instability as there is an increased chance of performing these two tests with the ankle plantarflexed (when the PTTL component of the DDL is lax). Gravity-stress radiographs especially appear to overestimate instability, and hence the need for operative treatment (15, 16). In contrast, weight-bearing stress radiographs have been shown to provide a reliable basis on which to base decisions regarding stability and non-operative treatment in isolated lateral malleolus fractures of the SER type, with excellent clinical and radiographic outcomes at short-term follow up.

Assessment of syndesmotic stability

Unless severe disruption to the syndesmosis is present, radiographs have been found to be a poor predictor of syndesmotic stability (17). A high index of suspicion is therefore required. Radiological measurements on a mortise view such as the tibio-fibular overlap (TFO) and the tibio-fibular clear space (TFCS) have been used to assess for syndesmotic stability (18) (Figure 15.8).

Less than 1 mm on a mortise view or less than 6 mm on an AP view are believed to be abnormal. However, 5% of normal ankles have no TFO and 8% have <1 mm overlap (19). This is likely due to radiographical acquisition

with varying degrees of ankle rotation and the fact that the size of Chaput tubercle can vary. The lack of TFO therefore does not define a syndesmotic injury.

The TFCS is likely to be a more reliable measurement as the TFCS is relatively more independent of ankle rotation (20). However, as variability for this measure also exists, the contralateral limb should also be examined, with a TFCS difference greater than or equal to 2 mm thought to be pathological (21).

Advanced imaging

CT scanning of ankle fractures adds to surgical planning with the more complex, high energy, fracture dislocations – particularly in cases where there is confirmed or suspected fracture of the posterior malleolus (22). Cross sectional imaging provides accurate assessment of all the fracture components and, in particular, any impaction or loose bodies within the fracture site thereby allowing the surgeon to plan appropriate strategies for reduction and fixation.

Management (non-surgical and surgical options)

Emergency management of all ankle fractures involves analgesia, appropriate reduction and splintage. The decision to treat the fracture with surgery will depend on stability assessment based on radiographs as described earlier. In general, the vast majority of Weber A-type fractures can be treated conservatively in a boot. In the case of isolated lateral malleolus fractures at the level of the syndesmosis, the Lauge-Hansen classification can guide treatment (Table 15.2).

If both the non–weight-bearing (NWB) and weight-bearing AP and mortise radiographs show no suspicion of widening of the MCS then this can be classed as a SER-2 fracture. These are stable injuries for which patients should be encouraged to fully bear weight as pain allows, with the support of a removable boot.

However, if the initial NWB radiographs suggest widening of the MCS, but the subsequent weight-bearing stress views do not, this can be classified as a SER-4a (Surrey Modification of the Lauge-Hansen classification) (5), which involves injury to the ATTL but preservation of all or part of the PTTL component of the deep deltoid ligament (DDL). In this injury, the PTTL is under tension when the ankle is plantigrade and loose when plantarflexed. Therefore, this fracture has the potential to be unstable if managed in a removable splint or boot. This is because, when the boot is off (for sleeping, bathing, etc.), the PTTL component of the DDL is lax, thereby allowing widening of the MCS and the potential for the DDL to heal at the wrong 'length'. This could potentially result in chronic instability and ultimate degeneration of the ankle joint. For this reason, it is suggested that treating these injuries in a formal cast with encouragement to bear weight as tolerated should continue for 6 weeks in order to hold position. Where both non–weight-bearing and weight-bearing radiographs show widening of the MCS then this is a SER-4b affecting both anterior and posterior portions of the DDL (ATTL and PTTL) and this details an injury which is unstable and therefore requires surgical fixation.

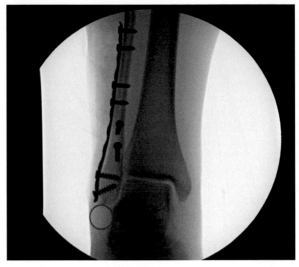

Figure 15.9 Dime/Penny sign. The dime is described on the AP view as an unbroken curve connecting the recess in the distal tip of the fibula and the lateral process of the talus when the fibula is out to length as demonstrated by the red circle.

All bi-malleolar and tri-malleolar fractures are, by definition, unstable and require internal fixation. Surgical treatment involving open reduction and internal fixation should adhere to the AO principles of fixation. The primary goal when treating ankle fractures is to restore the anatomical position of the talus within the ankle mortise and to hold this position until the fracture has united.

Lateral malleolus

Restoring length and rotational alignment of the fibula is the key to successful fixation of the lateral malleolus. In relation to fibula length, in addition to direct visualisation, the dime or penny sign on intra-operative AP imaging is often a good indicator of anatomical position (Figure 15.9).

Table 15.2 Suggested treatment for isolated fibula fractures according to the 'Surrey Modification' of the Lauge-Hansen classification system (5)

Fracture type	NWB radiograph	WB radiograph	Deep deltoid components	Treatment
SER-2	Stable	Stable	ATTL and PTTL intact	Boot/Brace and WB
SER-4a	Unstable	Stable	PTTL intact	WB Cast for 6 weeks
SER-4b	Unstable	Unstable	PTTL ruptured	ORIF

Abbreviations: ATTL, anterior tibiotalar ligament; NWB, non–weight-bearing; ORIF, open reduction internal fixation; PTTL, posterior tibiotalar ligament; SER, supination external rotation; WB, weight-bearing.

Lag screw fixation and neutralisation using a 1/3rd tubular plate is the most common technique for short oblique fractures of the fibula. Plate position can be lateral, posterolateral or posterior on the fibula depending on the approach used. Comminuted high fibula fractures, as often seen in PER injuries, where no interfragmentary screw fixation is possible (and hence no torsional control), require stronger bridging fixation with either low contact dynamic compression or reconstruction plates.

Locking plates have been shown to impart improved stability in osteoporotic bone during biomechanical tests. In clinical practice however, these plates have been associated with a higher infection rate when compared to standard techniques (23) and are a more costly intervention. For these reasons the use of locking plates should not be routinely employed for patients with good bone quality.

Intramedullary fixation of the fibula has also been described, especially for elderly patients with poor soft tissues. Reported outcomes of such devices have been mixed and their use has yet to be proven to be superior to traditional methods of fixation. Concerns have been raised highlighting difficulties in providing and maintaining reduction with these devices (24).

Medial malleolus

Various methods of fixation exist for fixing the medial malleolus. If the fragment is large enough, two parallel (solid or cannulated) partially threaded cancellous screws can be sited perpendicular to the fracture. However, it has been shown that in healthy bone, fully threaded cortical screws used with a lag technique are equal to or superior to partially threaded cancellous screws (25) and are the authors' preference. For comminuted medial malleolus fractures smaller gauge cortical screws (e.g., 2.7 mm) with small anatomical plates (if required) should be used in an attempt to reconstruct the fracture or, failing that, a tension band wire technique can be employed.

In vertical shear fracture patterns, as seen in SA type injuries, a plate used to buttress the fracture fragment is the most appropriate mode of fixation (Figure 15.10).

A lag screw through the plate can add compression if the fragment size and orientation of the fracture allow. Ensuring reduction and restoration of the impacted medial plafond is important with this pattern of injury.

Posterior malleolus

Posterior malleolus fractures that involve the PITFL (i.e., are seen on CT to extend into the incisura) (10, 11) they should be anatomically reduced and fixed to restore stability regardless of fragment size. A systematic review from 2016 showed that surgeons most commonly perform surgical fixation of the posterior

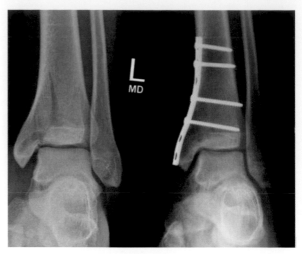

Figure 15.10 Radiographs showing a vertical shear medial malleolus fracture which has been surgically stabilised with plate fixation.

malleolus when the fragment exceeds 25% of the articular surface of the tibial plafond (26). The evidence base for this cut-off is rather insubstantial and anecdotal and more recent studies have shown that even smaller fragment posterior malleolus fractures are highly likely to affect syndesmotic stability (11). Fixation of the posterior malleolus is beneficial as it restores joint congruity and stability of the syndesmosis without the potential need for trans-syndesmotic screws or suture buttons (27).

Approaches to the posterior malleolus are best undertaken with the patient in a prone or sloppy lateral position (the latter negates the need for patient intubation) (28). Depending on the configuration of the fracture, approaches might include a combination of posterolateral and posteromedial approaches. Preoperative CT imaging is particularly useful in planning approaches to the posterior malleolus and also in identifying incarcerated fragments within the fracture which must be removed to allow reduction. The posterolateral approach has the additional benefit of allowing fixation of the fibula fracture through the same incision.

Once reduced, posterior malleolus fractures can often be held with a posteriorly sited 1/3rd tubular antiglide plate alone but the addition of a posterior-anterior screw perpendicular to the fracture can provide additional interfragmentary compression. Posterior malleolus fixation with anterior-posterior screws (with the exception of the very large posterolateral Bartoníček-Rammelt Type 4 fracture), risks damage to the anterior neurovascular structures and, more importantly, is associated with fracture malunion as the fracture cannot be anatomically reduced, especially if incarcerated fragments block reduction.

Stabilisation of the syndesmosis

Once fractures are fixed appropriately, an assessment of the syndesmosis with an intra-operative stress test should be performed. If diastasis is evident the syndesmosis should be stabilised by either restoring the attachment of the PITFL by fixing any posterior malleolus fracture as described earlier, thereby potentially negating the need for direct syndesmotic stabilisation or by trans-syndesmotic fixation. No consensus exists regarding the optimum method of syndesmosis stabilisation. No significant difference in outcomes has been reported between screw fixation and flexible suture devices, the use of small and large fragment screws (3.5 mm/4.5 mm) and whether three or four cortices are engaged (27, 29). However, siting the screws through a 2–3 hole 1/3rd tubular plate can serve to distribute compression more evenly and also, in osteoporotic bone, to reduce the risk of stress fracture.

There are, however, some important issues to be considered relating to syndesmotic screw fixation. The rate of syndesmotic mal-reduction is believed to be in the order of 30–52% following studies assessing syndesmotic mal-reduction with postoperative CT scanning (30–32). This may, in part, be due to anatomical variation of the incisura morphology (33). One strategy to reduce the risk of mal-reduction is to directly visualise the position of the fibula in the incisura either by performing an open reduction before fixation or, with arthroscopic evaluation. It is also crucial to note that closed reduction and stabilisation of the syndesmosis alone, particularly with fractures involving the middle and proximal 1/3rd fibula, does not compensate for lack of accuracy in restoring fibula length and rotation and, therefore, accurate fixation of the fibula fracture at whatever level in these cases is strongly recommended.

Syndesmotic screws should be placed following (preferably open) syndesmotic reduction. A large malleolar (or pelvic) clamp can be used with the tines of the clamp placed on the lateral fibula apex across to the anterior half of the medial malleolus (from postero-lateral fibula to anteromedial supra-malleolar area) (Figure 15.11). Evidence suggests that posterior positioning of the medial tine is associated with a greater rate of mal-reduction (34).

When tightening the clamp, there is a need to be careful so as not to over-compress and mal-reduce the syndesmosis into the incisura and to remember that these are position screws and not compression screws. Placement of the most distal screw should be at least 2 cm proximal to the joint line above the physeal scar. The need for subsequent removal of syndesmotic screws is debateable. Many surgeons advocate leaving the screws in situ for at least 3 months to allow adequate healing of the syndesmotic ligaments prior to removal, whereas some would remove them early at 6 weeks to reduce the

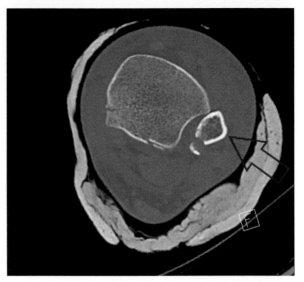

Figure 15.11 An axial CT slice of an ankle with syndesmotic instability. The red arrow shows the position of the lateral fibula apex, the ideal position for lateral tine placement.

chance of metal fatigue and breakage. Another surgical strategy, increasingly practiced, is to leave the screws in situ with the expectation that they may break but without significant detriment to the patient or limb function. There is a current lack of high quality evidence to support the routine removal of syndesmotic screws (35, 36). An alternative technique to screw fixation is the 'Tightrope' TM ('suture-button') device. However, no clear advantages are yet to be proven. The theoretical advantages are that the mobility of the suture allows normal rotational movement at the syndesmosis reducing stiffness that might occur with rigid fixation. Also, that use of these devices negates the need for a second operation to remove the hardware. A suture-button (SB) could also accommodate for inaccuracies of placement as it will allow a degree of self-reduction. Sanders et al, (37) compared syndesmotic stabilisation with screws and suture buttons and found that the SB group had a lower rate of mal-reduction (15% vs 39%). However, absolute mal-reduction was minimal and only visible on CT. Given that the functional outcome improved equally for both, one must question whether this difference was important. In fact, the only real difference was in re-operation rate, which was higher for the screw group, but again, given that there is ample evidence to support leaving the screws in situ, this difference may not be important.

The disadvantages of SBs lie with their cost as well as the fact that they cannot, and should not be used where there is a degree of vertical instability – such as multi-fragmented high Weber C-type/PER fibula fractures.

Also, a single SB does not adequately control sagittal plane instability in a severely disrupted syndesmosis (38). At least two SBs applied in a divergent fashion are required to afford stability in the sagittal plane (39). Adverse reactions to the tightrope device have also been reported.

Overall, although 'suture-button' devices certainly do have a role in the management of some syndesmotic injuries, they have not been proven to be superior to conventional screw fixation of the syndesmosis (4), especially when dealing with complex PER/Weber C-type fractures where there is a high likelihood of vertical and/or sagittal plane instability. More importantly, it is recognition of the potential for syndesmotic instability, and accurate reduction, that are more important than the choice between screws or suture button.

Other considerations

Ankle fractures in elderly patients or those with osteoporotic bone

Surgical management of ankle fractures in the elderly is technically challenging due to the high prevalence of osteoporosis combined with poor soft tissue condition and wound healing ability. Poor bone quality can result in suboptimal intra-operative fixation related to reduced screw purchase in bone, whilst medical conditions such as peripheral vascular disease and kidney disease are associated with delayed fracture healing (40). The advent of locking plate technology has revolutionised the treatment of fractures with osteoporotic bone. A more rigid fixation is achieved whilst preserving periosteal blood supply.

For frail patients, a trans-articular hindfoot nail device can be considered (Figure 15.12). Such an implant allows for decreased risk of wound complications when compared to traditional open reduction and internal fixation techniques and allows for the ability to bear weight immediately post surgery (41). Such an implant may benefit patients where the soft tissue envelope is of poor quality.

Operative fixation for diabetic patients with ankle fractures

Patients with diabetes mellitus have higher complication rates following both open and closed management of ankle fractures. Complications such as infection, wound complications and delayed union are increased further in such patients with concomitant neuropathy and vasculopathy (42, 43). Nonetheless, the same basic principles outlined earlier in this chapter should be followed to determine which fractures would benefit from surgical fixation. Should operative management be deemed appropriate, the use of a "super construct" approach has been proposed. This includes extending

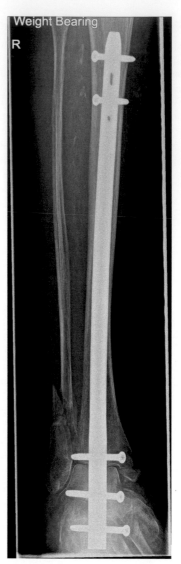

Figure 15.12 A radiograph demonstrating the use of a hindfoot nail in the treatment of an elderly patient.

fixation beyond the immediate zone of injury, planning incisions to allow for fixation placement in low-risk intervals for healing and utilisation of the strongest available fixation device (43). One possible method of increasing rigidity is the use of multiple four cortical syndesmotic screws. Diabetic patients may also require a longer period of immobilisation.

The incidence and the development of Charcot arthropathy in the setting of ankle fractures remain unclear. The early recognition and treatment of Charcot has been shown to be instrumental in preventing progressive deformity. If suspected in the context of an ankle fracture (unusual fracture pattern, comminution and abnormal bone quality), advanced imaging should be considered (44).

Complications

Complications following open reduction and internal fixation of ankle fractures are uncommon. A large study looking at over 57000 operated ankle fractures has reported a wound infection rate of 1.4%, symptomatic DVTs between 2–3% and a mortality rate of 1% within 90 days (45). The incidence of superficial peroneal nerve damage is generally underestimated. One study implies that this may be as high as 21% (46). Longer term, the rates of arthrofibrosis are unknown and have not been reliably estimated. With regards to post-traumatic osteoarthritis, the incidence of symptomatic osteoarthritis requiring treatment with ankle arthrodesis or arthroplasty is low (1%) at 5 years (45).

Take home messages

- Assessing stability is key in deciding the appropriate management of ankle fractures.
- Weight-bearing radiographs for isolated (Weber B/SER-type) lateral malleolus fractures are a good predictor of stability, and hence need for fixation.
- Stable fractures can safely be treated non-operatively, allowing the patient to bear weight as tolerated in a walking boot or cast.
- Unstable fractures require ORIF. Posterior malleolus fractures should have a pre-operative CT scan done for pre-operative planning and so as to exclude incarcerated fragments within the joint or fracture, which may block reduction.
- A high index of suspicion is required to ensure that syndesmotic injuries are not missed. All fractures treated surgically should be tested intra-operatively for syndesmotic stability.
- Patient co-morbidities such as diabetes and osteoporosis should be considered as these may affect choice of implant/surgical plan.

References

1. https://digital.nhs.uk/data-and-information/publications/statistical/hospital-admitted-patient-care-activity/2016-17
2. Gougoulias N, Khanna A, Sakellariou A, Maffulli N. Supination-external rotation ankle fractures: Stability a key issue. Clin Orthop Relat Res. 2010; 468:243–251.
3. Lloyd J, Elsayed S, Hariharan K, Tanaka H. Revisiting the concept of talar shift in ankle fractures. Foot Ankle Int. 2006; 27(10):793–796.
4. Solan MC, Davies MS, Sakellariou A. Syndesmosis stabilisation: Screws versus flexible fixation. Foot Ankle Clin. 2017; 22:35–63.
5. Gougoulias N, Sakellariou A. 'When is a simple fracture of the lateral malleolus not so simple? How to assess stability, which ones to fix and the role of the deltoid ligament. Bone Joint J. 2017; 99-B:851–855.
6. Lauge-Hansen N. Fractures of the ankle. III. Genetic roentgenologic diagnosis of fractures of the ankle. Am J Roentgenol Radium Ther Nucl Med. 1954; 71:456–471.
7. Lampridis V, Gougoulias N, Sakellariou A. Stability in ankle fractures: Diagnosis and treatment. EFORT Open Rev. 2018; 3(5):294–303.
8. Haraguchi N, Haruyama H, Toga H, Kato F. Pathoanatomy of posterior malleolar fractures of the ankle. J Bone Joint Surg [Am]. 2006; 88-A:1085–1092.
9. Bartoníček J, Rammelt S, Tuček M, Naňka O. Posterior malleolar fractures of the ankle. Eur J Trauma Emerg Surg. 2015; 41:587–600.
10. Bartoníček J, Rammelt S, Tuček M. Posterior malleolar fractures: Changing concepts and recent developments. Foot Ankle Clin. 2017; 22(1):125–145.
11. Mason LW, Marlow WJ, Widnall J, Molloy AP. Pathoanatomy and associated injuries of posterior malleolus fracture of the ankle. Foot Ankle Int. 2017; 38(11):1229–1235.
12. Costigan W, Thordarson DB, Debnath UK. Operative management of ankle fractures in patients with diabetes mellitus. Foot Ankle Int. 2007; 28:32–37.
13. Nasell H, Ottosson C, Tornqvist H, Linde J, Ponzer S. The impact of smoking on complications after operatively treated ankle fractures: A follow-up study of 906 patients. J Orthop Trauma. 2011; 25:748–755.
14. Weber M, Burmeister H, Flueckiger G, Krause FG. The use of weightbearing radiographs to assess the stability of supination-external rotation fractures of the ankle. Arch Orthop Trauma Surg. 2010; 130(5):693–698.
15. Dawe EJ, Shafafy R, Quayle J, Gougoulias N, Wee A, Sakellariou A. The effect of different methods of stability assessment on fixation rate and complications in supination external rotation (SER) 2/4 ankle fractures. Foot Ankle Surg. 2015; 21:86–90.
16. Seidel A, Krause F, Weber M. Weightbearing vs Gravity stress radiographs for stability evaluation of supination-external rotation fractures of the ankle. Foot Ankle Int. 2017; 38(7):736–744.
17. Nielson JH, Gardner MJ, Peterson MGE, Sallis JG, Potter HG, Helfet DL, Lorich DG. Radiographic measurements do not predict syndesmotic injury in ankle fractures: An MRI study. Clin Orthop Relat Res. 2005; (436):216–221.
18. Harper MC, Keller TS. A radiographic evaluation of the tibiofibular syndesmosis. Foot Ankle. 1989; 10(3):156–160.
19. Shah AS, Kadakia AR, Tan GJ, Karadsheh MS, Wolter TD, Sabb B. Radiographic evaluation of the normal distal tibiofibular syndesmosis. Foot Ankle Int. 2012; 33(10):870–876.
20. Pneumaticos SG, Noble PC, Chatziioannou SN, Trevino SG. The effects of rotation on radiographic evaluation of the tibiofibular syndesmosis. Foot Ankle Int. 2002; 23(2):107–111.
21. Del Buono A, Florio A, Boccanera MS, Maffulli N. Syndesmosis injuries of the ankle. Curr Rev Musculoskelet Med. 2013; 6(4):313–319.
22. Kumar A, Mishra P, Tandon A, Arora R, Chadha M. Effect of CT on management plan in malleolar ankle fractures. Foot Ankle Int. 2018; 39(1):59–66.
23. Schepers T, Van Lieshout EM, De Vries MR, Van der Elst M. Increased rates of wound complications with locking plates in distal fibular fractures. Injury. 2011; 42:1125–1129.
24. Gadham S, Leong E, McDonnell S, Molloy AI, Mason L, Robinson A. 'Fibular Nails – Is this the answer to ankle fracture fixation? In BOFAS Annual Scientific Meeting 2019 – Nottingham.

25. Parker L, Garlick N, McCarthy I, Grechenig S, Grechenig W, Smitham P. Screw fixation of medial malleolar fractures. Bone Joint J. 2013; 95:1662–1666.

26. Veltman ES, Halma JJ, de Gast A. Longterm outcome of 886 posterior malleolar fractures: A systematic review of the literature. Foot Ankle Surg. 2016; 22:73–77.

27. Hansen M, Le L, Wertherimer S, Meyer E, Haut R. Syndesmosis fixation: Analysis of shear stress via axial load on 3.5-mm and 4.5-mm quadricortical syndesmotic screws. J Foot Ankle Surg. 2006; 45:65–69.

28. Gougoulias N, Dawe EJ, Sakellariou A. The recovery position for posterior surgery of the ankle and hindfoot. Bone Joint J. 2013; 95-B:1317–1319.

29. Moore JA Jr., Shank JR, Morgan SJ, Smith WR. Syndesmosis fixation: A comparison of three and four cortices of screw fixation without hardware removal. Foot Ankle Int. 2006; 27:567–572.

30. Hamid N, Loeffler BJ, Brady W, Kellam JF, Cohen BE, Bosse MJ. Outcome after fixation of ankle fractures with an injury to the syndesmosis: The effect of the syndesmosis screw. J Bone Joint Surg BR. 2009; 91:1069–1073.

31. Gardner MJ, Demetrakopoulos D, Briggs SM, Helfet DL, Lorich DG. Malreduction of the tibiofibular syndesmosis in ankle fractures. Foot Ankle Int. 2006; 27(10):788–792.

32. Sagi HC, Shah AR, Sanders RW. The functional consequence of syndesmotic joint malreduction at a minimum 2-year follow-up. J Orthop Trauma. 2012; 26(7):439–443.

33. Cherney SM, Spraggs-Hughes AG, McAndrew CM, Ricci WM, Gardner MJ. Incisura morphology as a risk factor for syndesmotic malreduction. Foot Ankle Int. 2016; 37(7):748–754.

34. Cosgrove CT, Putnam SM, Cherney SM, Ricci WM, Spraggs-Hughes A, McAndrew CM, Gardner MJ. Medial clamp tine positioning affects ankle syndesmosis malreduction. J Orthop Trauma. 2017; 31(8):440–446.

35. Dingemans SA, Rammelt S, White TO, Goslings JC, Schepers T. Should syndesmotic screws be removed after surgical fixation of unstable ankle fractures? A systematic review. Bone Joint J. 2016; 98-B(11):1497–1504.

36. Boyle MJ, Gao R, Frampton CM, Coleman B. Removal of the syndesmotic screw after the surgical treatment of a fracture of the ankle in adult patients does not affect one-year outcomes: A randomised controlled trial. Bone Joint J. 2014; 96-B(12):1699–1705.

37. Sanders D, Schneider P, Taylor M, Tieszer C, Lawendy AR; Canadian Orthopaedic Trauma Society. Improved reduction of the tibiofibular syndesmosis with TightRope compared with screw fixation: Results of a randomized controlled study. J Orthop Trauma. 2019; 33(11):531–537.

38. Klitzman R, Zhao H, Zhang LQ, Strohmeyer G, Vora A. Suture-button versus screw fixation of the syndesmosis: A biomechanical analysis. Foot Ankle Int. 2010; 31(1):69–75.

39. Soin SP, Knight TA, Dinah AF, Mears SC, Swierstra BA, Belkoff SM. Suture-button versus screw fixation in a syndesmosis rupture model: A biomechanical comparison. Foot Ankle Int. 2009; 30(4):346–352.

40. Konopitski A, Boniello AJ, Shah M, Katsman A, Cavanaugh G, Harding S. Techniques and considerations for the operative treatment of ankle fractures in the elderly. J Bone Joint Surg Am. 2019; 101(1):85–94.

41. Baker G, Mayne AIW, Andrews C. Fixation of unstable ankle fractures using a long hindfoot nail. Injury. 2018; 49(11):2083–2086.

42. Wukich DK, Kline AJ. The management of ankle fractures in patients with diabetes. J Bone Joint Surg Am. 2008; 90(7):1570–1578.

43. Gandhi A, Liporace F, Azad V, Mattie J, Lin SS. Diabetic fracture healing. Foot Ankle Clin. 2006; 11:805–824.

44. Manway JM, Blazek CD, Burns PR. Special considerations in the management of diabetic ankle fractures. Curr Rev Musculoskelet Med. 2018; 11(3):445–455.

45. SooHoo NF, Krenek L, Eagan MJ, Gurbani B, Ko CY, Zingmond DS. Complication rates following open reduction and internal fixation of ankle fractures. J Bone Joint Surg Am. 2009; 91(5):1042–1049.

46. Redfern DJ, Sauve PS, Sakellariou A. Investigation of incidence of superficial peroneal nerve injury following ankle fracture. Foot Ankle Int. 2003; 24(10):771–774.

16 Lisfranc injuries

Nilesh Makwana

Introduction

Lisfranc injuries include a broad spectrum of injuries ranging from sprains and subluxations to grossly displaced fractures and fracture dislocations. The Lisfranc complex consists of the tarsometatarsal (TMT), intertarsal, proximal intermetatarsal joints and ligaments. The TMT complex should not be confused with injuries of the metatarsals and tarsal bones not including the TMT complex. Although these injuries are rare, missed injuries can result in significant pain, disability, deformity and post-traumatic degenerative joint changes, which may require further surgery. The standard of care is anatomical reduction and rigid stabilisation to obtain optimal outcome.

Lisfranc injury is named after Jacques L Lisfranc, a French gynaecologist and Napoleonic surgeon who described an amputation through the TMT joints on a soldier who had injured his midfoot falling from a horse (1). Cavalry troops in the Napoleonic era often trapped their foot in the stirrup resulting in a Lisfranc injury with a severe vascular insult (Figure 16.1)

Epidemiology

Acute Lisfranc injuries are relatively un-common injuries with an incidence of 0.2% of all fractures and are more common in men in the third decade. The reported incidence is 1 per 55,000 persons in the United States (2). Most injuries result from a direct high energy impact or an indirect injury such as a road traffic accident, fall from a height or from sports such as football. The annual incidence has been shown to be increasing (3) and this may be due to a true increase or better detection with modern imaging. Between 20% and 39% of Lisfranc injuries are missed due to distraction injuries, subtle presentations and lack of familiarity in recognising such an injury (3, 4).

Anatomy

The stability of the Lisfranc complex is due to osseous, ligamentous and soft tissue structures such as the capsule and surrounding tendons. The osseous components consist of the five metatarsals, cuneiform, and cuboid bones. The base of the metatarsals with the cuneiforms and cuboid form a transverse Roman arch that is more proximal laterally in the frontal plane (5). The apex of this arch corresponds to the 2nd TMT joint (Figures 16.2 and 16.3).

Additional stability is provided by the unique bony anatomy with the medial cuneiform protruding 8 mm and the lateral cuneiform 4 mm relative to the 2nd metatarsal (Figure 16.4). This creates the cuneiform mortise for the 2nd metatarsal base or "tenon". The lateral cuneiform is also recessed between the 2nd and 4th metatarsals thus creating a complex interlocking structure which, when disrupted, is usually with an associated fracture. Anatomical variations such as a short 2nd metatarsal or a shallow tenon have been identified as risk factors for Lisfranc injury (6).

The capsule of the Lisfranc complex consists of a fibrous membrane lined by synovium. The capsule divides the Lisfranc complex into three columns and forms the basis of the columnar classification for Lisfranc injury. The medial column includes the 1st TMT joint and medial cuneiform navicular joint; the middle column includes the 2nd and 3rd TMT joints as well as the articulation between the middle and lateral cuneiforms and the lateral column the 4th and 5th TMT joints (7). The lateral column is more flexible than the middle and medial column and is essential for gait on uneven surfaces. Every attempt should be made to maintain mobility of the lateral column. Arthrodesis of the lateral column can compromise the outcome (8).

The ligaments of the Lisfranc complex consist of dorsal, interosseous and plantar ligaments. The ligaments have longitudinal, transverse and oblique elements. The longitudinal ligaments connect the TMT joints whilst the transverse ligaments connect the intermetatarsal and intercuneiform bones. No intermetatarsal ligament exists between the 1st and 2nd metatarsal.

The dorsal ligaments are short flat ribboned structures which are weaker than the interosseous and

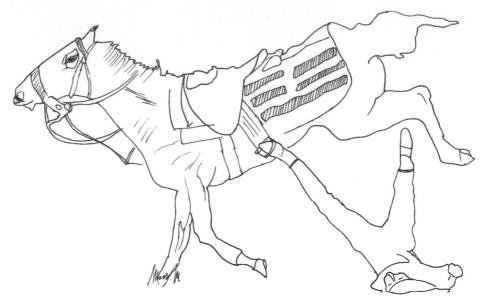

Figure 16.1 Modern day Lisfranc injury with the foot trapped in the stirrup.

plantar ligaments. As a result, they often fail first in tension following axial or indirect injuries.

The *interosseous ligaments* are the strongest with the Lisfranc ligament being the largest. It is 8–10 mm long and 5–6 mm thick. The ligament originates from the lateral side of the medial cuneiform and inserts onto the medial side of the base of the 2nd metatarsal. Most cases have a single bundle, but in some cases the ligament consists of two bundles (Figure 16.5). Following injury, an avulsion of the attachment of the Lisfranc ligament can occur, from either the metatarsal or cuneiform, which can be seen radiologically as a *"Fleck"* sign.

The *plantar ligaments* are better defined medially. The first cuneiform-metatarsal ligament is broad, and no plantar ligament exists between the middle cuneiform and 2nd metatarsal. The strongest, plantar ligament is the oblique ligament from the medial cuneiform to the 2nd and 3rd metatarsal bases (Figure 16.5). Recent studies have discovered a plantar ligament, the *lateral Lisfranc ligament* that spans from the 2nd to 5th metatarsal and this may explain the pattern of homolateral and divergent patterns of Lisfranc injury (9). The Lisfranc complex is also stabilised dynamically by muscle and tendons such as tibialis posterior, tibialis anterior and the plantar fascia. The dorsalis pedis artery

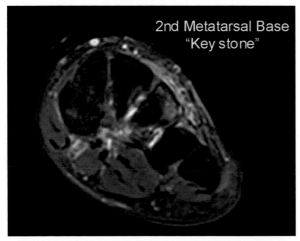

Figure 16.2 Coronal MRI scan at base of metatarsals. 2nd metatarsal forms the "Apex" of the Roman arch.

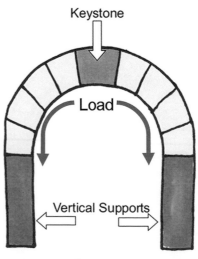

Figure 16.3 Principle of the Roman arch and *"Keystone"*.

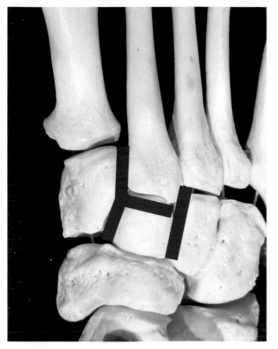

Figure 16.4 Cuneiform mortise with 2nd metatarsal base "tenon".

and deep peroneal nerve cross the TMT complex deep to extensor hallucis brevis. The artery passes between the 1st and 2nd metatarsal and gives a branch to the deep plantar artery which forms the plantar arch. Avulsion of the artery can occur following injury.

Classification

Quénu and Küss were the first to propose a classification based on the congruence and direction of the TMT joints (10). Hardcastle et al. further modified this classification based on their experience of 119 Lisfranc injuries (11). They classified injuries into *Type A – Total incongruity* of all TMT joints, *Type B – Partial Incongruity* and *Type C – divergent dislocation* (Figure 16.6). Myerson further modified this classification (7). More recently Chiodo and Myerson developed a *columnar*-based classification which is described earlier (7). This is a simple classification describing the columns as a unit. The *medial and middle columns* have relatively little mobility and can be sacrificed with a fusion. The *lateral column*, however, is more flexible and cannot be sacrificed easily without affecting gait.

A further classification has been proposed by Nunley and Vertullo, for subtle injuries in athletes. *Stage I* injuries are undisplaced injuries of the TMT complex with

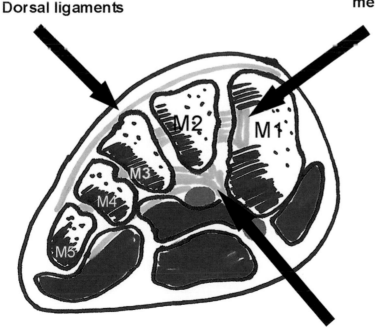

Dorsal ligaments

Lisfranc ligament, cuneiform to second metatarsal

Plantar Ligament. Cuneiform to 2nd and 3rd metatarsal base.

Figure 16.5 Illustration of the Lisfranc ligament complex.

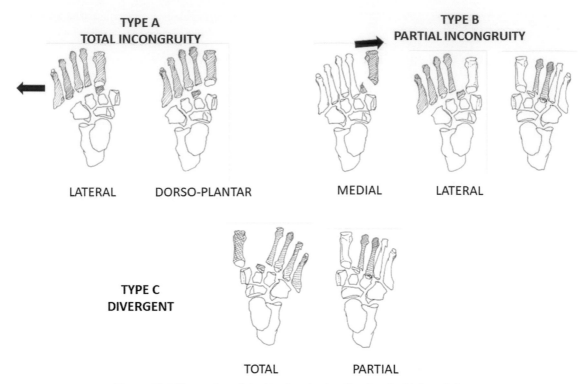

TYPE A
TOTAL INCONGRUITY

LATERAL   DORSO-PLANTAR

TYPE B
PARTIAL INCONGRUITY

MEDIAL   LATERAL

TYPE C
DIVERGENT

TOTAL   PARTIAL

Figure 16.6 Illustration of the Hardcastle classification for Lisfranc injury.

pain, local tenderness and a positive bone scan and normal x-rays. *Stage II* injuries show a 1st to 2nd intermetatarsal diastasis of 1–5 mm but no loss of arch height. *Stage III* shows a diastasis and loss of arch height (12). Although these classifications are useful for descriptive purposes, none have been shown to be reliable or predictive of outcome.

Mechanism of injury

Lisfranc injuries can result from high energy trauma with severe soft tissue compromise or, from less severe twisting injuries, resulting in sprains and subluxations. Road traffic accidents account for most cases, 43%, with 10% due to sports, 13% due to crush injury and 24% from falls, jumps or twisting injuries (13). They can be broadly grouped into *Direct* and *Indirect* injuries. *Direct* injuries are typically high energy trauma which are often compound, with significant soft tissue compromise and may be associated with compartment syndrome. *Indirect* injuries are typically seen with axial and/or rotational forces applied to a foot that is plantar flexed or stationary (Figure 16.7). In these cases, the dorsal ligament complex fails in tension resulting in dorsal displacement of the metatarsal with secondary medial or lateral displacement. The exact mechanism of injury, however, is not known due to the complex nature of the TMT complex.

Associated fractures include those of the cuboid, calcaneum, talus and the ankle. The most common are crush injuries to the cuboid and metatarsal fractures. Compartment syndrome may also occur, and a high index of suspicion should be maintained.

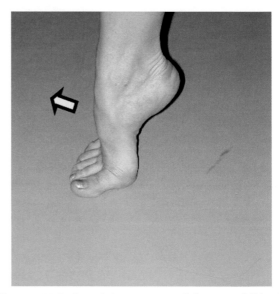

Figure 16.7 Indirect injury can occur following a fall leading to tension failure of the dorsal ligaments (arrow).

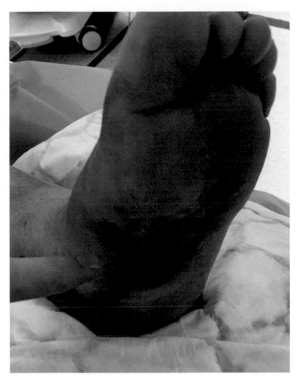

Figure 16.8 Plantar bruising indicative of a Lisfranc injury. (Courtesy of Consultant Orthopaedic Surgeon Jonathan Young.)

Symptoms and signs

In high energy injury the diagnosis is usually obvious. However, in subtle or indirect injuries, the diagnosis may not be so obvious. Patients may complain of midfoot pain whilst bearing weight or during strenuous activities. The midfoot may be swollen and some patients will present with bruising on the plantar aspect of the midfoot, a sign which is highly associated with a Lisfranc injury (Figure 16.8) (14).

Mild swelling and tenderness may be seen in athletes and the elderly. Provocative tests include dorsal and plantar translation, and passive abduction-rotation stress of the midfoot with the hindfoot stabilised. Single limb stance may also elicit pain in some patients.

Significant soft tissue swelling with or without fracture blisters may preclude early surgical intervention. In these cases, acute reduction of major deformity with temporary stabilisation using K-wires or external fixators will allow the soft tissue swelling to subside before definitive fixation is undertaken.

Investigations

Standard imaging should include *AP, lateral and 30° oblique views* of the foot and a high index of suspicion should be maintained. Between 20% and 39% of Lisfranc injuries are missed initially, especially in subtle injury (3). Normal parameters to look out for include:

1. The base of the 1st metatarsal lines up medially and laterally with the medial cuneiform (*AP view*)
2. The 1st intermetatarsal and intercuneiform distances are equal (*AP view*)
3. The medial border of the base of the 2nd metatarsal lines up with the medial border of the middle cuneiform (*AP view*)
4. The medial border of the 4th metatarsal lines up with the cuboid (*Oblique view*)
5. Dorsal or plantar displacement (*Lateral view*)

Contralateral images can be performed for comparison in difficult cases. Widening of the 1st intermetatarsal gap by more than 2 mm, more than 2 mm displacement of the TMT joints and/or dorsal displacement of the TMT joints on the lateral projection should raise the suspicion of a Lisfranc injury. An avulsion of the Lisfranc ligament may be seen in the 1st intermetatarsal space and is known as the *Fleck sign* (Figure 16.9) (15). In subtle injuries, weight-bearing images of both feet may reveal a diastasis of the 1st intermetatarsal space (Figure 16.10).

In patients where the mechanism of injury and the clinical signs and symptoms suggest a Lisfranc injury, but the x-rays are not conclusive, then advanced imaging such as a CT scan or MRI is indicated. A CT scan is useful for confirming a Lisfranc injury and it will also detect fractures around the TMT complex as well as fractures to other bones in the foot. For complex, high energy trauma, CT scans help with planning definitive

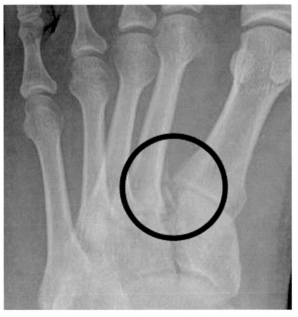

Figure 16.9 *Fleck sign* (circled).

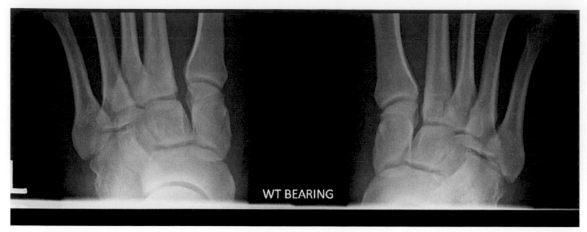

Figure 16.10 Bilateral weight-bearing AP x-rays of the foot showing an increased 1st-2nd intermetatarsal space (Left).

surgery. It should be noted that in purely ligamentous injury, a CT scan may not be useful as it is a static non–weight-bearing imaging modality. However, weight-bearing CT scan might change this in future.

MRI is valuable in detecting subtle and purely ligamentous Lisfranc injuries. MRI has been shown to be superior to plain x-rays in detecting TMT injuries in hyperflexion injuries. Here, 50% of the injuries were missed by plain x-ray (16). MRI can detect the continuity of the Lisfranc ligament which is seen as a hypointense band-like structure between the medial cuneiform and base of 2nd metatarsal (Figure 16.11).

Principles of treatment

Non-surgical treatment for Lisfranc injuries is reserved for stable injuries that do not displace on dynamic weight-bearing. This may be determined by weight-bearing x-rays in subtle cases and compared with the normal side. Weight-bearing CT may eventually negate the need for weight-bearing plain x-rays. If suspicion or doubt remains, despite further imaging, then examination under anaesthesia with stress testing is recommended. Stress views under regional or general anaesthetic can be performed with abduction and pronation stressing of the TMT joint with the hindfoot stabilised or with compression and distraction of the 2nd TMT joint. The normal side can be used for comparison. Displacement in the transverse plane, greater than 2 mm between the 1st intermetatarsal and intertarsal space or, in the dorsoplantar plane, indicates an unstable Lisfranc complex.

Stable injuries can be treated in a plaster cast or a controlled ankle motion (CAM) boot. Non–weight-bearing for 6–8 weeks followed by protected weight-bearing for a further period of 4–6 weeks is recommended. Weight-bearing repeat x-rays are useful for the detection of any interval diastasis or displacement. A high rate of displacement in minimally displaced Lisfranc injuries treated conservatively has been reported. Subsequent surgery, however, resulted in similar outcomes compared to those that did not displace (17).

Unstable, displaced fractures require anatomical reduction and surgical stabilisation to obtain a stable plantigrade foot that is relatively pain free with a good functional outcome.

In high energy injuries with gross displacement and soft tissue compromise, definitive surgical reconstruction with multiple incisions may not be possible without

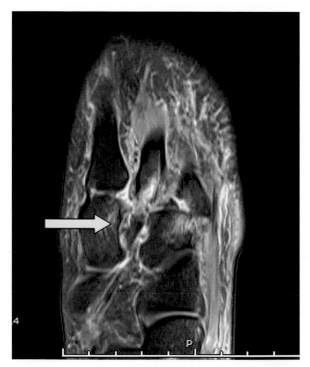

Figure 16.11 MR scan showing the Lisfranc ligament (arrow).

risking infection and skin necrosis. Initial management, with closed reduction of the deformity and temporary stabilisation with 2.0 mm K-wires, can allow the soft tissue to settle before definitive surgery is undertaken. (18) External fixators have also been used to maintain temporary alignment. Open injures will require early debridement and temporary stabilisation and if there is severe soft tissue injury plastic surgical reconstruction may also be indicated. An algorithm for the management of Lisfranc injuries is shown in Figure 16.12.

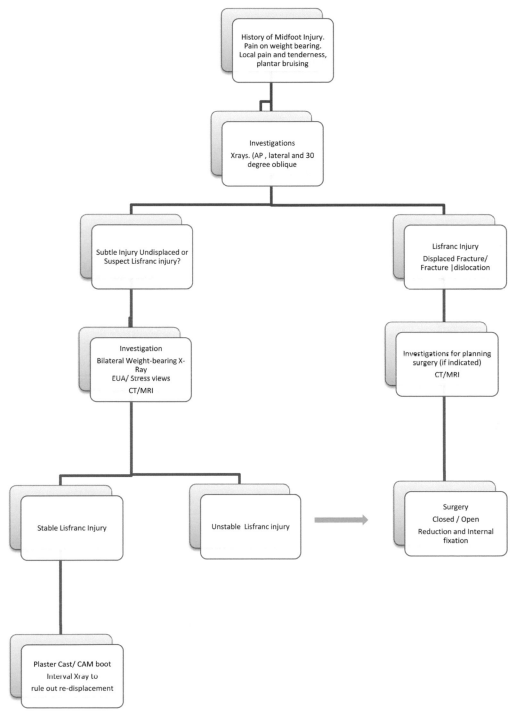

Figure 16.12 An algorithm for the management of a Lisfranc injury.

Surgical treatment

Surgical techniques of reduction and stabilisation include closed reduction and K-wire or screw stabilisation, open reduction and internal fixation with screws and/or plates and primary fusion.

Closed reduction and K-wire stabilisation has been used with the K-wires removed at 6–8 weeks. In pure ligamentous injury this may not be sufficient for the ligaments to have healed fully and re-displacement can occur. Other complications include wire breakage, migration and infection. However, good outcomes have been reported in the literature and the main determinate of outcome appears to be early anatomical reduction and stabilisation.

Percutaneous screw fixation has been advocated. A systematic review of the literature showed good outcomes with this technique. The review did emphasise that anatomical reduction must be obtained; if not, then conversion to an open reduction should be undertaken (19). Inability to reduce closed could be due to soft tissue interposition such as entrapment of the tibialis anterior tendon between the medial cuneiform and 1st metatarsal or, due to fracture fragments. Displacement greater than 2 mm between the medial and middle cuneiforms, a talar-metatarsal angle greater than 15° or any coronal displacement is associated with a poor outcome (15).

Open reduction and internal fixation are performed with the patient supine with a bolster under the ipsilateral hip on a radiolucent table. Incisions will need to consider the soft tissue injury, but generally reduction can be performed through two or three incisions. Care should be taken to leave an adequate bridge to prevent skin necrosis. The medial incision is placed over the 1st

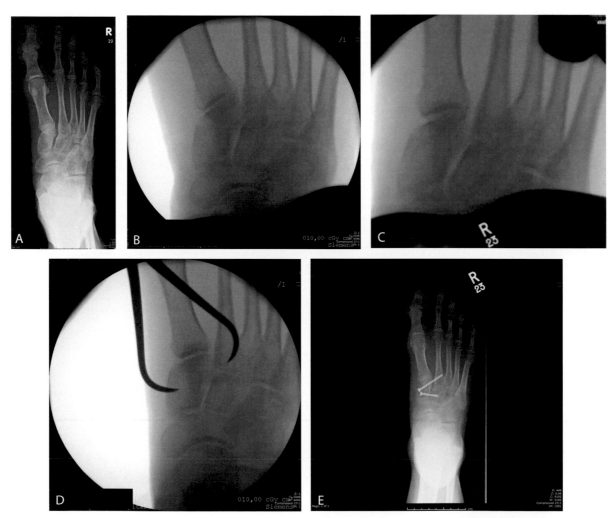

Figure 16.13 Case 1: 23-year-old male with a crush injury. (A) 1st–2nd intermetatarsal and intertarsal diastasis, (B) fluoroscopic view before stress applied, (C) stress views demonstrating diastasis. (D) Closed reduction and (E) percutaneous reduction and stabilisation.

intermetatarsal space. This allows identification of the neurovascular bundle which lies deep to extensor digitorum brevis and allows access to the 1st and 2nd TMT joints. The second incision is placed over the 4th metatarsal which gives access to the 3rd to 5th TMT joints. A third incision may be necessary to address fractures of the cuboid, cuneiform, naviculum or metatarsals.

The suggested order of reduction is the medial, middle and then the lateral column. Anatomical reduction with joint congruity must be achieved. Large intra-articular fractures can be stabilised first prior to joint reduction and then the TMT joint can be stabilised with trans-articular screws or bridging plates. Trans-articular screws can arguably further damage the

articular surface. Highly comminuted intra-articular fractures may need to be treated by fusion. Care should be taken to reduce the inter-cuneiform joints also, as it is not uncommon for diastasis to occur at this level. The lateral column can be similarly reduced and stabilised with K-wires, which can be removed later to maintain lateral column mobility.

Cuboid crush injuries with shortening of the lateral column may need to be treated with dis-impaction and bone grafting, with stabilisation using a small plate, or a bridging plate from the calcaneum to the 4th metatarsal. External fixators have been used to maintain the lateral column length. Cases to illustrate the techniques are shown in Figures 16.13 and 16.14 (Cases 1 and 2).

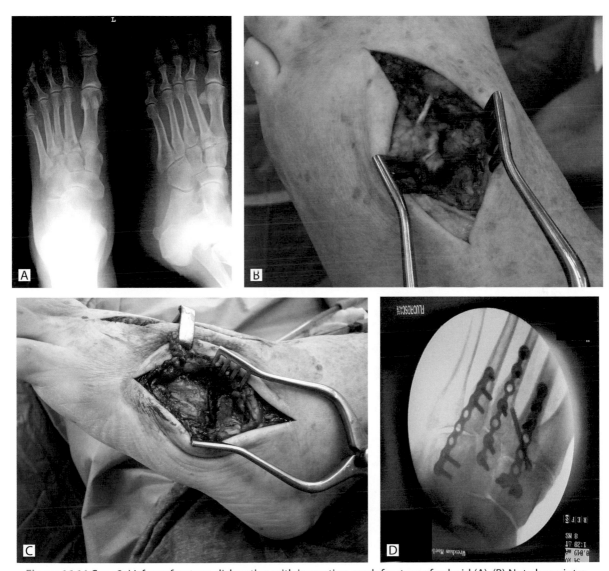

Figure 16.14 Case 2: Lisfranc fracture-dislocation with impaction crush fracture of cuboid (A). (B) Note large intra-articular fragment of the 2nd metatarsal. (C) Impaction fracture cuboid. (D) Open reduction and internal fixation with dis-impaction of the cuboid and bridging plates across the TMT complex.

Surgery should be performed within 24 hours if possible, as this reduces the risk of vascular compromise and facilitates anatomical reduction. After 24 hours the soft tissue may become too swollen and surgery will need to be delayed until the soft tissue swelling is reduced. Hardcastle (11) reported poor results if the reduction was performed after 6 weeks.

Current controversies

Open reduction and internal fixation or primary arthrodesis

Traditionally, primary arthrodesis was a salvage procedure but more recently, it has been advocated for pure ligamentous injuries. Improved functional outcome, less pain and higher return to pre-injury level compared to ORIF in 41 patients was reported (20). A systematic meta-analysis, however, concluded no difference in patient reported outcome, need for revision surgery, and anatomic reduction. Significantly more hardware removal was found in the ORIF group (21). A recent systematic meta-analysis looked at the most recent randomised control trials, including retrospective and prospective studies. This review also found no difference in the complication rate, outcome score, return to work, unplanned return to theatre and in-patient satisfaction. The study did find a significantly higher need for removal of metalwork in the ORIF group (22). This is likely to be due to a standard protocol of metalwork removal to allow movement and to prevent metalwork breakage.

Trans-articular screws or bridging plate

Trans-articular screws have become popular for fixing the TMT complex as this technique avoids the need for percutaneous K-wires, which require subsequent removal. However, trans-articular screws can disrupt up to 6% of the articular surface and potentially risk osteoarthritis (23). Bridging plates that span the joint can provide rigid fixation and avoid this. Biomechanical studies demonstrate that bridging plates have better stiffness and less displacement than screws. Midterm studies have shown no significant difference regarding functional outcome, pain and osteoarthritis between trans-articular screws and joint sparing techniques (24). Bridging plates do require more dissection compared to percutaneous screw fixation and some surgeons routinely remove the plate at 3–6 months.

Complications

Early complications include wound infection, nerve injury, re-displacement, vascular injury, compartment syndrome and complex regional pain syndrome. Amputation due to ischaemia and vascular compromise has been reported especially with high energy injury. A

high index of suspicion should be maintained for compartment syndrome.

Late complications include post-traumatic osteoarthritis, deformity, prominent osteophytes, chronic pain, non-union and late displacement. Arthrodesis is indicated for neglected or misdiagnosed Lisfranc injury. Corrective arthrodesis for deformity has also been shown to give good results in terms of pain and function.

Outcome

Anatomical reduction and stable rigid fixation have been shown to be a prerequisite for a good outcome. This does not, however, guarantee a good outcome. A long-term review of the clinical outcome of 61 patients at an average of 10.9 years found most patients were able to return to their previous level of function and employment. A high number (72%) developed radiographic osteoarthritis of which 54% were symptomatic (25).

Several studies have looked specifically at return to sports following Lisfranc injury. Most have found that return to training and competition sport is possible but may take up to a year to occur. Return to soccer was found to be faster than return to rugby. Not all patients return to pre-injury levels.

Take home messages

- Lisfranc complex injuries range from subtle injuries or sprains with pure ligamentous injury, to grossly displaced fracture dislocations.
- Missed or neglected injuries are associated with a poor outcome.
- Salvage surgery often requires arthrodesis of the TMT joints.
- The Gold Standard for optimal outcome remains with early anatomical reduction and rigid stable fixation.
- Most patients can anticipate a good outcome with a return to pre-injury levels of activity. Post-traumatic osteoarthritis is common but this does not appear to correlate with the clinical outcome.

References

1. Cassebaum WH. Lisfranc fracture dislocations. *Clin Orthop.* 1963;30:116.
2. English TA. Dislocation of the metatarsal bone and adjacent toe. *J Bone Joint Surg.* 1964;46B:700.
3. Vuori JP, Hannu TA. Lisfranc Joint injuries: Trauma mechanisms and associated injuries. *J Trauma.* 1993;35(1):40–5.
4. Goosens M, DeStoop N. Lisfrancs fracture dislocation: Etiology, radiology and results of treatment. *Clin Orthop Rel Res.* 1983;176:154–62.
5. Sarrafian SK. *Anatomy of the Foot and Ankle. Descriptive Topographic Functional.* 2nd ed. JB Lippincott. 1993.
6. Gallagher SM, Rodriguez NA, Anderson CR, Granberry WM, Panchbhavi VK. Anatomic predisposition to ligamentous

Lisfranc injury. A matched case-control study. *J Bone Joint Surg Am*. 2013;95(22):2043–7.

7. Chiodo C, Myerson MS. Developments and advances in the diagnosis and treatment of injuries to the tarsometatarsal joint. *Orth Clin North Am*. 2001;32(1):11–20.

8. Nadaud JP, Parks BG, Schon LC. Plantar and calcaneocuboid joint pressure after isolated medial column versus medial and lateral column fusion: A biomechanical study. *Foot Ankle Int*. 2001;32(11):1069–74.

9. Mason L, Malwattage LTJ, Fisher A, Swanton E, Molloy A. Anatomy of the lateral plantar ligament of the transverse metatarsal arch. *Foot Ankle Int*. 2020;41(1):109–14.

10. Quénu E, Küss G. Etude sur les luxations du metatarse. *Reb Chir*. 1909;39:281–336.

11. Hardcastle PH, Reschauer R, Schoffmann W. Injuries to the tarsometatarsal joint. *J Bone Joint Surg*. 1982;64-B:349–56.

12. Nunley JA, Vertullo CJ. Classification, investigation and management of midfoot sprains. Lisfranc injuries in the athlete. *Am J sport Med*. 2002;30(6):871–8.

13. Lievers WB, Frimenko RE, Crandell JR, Kent RW, Park JS. Age, sex, casual and injury patterns in tarsometatarsal dislocations: A literature review of over 2000 cases. *Foot*. 2012;22(3):117–24.

14. Ross G, Cronin R, Hauzenbias J, Juliano P. Plantar ecchymosis sign: A clinical aid to diagnosis of occult Lisfranc tarsometatarsal injuries. *J Orthop Trauma*. 1996;10(2):119–22.

15. Myerson MS, Fisher RT, Burgess AR, Kenzora JE. Fracture dislocation of the tarsometatarsal joints. End results correlated with pathology and treatment. *Foot Ankle Int*. 1986;6(5):225–52.

16. Preidler KW, Peicha G, Lajtai G, Seibert FJ, Fock C, Szolar DM, Raith H. Conventional radiography, CT and MR imaging in patients with hyperflexion injuries of the foot: Diagnostic accuracy in the detection of bony and ligamentous changes. *AJR*. 1999;173.1673–7.

17. Chen P, Ng N, Snowden G, Mackensie S, Nicholson J, Amin A. Rates of displacement and patient-reported outcomes following conservative treatment of minimally displaced Lisfranc injury. *Foot Ankle Int*. 2020;41(4):387–91.

18. Herscovici D, Scaduto JM. Acute management of high-energy Lisfranc injuries: A simple approach. *Injury*. 2018;49: 420–4.

19. Stavrakakis IM, Magarakis GE, Christoforakis Z. Percutaneous fixation of Lisfranc injuries: A systematic review of the literature. *Acta Orthopaedica et Traumatologica Turcica*. 2019;53:457–62.

20. Ly TV, Coetzee JC. Treatment of primary ligamentous Lisfranc joint injuries: Primary arthrodesis compared with open reduction and internal fixation. A prospective randomised study. *J Bone Joint Surg Am*. 2006;88:514–20.

21. Smith N, Furrey A. Does open reduction and internal fixation versus primary arthrodesis improve patient outcomes for Lisfranc trauma? A systematic review and meta-analysis. *Clin Orthop Relat Res*. 2016;474:1445–52.

22. Alcelik I, Fenton C, Hannant G, Abdelrahim M, Jowett C, Budgen A, Stanley J. A systematic review and meta-analysis of the treatment of acute Lisfranc injuries: Open reduction and internal fixation versus primary arthrodesis. *Foot Ankle Surg*. 2019, https://doi.org/10.1016/j.fas.2019.04.003.

23. Alberta FG, Aronow MS, Mauricio M, Barrero M, Diaz-Doran V, Sullivan RJ, Adams DJ. Ligamentous Lisfranc joint injuries: A biomechanical comparison of dorsal plate and transarticular screw fixation. *Foot Ank Int*. 2005;26:462–73.

24. Hu SJ, Chang SM, Li XH, YU GR. Outcome comparison of Lisfranc injuries treated through dorsal plate fixation versus screw fixation. *Acta Orth Bras*. 2014;22:315–20.

25. Dubois-Ferriere V, Lubbeke A, Chowdary A, Stern R, Dominquez D, Assal M. Clinical outcomes and development of symptomatic osteoarthritis 2-24 years after surgical treatment of tarsometatarsal joint complex injuries. *J Bone Joint Surg Am*. 2016;98:713–20.

17 Fractures of the talus

Hiro Tanaka and Lyndon Mason

Introduction

Fractures of the talus comprise a heterogeneous group of injuries ranging from those presenting as an ankle sprain when radiologic diagnosis can be difficult to the severe, resulting from car accidents or falls from a height, when limb preservation becomes paramount and surgery is technically demanding.

These fractures are best considered according to their anatomic locations which include the talar neck, body, head and the lateral/posterior processes.

This chapter covers the basic science knowledge necessary to understand the principles of surgical management, the important clinical and radiological assessment tools to establish correct diagnosis, the higher order decision-making process for optimal treatment and the things to look out for postoperatively.

Basic science

There are three reasons why a thorough understanding of the structural anatomy of the talus is essential in the management of these injuries.

1. Since the talus is largely an articular bone being 60% covered by articular cartilage, many fractures may be intra-articular and knowing which one is involved is important.
2. Anatomic surgical reconstruction and placement of hardware requires an understanding of the morphology of the bone.
3. Due to a tenuous bloody supply, the talus is prone to avascular necrosis, and therefore the surgical approach must take into consideration the vascular network to minimise this risk and prevent iatrogenic damage.

The talus consists of three main parts, the body, neck and head. The body articulates with the tibia at the ankle joint superiorly and subtalar joint inferiorly. It is widest anteriorly which confers bony stability to the ankle joint when dorsiflexed and causes external rotation of the fibula. The neck faces anteromedially and is the weakest part of the bone. The head is entirely covered with articular cartilage, articulates with the navicular and is supported by the calaneonavicular or "Spring" ligament, which maintains the arch of the foot.

Figure 17.1 demonstrates the superior view of the talus. This shows the lateral process of the talus which articulates with the lateral malleolus in the lateral gutter of the ankle joint as well as the subtalar joint inferiorly. Posteriorly, on either side of the flexor hallucis longus (FHL) tendon are the medial and lateral posterior tubercles. An os trigonum is an accessory bone found in 10% of individuals and is attached by a fibrous band to the posterior part of the talus. It is usually an incidental finding but can be mistaken for a posterior process fracture. Each of these anatomic parts may be fractured individually or in combination.

Figure 17.2 demonstrates the inferior view showing the three separate articulations with the subtalar joint. The posterior facet is separated by the tarsal canal with the middle facet, which articulates with the sustentaculum tali and the anterior facet. It is useful to note the areas of the talus which are not covered with articular cartilage as these are the areas optimal for the placement of hardware.

The blood supply to the talus was described by Haliburton in 1958 (1). It was originally thought that most of the talar body receives most of its blood supply in a retrograde fashion through anastomoses around the talar neck. These vessels are made up of branches from the anterior tibial (36%), perforating peroneal (47%) and posterior tibial arteries (17%). Recent cadaveric studies have demonstrated a more robust anterograde blood supply, which might explain why not all fractures develop avascular necrosis (2).

The vessels enter the bone at five non-articulating sites (Figure 17.2).

1. Superior neck of talus – Anterior tibial artery
2. Inferior neck of talus – Anastomosis between tarsal sinus and tarsal canal artery

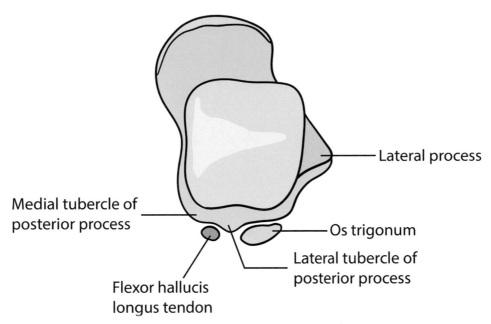

Figure 17.1 Superior view of the talus.

3. Sinus tarsi
4. Medial body – Deltoid branches
5. Posterior body – Posterior anastomosis

The clinical implication of this vascular supply is that whilst an undisplaced talar neck fracture will disrupt the intraosseous supply from the tarsal sinus and tarsal canal, the major vascular sling remains intact. With a displaced fracture however, the whole network is prone to rupture and the only remaining supply may be the direct perforating branches from the deltoid and posterior branches. It is therefore essential to preserve what remaining supply is present to minimise the risk of avascular necrosis.

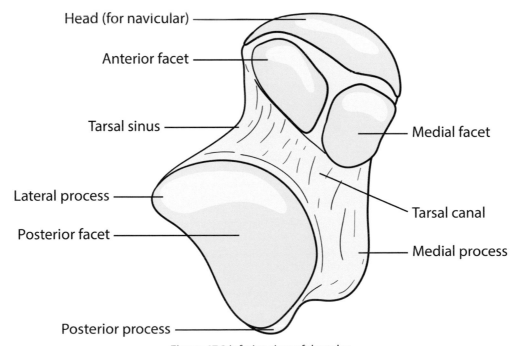

Figure 17.2 Inferior view of the talus.

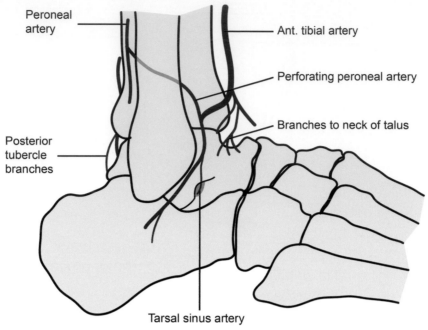

Peroneal artery

Ant. tibial artery

Perforating peroneal artery

Branches to neck of talus

Posterior tubercle branches

Tarsal sinus artery

Figure 17.3 Lateral view of blood supply.

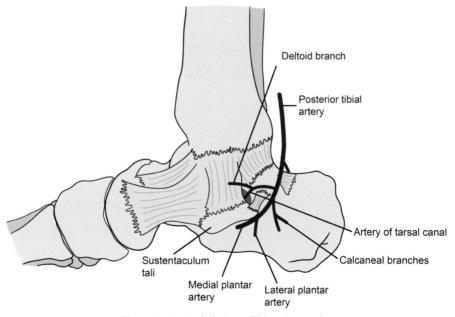

Deltoid branch

Posterior tibial artery

Artery of tarsal canal

Calcaneal branches

Sustentaculum tali

Medial plantar artery

Lateral plantar artery

Figure 17.4 Medial view of bloody supply.

Learning Point

In a displaced talar neck fracture, the only remaining blood supply may be the perforating deltoid and posterior branches. They must not be damaged in the surgical approach.

Talar neck fractures

These injuries are the most common accounting for 50% of talar fractures and typically are the result of high energy injuries such as falls from a height or car accidents. The neck is the apex of the medial longitudinal arch, and the structure is at risk with forced dorsiflexion of the ankle. The fracture occurs as a result of the neck

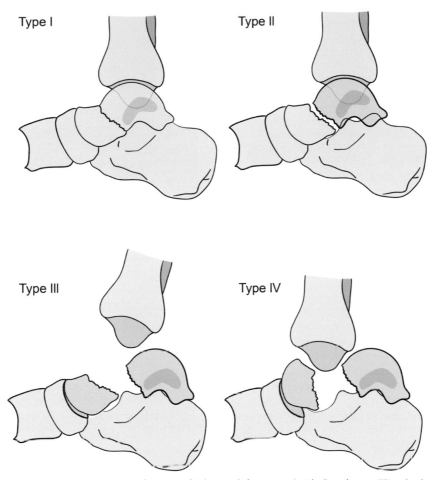

Figure 17.5 Hawkins Classification of talar neck fractures (with Canale modification).

being forced against the distal tibia. This was the mechanism first described by Anderson in 1919 who coined the term "Aviator's Astragalus".

It is important to appreciate the degree of force required to cause this injury as there is a high probability of other life threatening injuries as well as injuries to the ipsilateral limb, compartment syndrome, neurovascular compromise and severe soft tissue damage.

Classification

Hawkins originally described a classification system in 1970 modified by Canale in 1978 and this remains a useful standard since there is a direct relationship with the risk of avascular necrosis (AVN) (3, 4). Recent systematic reviews have reported significant variances in the AVN rates; however, most have low patient numbers and variable treatment, which may account for the differences (5–7). Vallier proposed the addition of Types IIa and IIb which further improves the utility of the system as they noted a significant difference in AVN rates with subtalar dislocation as opposed to subluxation (8).

Imaging

Plain radiographs including AP, lateral and mortise views of the ankle will identify severe talar neck fractures; however, undisplaced fractures can be subtle and

Table 17.1 Hawkins Classification of talar neck fractures (with Canale modification)

Type	Description	AVN rate
Hawkins I	Undisplaced	0–5.7%
Hawkins II	Subtalar dislocation	15.9–20.7%
Hawkins III	Subtalar and talonavicular dislocation	38.9–44.8%
Hawkins IV	Subtalar, talonavicular and tibiotalar dislocation	12.1–55%
Vallier IIa	Subtalar subluxation	0%
Vallier IIb	Subtalar dislocation	25%

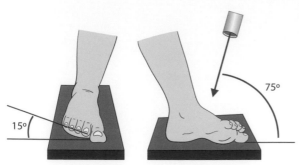

Figure 17.6 Canale view of the talar neck.

there must be a high index of suspicion based on the mechanism of injury and clinical presentation. Canale described a useful oblique view of the talar neck and it is taken with the foot fully plantarflexed with 15 degrees of foot pronation. The foot is placed on the x-ray plate and the beam is centered over the talar neck angled 75 degrees cephalad (4).

Whether there is a suspected injury, confirmed undisplaced fracture or a fracture that requires surgical fixation, CT scanning should be performed. CT not only helps in the diagnosis of subtle injuries but will also provide additional information such as degree and location of comminution, articular involvement, displacement not visible on a plain x-ray and other tarsal injuries. These factors will affect the decision-making process for treatment.

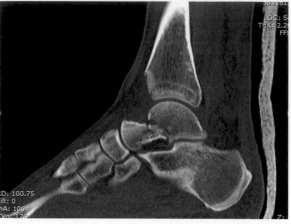

Figure 17.8 CT confirms a comminuted displaced Type IIa talar neck fracture with medial malleolar fracture.

Non-surgical management

Since the talus is largely an articular bone, anatomic restoration and stability are essential to maintain function and minimise the risk of post-traumatic osteoarthritis (PTA). Therefore, there is limited scope for non-surgical management even for undisplaced Type I fractures unless articular congruity can be confirmed on CT or the patient is either medically unfit for surgery or not mobile.

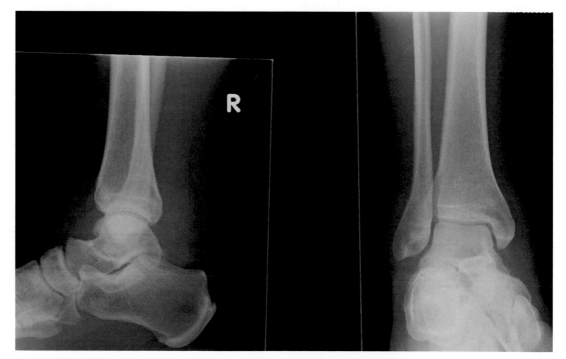

Figure 17.7 Radiograph of 34-year-old male patient involved in a road traffic accident with subtle findings.

Where there is no articular surface displacement, a trial of non-surgical management with a non-weight-bearing below knee plaster for a period of 6 weeks with progressive weight-bearing for 6 weeks can be attempted. Patients should be monitored closely for any evidence of displacement (9).

> ### Learning Point
>
> Undisplaced Type I fractures can be treated non-surgically; however, it is essential to confirm that there is no displacement with a CT and with early follow-up to ensure it does not displace.

Surgical management

Due to the high energy nature of displaced talar neck fractures, up to a third of patients present with an open injury and over 50% of patients will have other fractures. Major ligamentous disruption can result in complete extrusion of the talus. Despite the severe bony injury, it is the extent of soft tissue damage in the form of open wounds, severe swelling, fracture blisters (particularly sanguineous) and contamination which dictates the surgical planning.

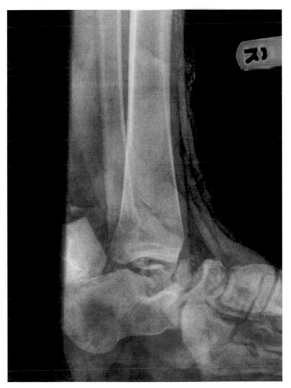

Figure 17.9 Open talar extrusion from a motorbike accident. The soft tissue injury is the priority.

> ### Learning Point
>
> The degree of soft tissue injury is the primary determinant and priority in surgical management.

Surgical timing

Reduction of closed displaced fractures should be performed immediately where possible to protect the soft tissues and prevent neurovascular injury in the emergency department. Open fractures, irreducible dislocations and talar extrusions will require urgent surgical management. Open fractures should be debrided and reduced. Talar extrusions rarely reduce with closed ligamentotaxis, and therefore the surgeon should be prepared to undertake an open reduction via one of standard talar neck approaches. Open reduction is often technically demanding due to tendon interposition (e.g., tibialis posterior) and the surgeon should be familiar with the approach before attempting it.

In the presence of significant soft tissue injury, the injury should be stabilised with a standard spanning external fixator.

Definitive fixation of closed talar neck fractures was historically treated with the same degree of urgency as it was theorised that early stabilisation of the fracture would preserve the blood supply and lower the risk of AVN (10). However, recent evidence supports that the time to definitive fixation does not correlate to AVN risk (11). Therefore, as long as the fracture and the joints are reduced, delayed fixation should be performed once the soft tissues have settled, which may take up to 3 weeks (12).

> ### Learning Point
>
> Closed, displaced fractures should be reduced immediately. For irreducible dislocations, open reduction may be necessary, and for open fractures a spanning fixator allows soft tissue resuscitation. Definitive fixation may be delayed until the soft tissues settle without increasing the risk of AVN.

Surgical approaches

Combined anteromedial and anterolateral approaches are the classic approaches, which give optimal visualisation of the entire talar neck and allow direct anatomic reduction. The tolerance of the talus for malunion is slight and even a 3-degree varus malunion would result in subtalar joint dysfunction and stiffness (13). Therefore, notice should be taken of any evidence of comminution of the medial wall of the neck on CT as this makes reduction and fixation technically more difficult.

If there is significant dorsomedial wall comminution, it is not always possible to confirm reduction from the medial side and the lateral side may be the only reference point.

These approaches can be combined with medial and lateral malleolar osteotomies for access to the whole of the talar body except for the posterolateral corner. The anterior talar fibular ligament and calcaneofibular ligament can be released through an anterolateral approach to give access to most of the talus (except the posteromedial corner). Posterolateral and posteromedial approaches are small windows but maybe required depending on the location of the displaced talus.

Ultimately, the choice of surgical approach must be determined by the soft tissue envelope and any other bony injuries requiring fixation.

The patient should be positioned supine on the operating table with a sandbag under the ipsilateral buttock to bring the foot into a neutral position.

Anteromedial approach

The anteromedial incision is centered over the tip of the medial malleolus and extends in the intermuscular plane between tibialis anterior and tibialis posterior towards the medial talonavicular joint. The intact fibres of the deltoid ligament should be protected and dissection limited on the posterior aspect to prevent further injury to the remaining blood supply from the branches of the posterior tibial artery. This exposes the anteromedial talar body, the medal talar neck and the head.

If a medial malleolar osteotomy is required, it is easier to first insert two guidewires perpendicular to the osteotomy, drill and insert two partially threaded cancellous screws which pre-taps the final fixation and prevents shear of the osteotomy.

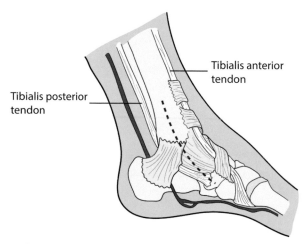

Figure 17.10 Anatomy for the anteromedial approach.

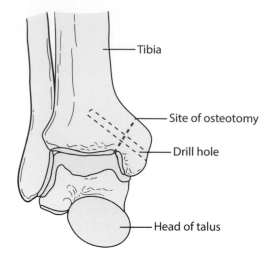

Figure 17.11 Line of the medial malleolar osteotomy and predrill holes.

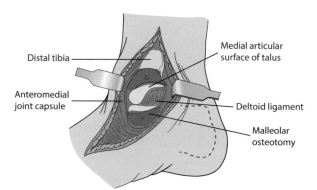

Figure 17.12 Anteromedial approach with malleolar osteotomy reflected.

The osteotomy should be performed with a microsagittal saw aiming to exit at the medial corner of the tibial plafond. Exiting too medially in the gutter is problematic as it will limit visualization and it is useful to insert a K-wire to radiologically check the exit point. The osteotomy should be completed with a thin osteotome to prevent damage to the talar articular surface and irregular fracture of the subchondral bone.

Once the osteotomy is complete, it can be carefully retracted distally on the deltoid ligament, preserving the deltoid vascular branches.

Anterolateral approach

The anterolateral incision extends from the tip of the lateral malleolus towards the fourth ray terminating at the talonavicular joint. The superficial peroneal nerve may cross the incision proximally and should be protected. The dissection is carried out sharply and full thickness flaps maintained. The extensor retinaculum is incised to

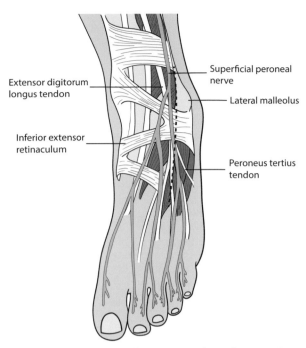

Extensor digitorum longus tendon

Inferior extensor retinaculum

Superficial peroneal nerve

Lateral malleolus

Peroneus tertius tendon

Figure 17.13 Anatomy for the anterolateral approach.

allow medial retraction of peroneus tertius and extensor digitorum brevis inferiorly.

This exposes the anterolateral talar body, lateral talar neck, lateral process and subtalar joint.

The use of a lateral malleolar osteotomy is rarely indicated and involves a two-plane osteotomy to preserve the attachments of the lateral ligament complex of the ankle. Releasing the ATFL and CFL allows anteromedial talar rotation giving access to a large portion of the talus, except the posteromedial corner of the talar body.

> ### Learning Point
>
> Most displaced talar neck fractures will require a combined anteromedial and anterolateral surgical approaches to ensure anatomic reduction. Care must be taken to ensure that the medial neck is out to length to prevent varus malunion.

Fixation

The principle of fixation is to achieve anatomic reduction and rigid fixation to facilitate early range of motion. The decision of what implant to use is primary determined by the configuration of the fracture pattern.

Lag screw fixation with two screws to control rotational forces is satisfactory for simple fracture patterns without comminution. They can be inserted anterograde, retrograde or, in combination, however retrograde fixation can have a propensity to flex and superiorly displace the head (14).

There are a few things to be aware of when using just screws.

1. Compression with lag screws will cause collapse and malunion if there is wall comminution.
2. They should be countersunk to prevent impingement at the talonavicular joint or headless screws can be used.
3. Anterograde screws are mechanically superior but can cause problems with penetration of the subtalar joint, damage to the FHL tendon, injury to the peroneal artery and screw head impingement (15).

Lateral plating has become a popular and effective fixation method especially with the development of customised implants. Plates act as a bridging construct and prevent collapse of the neck. They can be used in combination with a screw which would provide compression. This method is biomechanically as stable as two screws and allows a more accurate reduction (16).

The lateral plate sits in a sulcus above the sinus tarsi and is fixed with mini-fragment (2–2.7 mm) locking screws. Addition of a fully threaded positional screw down the medial column can increase the strength in severe comminution.

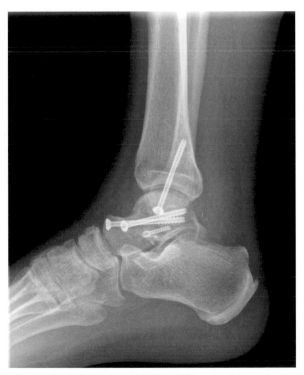

Figure 17.14 Type II talar neck fracture with two screw fixation.

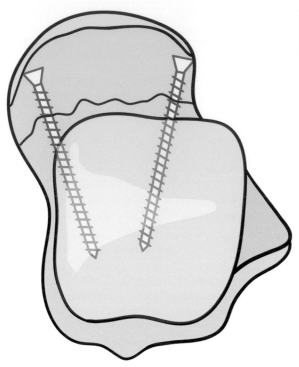

Figure 17.15 Ideal positioning of screws.

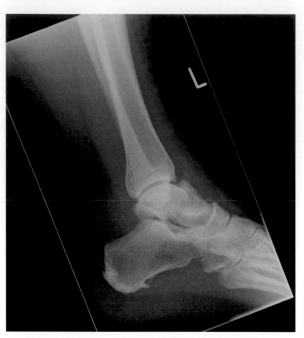

Figure 17.16 A 51-year-old female patient with a Type III talar neck fracture from a road traffic accident.

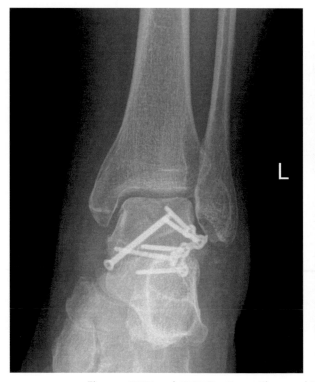

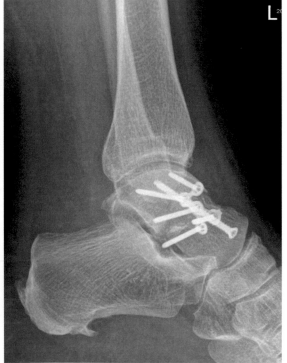

Figures 17.17 and 17.18 Fixation with a combination of screw and lateral plate fixation.

Bone grafting is not usually necessary but can be selectively utilised if there is a significant bone defect or there is concern regarding union.

Learning Point

Anterograde two screw fixation for fractures with a stable reduction is the easiest option. Posterior to anterior screws are fraught with problems due to the technical challenge of correct hardware positioning. For comminuted fractures, a lateral locking plate provides anatomic restoration without the risk of collapsing the neck with screw compression.

Postoperative care

The aims of postoperative care are to allow the surgical wound to heal, soft tissue injury to resolve, initiate early active motion and prevent weight-bearing until there is evidence of union and revascularisation of the bone.

A below knee non-weight-bearing plaster is recommended for 2 weeks or until the wounds have satisfactorily healed. Active motion can commence with a boot, but weight-bearing should be avoided for a minimum period of 6 weeks. Thereafter, progressive weight-bearing can be allowed over the next 6 weeks.

AVN of the talus can be identified using Hawkins sign. This is seen as a radiolucent line on an x-ray 6–8 weeks following the injury (Figure 17.19) and

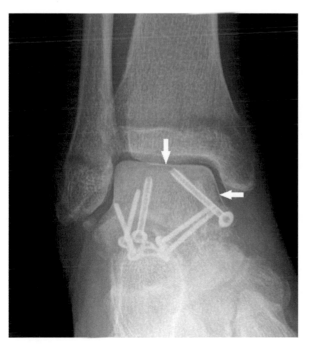

Figure 17.19 X-ray 6 weeks following fixation of Hawkins III fracture. White arrows demonstrating Hawkins sign.

indicates that the talus is unlikely to develop AVN. It is due to subchondral atrophy with a similar mechanism to disuse osteoporosis. It is a reliable test with a high sensitivity (17).

Learning Point

Hawkins sign seen after 6 weeks following injury is a positive sign that the patient is unlikely to develop AVN. The absence of the sign does not mean that the patient will develop AVN.

Complications

Infection and soft tissue problems

Deep infection is a significant concern and rates as high as 21% have been reported for closed injuries (5) and 38% for open fractures (18).

The risk of deep infection and soft tissue problems are minimised by following the key principles of surgical management. Emergency reduction of displaced fractures to protect the soft tissues, early surgical management of open or irreducible fractures and stabilisation with an external fixator. Otherwise, closed fractures should be managed when the soft tissues have recovered.

Avascular necrosis

In the original study, Hawkins reported overall AVN rates of 0%, 42% and 91% for Type I, II and III, respectively. However, this is a historical study which recommended practices such as deltoid release that have now been abandoned. In recent systematic reviews, the overall rates have improved and this reflects the shift in modern management with the use of CT, more favourable approaches and better fixation methods. The factors contributing to the risk relates to the severity of the injury, presence of comminution, open fractures and the presence of subtalar dislocation (8).

The radiographic definition of AVN in the literature is poor and most have reported incidence based on plain radiographic findings. Increased radiodensity compared to the contralateral side is the most common criteria appearing anywhere from 4 weeks to 6 months following the injury (9). MRI has limited utility in diagnosis since the images will be affected by the presence of metalwork, unless they are removed.

It is important to note that more than half of patients with radiographic changes of AVN will be asymptomatic and treatment should be based on clinical symptoms. Observation and activity modification with offloading should be considered for symptomatic patients; however, this has not been shown to affect the risk of talar dome collapse. In a third of patients, the talus will revascularise without collapse and this may take up to 2 years (19).

Malunions and non-unions

The rate of non-union is rare with an incidence of 5% (5). A more common problem is varus malunion at the talar neck (17%) and the key to avoiding this problem is careful planning to fix the fracture anatomically at the time of index surgery. Varus malunion results in pain, poor function of the subtalar joint and PTA (13). There should be a low threshold for CT scans postoperatively with a suspected malunion and it can be treated with a medially based opening wedge osteotomy.

Post-traumatic osteoarthritis (PTA)

PTA is the most common complication and affects any of the peritalar joints, the subtalar joint being the most commonly involved. Patients should be informed of this risk during consent. Whilst there may be radiographic evidence of OA, not all patients will be symptomatic and therefore conservative management options should always be tried first.

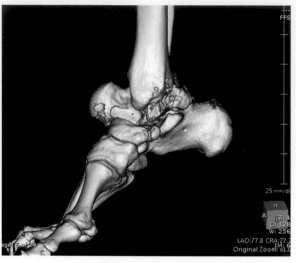

Figure 17.20 A 43-year-old male motorcyclist with a closed comminuted talar body fracture.

Learning Point

Complications are common following a talar neck fracture and patients should be informed of these risks pre-operatively. Major risks can be mitigated with good early soft tissue management, anatomic reconstruction and early mobilisation. AVN may develop over several months in the absence of Hawkins sign and follow-up is necessary to watch for talar collapse.

Talar body fractures

These fractures account for 20% of all fractures of the talus and are rarely an isolated injury. Boyd classified the injury according to the plane of fracture (20). A Type I is a coronal or sagittal plane fracture due to axial loading of the talus such as in a fall from a height and is the most common. A Type II fracture is a horizontal plane fracture. It has a similar mechanism to talar neck fractures and because of the involvement of the articular surfaces of the ankle and subtalar joints, they are almost always treated operatively.

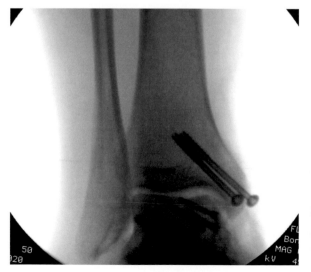
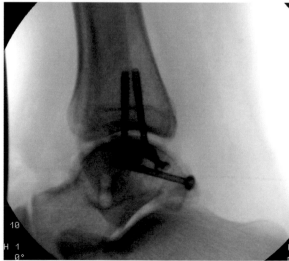

Figures 17.21 and 17.22 The fracture was irreducible therefore early fixation performed with medial malleolar osteotomy and headless screws.

Undisplaced or minimally displaced fractures can be difficult to detect radiographically and can be missed. CT should be performed with a high index of suspicion.

The same principles of initial management of talar neck fracture apply but internal fixation often requires the use of malleolar osteotomies to achieve direct visualisation of the talar body. Headless compression screws are often required for fixation.

Talar body fractures have been associated with a high incidence of complications including AVN and OA of the ankle and subtalar joints (21).

Talar head fractures

The talar head is the least commonly fractured part and is sustained when the foot is plantarflexed and an axial load applied to it. They are often intra-articular and may present as part of a high energy talar neck injury or undergo insufficiency fracture in elderly patients (22).

The key difference is that the talar head receives a good blood supply, and therefore is much less prone to AVN.

The aim of treatment is to maintain congruity and stability of the talonavicular joint and an isolated undisplaced or impacted fracture without disruption of the joint can be managed non-operatively.

In a displaced fracture, fixation is advised. Where direct fixation with headless screws is not possible, the talonavicular joint may need to be bridged with a locking plate to hold the joint out to length.

Talar process fractures

Fractures of the talar processes are uncommon and are frequently missed due to a low level of suspicion and difficulty in diagnosis with plain radiographs. Early diagnosis and management is important to prevent long-term complications such as non-union, malunion and subtalar joint OA.

Lateral process fractures

Despite being the second most common fracture of the talus, they are frequently misdiagnosed as ankle sprains. Since it was first reported in 1943, the fracture has recently been termed "Snowboarder's ankle". This relates to the high-energy mechanism of injury where there is forced impact upon a dorsiflexed ankle with the foot everted.

The fracture is best seen on a mortise view of the ankle and the extent of involvement of the subtalar joint can be visualised using a Broden's view. Van Knoch described the "V-sign" where on the lateral x-ray the lateral process normally produces a distinct V shape above the angle of Gissane and this is disrupted with a fracture (23). The involvement of the subtalar joint is often underestimated radiographically, and therefore CT is considered the gold standard investigation.

Hawkins first classified these injuries into three types (24). Bladin reordered the original classification to reflect the severity of the injury and this is mistakenly referred to as Hawkins classification and is in use today (25).

- Type I – Chip fracture
- Type II – Simple large fragment
- Type III – Comminuted fracture

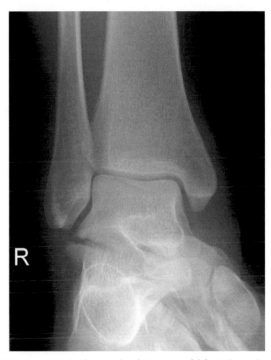

Figure 17.23 Radiograph of 36-year-old female with a displaced Type II fracture.

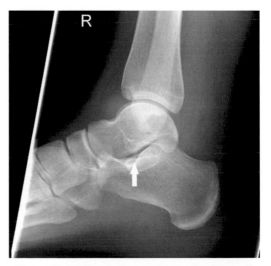

Figure 17.24 White arrow indicates the "V-sign".

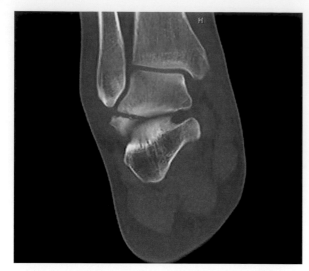

Figure 17.25 CT confirms incongruity of the subtalar joint.

Treatment depends upon the size, degree of displacement and comminution. The aim is to achieve union with congruence of the subtalar joint as well as competence of the talocalcaneal ligament.

Type I fractures are extra-articular, and therefore can be treated with a short period of immobilisation and early motion.

Type II fractures are dependent upon the size of the fragment and degree of displacement at the subtalar joint. Small undisplaced fragments <1 cm with <2 mm displacement can be treated with non-weight-bearing immobilisation for 4–6 weeks. Larger fragments >1 cm or those displaced >2 mm can cause instability of the subtalar joint and incompetence of the talocalcaneal ligament, and therefore fixation with headless screws is recommended.

Type III fractures can be technically challenging to fix. Those that defy internal fixation can be managed with immobilisation with subsequent excision of loose fragments. It is preferable however to achieve stability with screws or a buttress plate with excision of loose fragments acutely (25).

The surgical approach is the anterolateral approach as described previously (talar neck fracture).

> ### Learning Point
> Lateral talar process fractures are often difficult to diagnose radiographically, and missed fractures are prone to non-union, subtalar instability and OA. Displaced fractures should be reduced and fixed to restore congruity of the subtalar joint.

Posterior process fractures

The posterior process of the talus consists of medial and lateral tubercles separated by the groove for the FHL tendon. It articulates with the posterior facet of the subtalar joint. The lateral tubercle lies posteriorly and provides the attachment for the posterior talofibular and talocalcaneal ligaments. The medial tubercle provides the attachment for the deltoid and talocalcaneal ligaments.

Fractures of the entire posterior process are rare and these injuries usually involve the posterolateral process called Shepherd's or Steida process fracture. The posteromedial process is called Cedell's fracture from the original description (26).

Both present in a similar manner to an ankle sprain and are often missed or misdiagnosed as an os trigonum. The mechanism is most likely due to forced plantarflexion resulting in a "nutcracker" effect between the tibial plafond and the calcaneum. The os trigonum itself may also fracture, which highlights the importance of careful clinical examination. Patients will present with posterior ankle tenderness with pain on passive movement of the subtalar joint and on passive movement of the FHL tendon.

A high index of suspicion should be kept, and an urgent CT scan requested to delineate the size, displacement and comminution of the fragment.

Small fragments may be treated non-operatively; however, larger fragments should be reduced and fixed using either the posteromedial or posterolateral approaches described previously (ankle fracture).

> ### Learning Point
> Posterior process fractures are often mistaken for an os trigonum which is only present in 10% of individuals. There should be a high index of suspicion for fractures and clinical examination should determine the need for further investigation with a CT.

Take home messages

- Due to a tenuous bloody supply, the talus is prone to avascular necrosis and therefore the surgical approach must take into consideration the vascular network to minimise this risk.
- Due to the high energy nature of displaced talar neck fractures, up to a third of patients with present with an open injury.
- Hawkins sign seen after 6 weeks following injury is a positive sign that the patient is unlikely to develop AVN.
- Internal fixation of talar head fractures often requires the use of malleolar osteotomies to achieve direct visualisation of the talar body.

- Fractures of the talar processes are uncommon and are frequently missed due to a low level of suspicion and difficulty in diagnosis with plain radiographs.

References

1. Haliburton RA, Sullivan CR, Kelly PJ, Peterson LF. The extra-osseous and intra-osseous blood supply of the talus. J Bone Joint Surg Am. 1958; 40(5):1115–1120.
2. Miller AN, Prasarn ML, Dyke JP, Helfet DL, Lorich DG. Quantitative assessment of the vascularity of the talus with gadolinium-enhanced magnetic resonance imaging. J Bone Joint Surg. 2011; 93(12):1116–1121.
3. Hawkins L. Fractures of the neck of the talus. J Bone Joint Surg Am. 1970; 52(5):991–1002.
4. Canale ST, Kelly FB. Fractures of the neck of the talus. Long-term evaluation of seventy-one cases. J Bone Joint Surg Am. 1978; 60(2):143–156.
5. Halvorson JJ, Winter SB, Teasdall RD, Scott AT. Talar neck fractures: A systematic review of the literature. J Foot Ankle Surg. 2013; 52(1):56–61.
6. Dodd A, Lefaivre KA. Outcomes of talar neck fractures: A systematic review and meta-analysis. J Orthop Trauma. 2015; 29(5):210–215.
7. Jordan RK, Bafna KR, Liu J, Ebraheim NA. Complications of talar neck fractures by Hawkins classification: A systematic review. J Foot Ankle Surg. 2017; 56(4):817–821.
8. Vallier HA, Reichard SG, Boyd AJ, Moore TA. A new look at the Hawkins classification for talar neck fractures: Which features of injury and treatment are predictive of osteonecrosis? J Bone Joint Surg Surg Am. 2014; 96(3):192–197.
9. Buza JA, Leucht P. Fractures of the talus: Current concepts and new developments. Foot Ankle Surg. 2018; 24(4):282–290.
10. Grear BJ. Review of talus fractures and surgical timing. Orthop Clin North Am. 2016; 47(3):625–637.
11. Vallier HA. Fractures of the talus: State of the art. J Orthop Trauma. 2015; 29(9):385–392.
12. Patel R, Van Bergeyk A, Pinney S. Are displaced talar neck fractures surgical emergencies? A survey of orthopaedic trauma experts. Foot Ankle Int. 2005; 26(5):378–381.
13. Daniels TR, Smith JW, Ross TI. Varus malalignment of the talar neck. Its effect on the position of the foot and on subtalar motion. J Bone Joint Surg Am. 1996; 78(10):1559–1567.
14. Abdelkafy A, Imam MA, Sokkar S, Hirschmann M. Antegrade-retrograde opposing lag screws for internal fixation of simple displaced talar neck fractures. J Foot Ankle Surg. 2015; 54(1):23–28.
15. Beltran MJ, Mitchell PM, Collinge CA. Posterior to anteriorly directed screws for management of talar neck fractures. Foot Ankle Int. 2016; 37(10):1130–1136.
16. Attiah M, Sanders DW, Valdivia G, Cooper I, Ferreira L, MacLeod MD, Johnson JA. Comminuted talar neck fractures: A mechanical comparison of fixation techniques. J Orthop Trauma. 2007; 21(1):47–51.
17. Tezval M, Dumont C, Stürmer KM. Prognostic reliability of the Hawkins sign in fractures of the talus. J Orthop Trauma. 2007; 21(8):538–543.
18. Marsh JL, Saltzman CL, Iverson M, Shapiro DS. Major open injuries of the talus. J Orthop Trauma. 1995; 9(5):371–376.
19. Maher MH, Chauhan A, Altman GT, Westrick ER. The acute management and associated complications of major injuries of the talus. J Bone Joint Surg Rev. 2017; 5(7):1–11.
20. Boyd HB, Knight RA. Fractures of the astragalus. South Med J. 1942; 35:160–167.
21. Vallier HA, Nork SE, Benirschke SK, Sangeorzan BJ. Surgical treatment of talar body fractures. J Bone Joint Surg Am. 2003; 85(9):1716–1724.
22. Long NM, Zoga AC, Kier R, Kavanagh EC. Insufficiency and nondisplaced fractures of the talar head: MRI appearances. AJR Am J Roentgenol. 2012; 199(5):613–617.
23. Von Knoch F, Reckord U, Von Knoch M, Sommer C. Fracture of the lateral process of the talus in snowboarders. J Bone Joint Surg Br. 2007; 89(6):772–777.
24. Hawkins LG. Fracture of the lateral process of the talus. J Bone Joint Surg Am. 1965; 47:1170–1175.
25. Bladin C, McCrory P. Snowboarding injuries: An overview. Sports Med. 1995; 19:358–364.
26. Cedell CA. Rupture of the posterior talotibial ligament with the avulsion of a bone fragment from the talus. Acta Orthop Scand. 1974; 45:454–461.

18 | Calcaneal fractures

Devendra Mahadevan and Adam Sykes

Introduction

Fractures of the calcaneum have a reported yearly incidence of around 12 per 100,000 population, with fractures occurring 2–3 times more often in males and at a younger average age compared to their female counterparts. The most common mechanism for the injury is due to a fall and this is most often from heights of over 6 feet. Due to this, there is a strong association between calcaneal fractures and people who work at height, such as scaffolders and roofers. However, there are many other high-risk activities that contribute to the number of calcaneal fractures presenting to the Emergency Department. The mechanism of axial loading through the calcaneum will also transmit energy higher up in the musculoskeletal system and so there are several commonly associated injuries, including ipsilateral lower limb fractures (especially of the tibial plateau) and fractures of the vertebrae. These should be actively examined for when a calcaneal fracture has been found (1, 2).

Anatomy of the calcaneum (Figure 18.1)

The calcaneum is a complex, irregular bone in appearance, with several prominences and articular surfaces.

The main bulk of the bone, known as the body, is ovoid in cross-section with densely packed cancellous bone and comparatively thin cortical walls. This gives it a degree of flexibility to act as a shock absorber when the heel strikes the floor.

Posteriorly sits the calcaneal tuberosity which represents the attachment point for the Achilles tendon. The plantar continuation of the tuberosity splits into a medial and lateral process. The medial side is the origin of the plantar fascia and flexor digitorum brevis muscle and transmits the force of the gastrocsoleus complex forward into the foot. The lateral process is comparably smaller and acts as the origin of the abductor digiti minimi muscle.

A flat process called the sustentaculum tali projects medially and acts like a shelf to support the middle facet of the subtalar joint. Underneath it sits the flexor hallucis longus tendon which uses the process as a pulley as it changes direction moving forwards into the foot. The sustentaculum tali has strong attachments to the medial malleolus via the deltoid ligament and the navicular via the spring ligament. Due to this, it is held in place when the calcaneum is fractured and is therefore often referred to as the "constant fragment" which can subsequently be used to rebuild the calcaneum around.

The anterior process of the calcaneum projects forward into the foot from the body until it forms the calcaneocuboid joint. The bifurcate ligament connects the superior part of the anterior process to the cuboid and the navicular. On the superomedial surface of the anterior process sits the anterior facet of the subtalar joint which is widened by a fibrocartilaginous plate. It provides further support to the head of the talus and creates the ball and socket appearance of the talocalcaneonavicular (TCN) joint.

The anterior and middle facets of the subtalar joint are joined by the posterior facet that sits on the anterosuperior surface of the body of the calcaneum. Together they cradle the talus and allow the subtalar motion that ranges from an inverted/plantarflexed position to an everted/dorsiflexed position.

The blood supply to the calcaneum comes from both the posterior tibial and peroneal arteries. On the medial side, the posterior tibial first gives off a posterior branch to supply the body of the calcaneum, followed by the artery of the tarsal canal. It then loops under the sustentaculum tali and splits into the medial and lateral plantar arteries, giving off branches along the way to the sustentaculum tali itself and the anterior process. On the lateral side the peroneal artery gives off multiple small branches to the lateral side of the calcaneum as well as the artery of the sinus tarsi, which anastomoses with the artery of the tarsal canal (3).

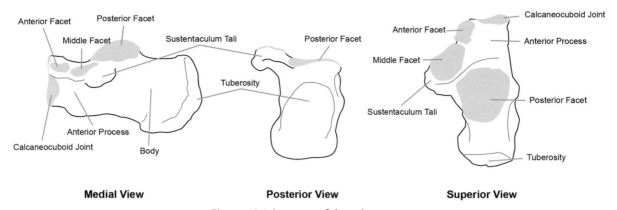

Figure 18.1 Anatomy of the calcaneum.

Types of fracture and classification systems

Fractures of the calcaneum can broadly be divided into fractures, which involve the posterior facet of the subtalar joint and fractures that do not (4). Each of these divisions can then be further sub-classified.

Fractures involving the posterior facet

Around 75% of calcaneal fractures involve the posterior facet of the subtalar joint. They result from axial loading injuries which drive the wedge shape of the lateral process of the talus into the corresponding v-shaped recess that makes up the floor of the sinus tarsi.

Essex Lopresti described two types of fracture from plain lateral radiographs: tongue- and depression-types. In both types, a vertical fracture is seen on the lateral radiograph that detaches the anterior process from the rest of the calcaneum. A second fracture line is also seen running in a more horizontal plane (Figure 18.2).

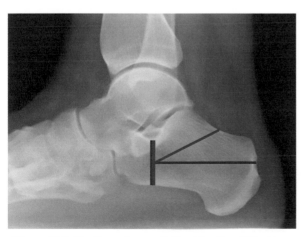

Figure 18.2 The Essex-Lopresti Classification. This demonstrates the tongue-type (red) and depression-type (blue) fracture lines as described from plain radiographs.

In depressed-type fractures, this second fracture line exits the superior part of the body of the calcaneum, thus detaching the posterior facet was from the rest of the bone. In tongue-type fractures, the horizontal fracture exits more posteriorly through the tuberosity itself, creating a shelf of bone.

Computerised tomography (CT) revolutionised the understanding of the complexity of calcaneal fracture patterns. The horizontal fracture lines seen on radiographs are in fact oblique in both the axial and coronal planes on CT. This obliquity determines whether or not a fracture line exits through the articular surface of the subtalar joint (5). Furthermore, fragmentation at the posterior facet was frequently observed. Sanders developed a CT based classification of calcaneal fractures that describes the number of articular surface fragments that are displaced by more than 2 mm (Figure 18.3) (6).

Fractures not involving the posterior facet

Anterior process fractures

Fractures of the anterior process occur when there is either a plantarflexion and inversion or dorsiflexion and eversion force applied to the foot. With plantarflexion and inversion the bifurcate ligament causes an avulsion fracture of its insertion on the superior aspect of the anterior process. These fragments are usually small and easily missed on plain radiographs, and do not involve a significant portion of the articular surface. As the mechanism, presentation and bruising are similar, they are often associated with or mistaken for lateral ankle sprains. Dorsiflexion and eversion of the foot creates a compression force through the lateral column of the foot, often referred to as a 'Nutcracker' injury. These are high energy injuries that result in fractures involving the anterior process of the calcaneum and the cuboid and may even have associated disruption or subluxation of the entire Chopart joint (7).

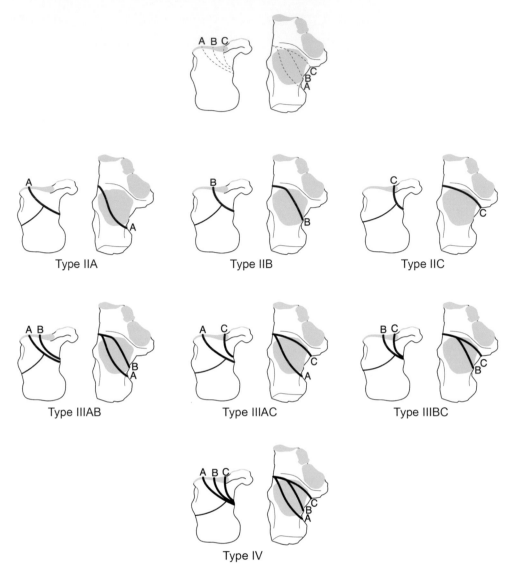

Figure 18.3 The Sanders Classification represented by axial and coronal diagrams of the calcaneum. A, B and C represent the potential fracture lines for fractures involving the posterior facet. Fragments are only counted as separate if they are displaced by more than 2 mm. Type I fractures have no displaced fragments. Type II and III fractures have two or three fragments, respectively. Type IV fractures have four or more fragments.

Sustentaculum tali fractures

Isolated fractures of the sustentaculum tali are rare, and therefore there is little literature written about them. The mechanism is thought to be through axial loading with the foot inverted. The fractures that occur will have a varying degree of displacement depending on the amount of energy transferred and may or may not involve the middle facet of the subtalar joint. As the sustentaculum tali is a vital load-bearing structure that supports the medial arch, fractures involving it may have significant consequences for future foot shape and hindfoot function if they are not appropriately managed. On plain AP and lateral radiographs of the ankle and foot, this injury may be missed, and therefore CT imaging should be used if there is significant clinical suspicion (8).

Tuberosity fractures

Tuberosity fractures account for 1–2% of all calcaneal fractures and represent a type of avulsion fracture that defunctions all or part of the Achilles tendon. They usually occur in patients with poor bone quality and are therefore associated with osteoporosis, diabetes and peripheral neuropathy. The most accepted classification of these fractures is by Lee et al. (9) (Figure 18.4).

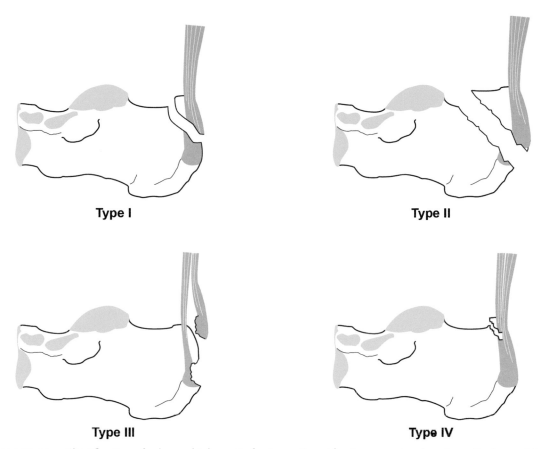

Type I

Type II

Type III

Type IV

Figure 18.4 Lee Classification of calcaneal tuberosity fractures. Type I fractures are simple extra-articular avulsion of the whole Achilles insertion. Type II fractures involve a 'beak' of bone and may threaten the overlying skin. Type III and IV fractures are an avulsion of only the superficial and deep fibres, respectively.

Presentation and examination

Patients with calcaneal fractures will present with pain and swelling around the hindfoot with difficulty or complete inability to bear weight through the affected limb. The mechanism of injury may give clues to the type of fracture that has occurred and any other potential injuries. A focused history detailing their level of activity, occupation, co-morbidities and smoking status will help to guide the appropriate treatment path for the individual.

The bruising found may be extensive and fracture blisters are common, especially if there is any delay in presentation. It is important to examine the integrity of the overlying soft tissues as the bony deformity may create open fractures or threaten the vascularity to the skin, particularly in beak-type tuberosity fractures.

Knowledge of the anatomy of the hindfoot is essential to determine which structures are tender, and therefore may be damaged. The anterior process of the calcaneum lies more anteriorly in the foot to the anterior talo-fibular ligament (ATFL) and so tenderness here

after an inversion injury should alert the examiner to the possible presence of a fracture (7). There is also an association between calcaneal fractures and peroneal sheath injuries resulting in tendon subluxation (10), and therefore tenderness and swelling posteriorly to the distal fibula should raise suspicion of this injury. A palpable defect or swelling and tenderness at the Achilles tendon insertion may alert to the presence of a tuberosity fracture. Sustentaculum tali fractures produce extensive bruising and swelling in the medial arch, extending into the plantar aspect of the foot.

It is important to assess and document the neurological and vascular status of the foot. Doppler assessment of the dorsalis pedis and posterior tibial arteries may be required when the swelling is significant. A good blood supply will be essential for the foot to heal if any operative intervention is undertaken and may guide towards non-operative management if there are concerns. Compartment syndrome of the foot is said to occur in up to 10% of all calcaneal fractures and should be suspected in a foot that is tensely swollen with increasing pain not responding to analgesia (11).

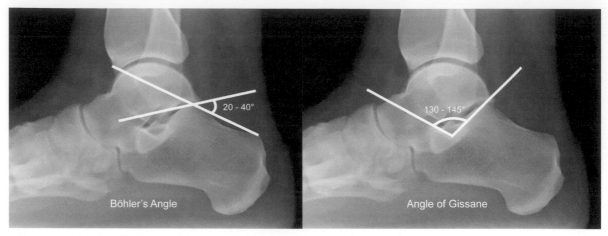

Figure 18.5 Angles of Böhler and Gissane. These angles represent the normal anatomy. A Böhler's angle of less than 20 degrees or an angle of Gissane of less than 120 degrees suggests a depression of the posterior facet of the subtalar joint in keeping with a fracture.

Imaging

Plain radiographs

If a calcaneal fracture is suspected then an anterior to posterior (AP) and a lateral view of the ankle may be enough to confirm the diagnosis. The AP view can give an idea of the width (lateral wall displacement) and to a lesser degree the varus or valgus angulation of the calcaneum. The lateral view will allow for measurement of the angles described by Böhler and Gissane (Figure 18.5). These angles help to show the severity of depression of the posterior facet.

In addition, calcaneal axial and Broden's views can give further information about the fracture pattern. A calcaneal axial view is taken with the ankle in maximal dorsiflexion; the x-ray is beamed at a 40-degree angle to the plantar surface of the foot (Figure 18.6). This gives good visualisation of the body and tuberosity and will show if the heel appears widened. It is also one of the best views for imaging isolated sustentaculum tali fractures.

Before the advent of CT, Broden's views were the best method of imaging the posterior facet of the subtalar joint. They are still commonly used in theatre to

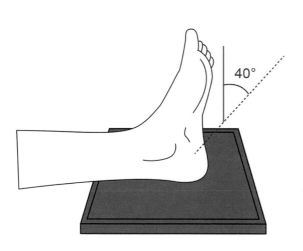

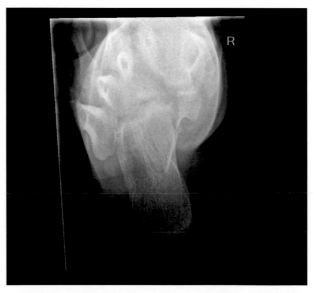

Figure 18.6 Calcaneal axial view. The red dotted line represents the beam of the x-rays which should be at 40 degrees to the sole of the foot. The radiograph shows the view that this creates and a sustentaculum tali fracture is demonstrated.

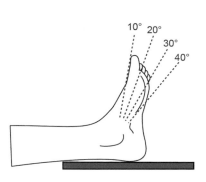 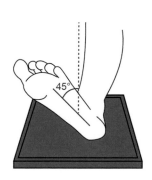 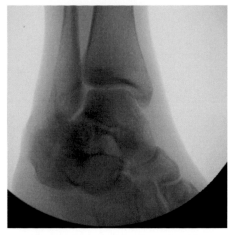

Figure 18.7 Broden's views. The solid red line shows the foot internally rotated by 45 degrees. The dotted red lines represent the x-ray beam angles. The image intensifier capture shows an intra-operative view demonstrating the posterior facet of the subtalar joint in this fracture.

assess reduction of the posterior facet. Starting with the image intensifier in the vertical position and the patient supine, the knee is first slightly flexed. With the ankle in a neutral position, the entire leg is internally rotated by 45 degrees. The beam is then angled and images are taken at 10-degree increments between 10 and 40 degrees of cephalic tilt to show the congruity of the posterior facet from the posterior to the anterior portions of the curved surface (Figure 18.7).

Computerised tomography (CT)

Modern helical scanners are able to take multiple fine slices through the bone to allow high resolution images and reliable reconstructions in any plane. The ankle, if uninjured, is typically used as a reference to determine the axial, sagittal and coronal planes for reformatting. Furthermore, digital subtraction can allow for three-dimensional modelling, further enhancing the surgeon's understanding of the fracture. This information helps to guide the treatment options and provide the patient with an idea of future prognosis.

Magnetic resonance imaging (MRI)

MRI is rarely required in the acute setting of calcaneal fractures as most injuries will be found with the other imaging modalities. It may be useful in looking for soft tissue injuries around the hindfoot. In subacute heel pain without trauma, it is the best method for diagnosing stress fractures of the calcaneum (see Chapter 10).

Management

Initial management

The initial management of calcaneal fractures should focus on the assessment and protection of the overlying soft tissues. Tongue-type and tuberosity fractures can put significant pressure on the skin overlying the posterior heel, causing ischaemia and necrosis. If the soft tissues appear under threat, then emergent reduction of the fracture should be undertaken. This can either be through manipulation and splintage in an equinus position, or, ideally if the expertise are available, through percutaneous reduction and fixation.

Open fractures should be managed in line with the guidance from the British Orthopaedic Association Standards for Trauma (BOAST) (12). Wounds should be photographed for medical records before being covered with saline soaked gauze and an occlusive dressing before any splintage is applied. Surgical management should be undertaken in a centre that is able to provide combined orthopaedic and plastics expertise. Early surgical debridement should be undertaken with fixation and definitive soft tissue coverage at the same time if possible and certainly within 72 hours.

If no immediate threat or compromise to the skin is present, then high elevation and rest will help to reduce swelling, and therefore diminish the chance of forming fracture blisters. The application of ice or a cooling device can also be of benefit in achieving this.

Decision-making in surgical versus non-surgical management

A tailored approach to calcaneal injuries should be used in order to take into account the nature of the fracture and the rest of the patient that surrounds it. Early counselling regarding the severity of the injury and their involvement in the decision-making process will help to keep the patient informed of their likely prognosis and outcome after treatment. Poor wound healing and subsequent infection are the most common complications after surgical management and so smoking status, diabetes and peripheral vascular disease may guide towards a non-operative route. The surgeon should also be wary of patients who may not be compliant with postoperative instructions, as rest and elevation are the most reliable ways of ensuring that the wounds heal promptly.

The goal of treatment is to retain the mobility and function of the hindfoot as much as possible and produce a foot that is able to fit into shoes after treatment. The reduction of intra-articular fractures will also hopefully reduce the chance of post-traumatic arthritis and ongoing pain.

Minimally displaced intra-articular posterior facet fractures and extra-articular fractures without significant deformation of the shape of the heel have good outcomes with non-operative management. Fractures involving the attachment of the Achilles tendon can be managed non-operatively providing there is minimal displacement and should be monitored to ensure there is no late displacement due to the pull of the gastrocsoleus complex (13). Fractures involving the anterior process of the calcaneum in isolation can also be treated without surgery and should expect a good outcome (14).

The management of displaced fractures involving the posterior facet of the subtalar joint has been debated for some time. Sanders (6) showed excellent or good clinical outcomes following surgery in 73% of Type II and 70% of Type III fractures, but only 9% of Type IV fractures.

Buckley et al. in their randomised controlled trial showed that surgical management led to better outcomes in a subgroup of patients (e.g., not receiving worker's compensation, female, younger patients <29 years old) (15).

In 2014, the UK Heel Fracture Trial reported similar 2-year results in calcaneal fractures treated with either operative or non-operative management (16). There was a trend towards better outcomes for patients treated surgically with Sanders II fractures; although the study was inadequately powered to formally assess this difference. There were higher complication rates in both the surgically treated groups (15, 16).

In the two randomised controlled trials discussed earlier (15, 16), an extensile lateral surgical approach and plating fixation techniques were used. Although this is the established method for fixation, there have been advances in minimally invasive techniques. These have been shown to have favourable results, albeit with a steep learning curve (17, 18). They are associated with a significantly lower complication rate than the extensile approach.

In all studies, Sanders Type IV fractures demonstrated poorer outcomes compared to the less fragmented fractures, regardless of management strategy. There have been several small studies assessing the feasibility of a primary subtalar fusion for these injuries, working on the assumption that they will develop painful subtalar arthritis in the future as a result of the injury. A small randomised controlled trial by Buckley et al. (19) compared the traditional open reduction and internal fixation approach to primary subtalar arthrodesis. They found that the functional outcomes at 2 years were the same for both groups and concluded that in the right patient, the fusion procedure may be the correct choice.

Non-surgical management

If a non-surgical plan is chosen, a period of immobilisation is undertaken to allow the soft tissues to settle. This is usually in the form of a backslab or boot to allow for post-injury swelling. In fractures involving the insertion of the Achilles tendon this should be in an equinus position to remove the tension from the pull of the gastrocsoleus complex and help to prevent late displacement (13). In all other cases this should be in a neutral ankle position to prevent contracture of the Achilles tendon. Patients should be reassessed after 1–2 weeks once the soft tissues have settled and early range of motion should be commenced of the ankle and subtalar joint to prevent stiffness. Non–weight-bearing should be undertaken for at least 6 weeks where possible to prevent further displacement of the fracture, followed by a progressive increase in weight-bearing thereafter (15, 16).

Surgical techniques for fractures involving the posterior facet

Open reduction and internal fixation (Figure 18.8)

Calcaneal fractures have traditionally been approached and fixed through an extended, lateral approach with an L-shaped incision that was first described by Zwipp et al. in 1988 (20). The incision has a vertical limb positioned midway between the posterior edge of the fibula and the edge of the Achilles tendon and a horizontal limb at the junction between the plantar and dorsal skin of the foot. The two limbs are joined by a curve to prevent necrosis of the tip of the flap (Figure 18.9).

A full thickness flap is raised through this incision all the way down to the calcaneum, including the periosteum in order to maintain the blood supply through the lateral calcaneal artery. At the proximal and distal ends of the incision, there is a risk of iatrogenic injury to the sural nerve and so careful dissection should be undertaken. The flap can be sharply elevated and the calcaneofibular ligament divided to expose the posterior facet of the subtalar joint, the sinus tarsi and the calcaneocuboid joint allowing an excellent view for fixation. The peroneal tendons should be retracted superiorly with the flap.

The approach allows direct visualisation and reduction of the fracture fragments onto the "constant"

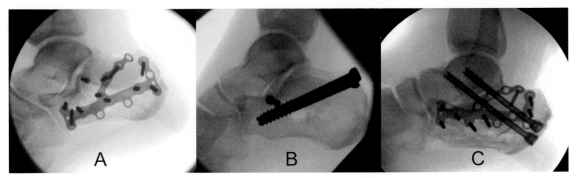

Figure 18.8 Intra-operative imaging. Showing the position after an extensile approach and plate fixation (A), minimally open fixation (B) and extensile approach, plate fixation and primary subtalar fusion (C).

sustentaculum tali fragment. Fixation can be through individual screw placement or plating to support the posterior facet, maintain hind foot alignment and compress the lateral wall.

Minimally invasive fixation (Figure 18.8)

Due to the wound complications seen with the traditional open approach, minimally invasive procedures have been popularised to reduce the soft tissue insult from surgery. Through a combination of percutaneous

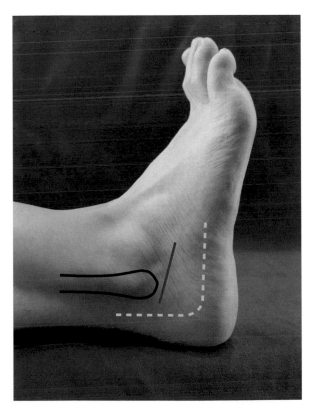

Figure 18.9 Incisions for an extensile lateral approach (blue dotted line) and sinus tarsi approach (red line).

and mini-open approaches it is possible to reduce the fracture fragments, assess the reduction where necessary and place fixation to hold the fragments in place. The use of image intensifier guidance is of paramount importance in positioning screws and assessing the reduction.

Arthroscopically assisted fixation

The use of an arthroscope to assess the congruency of the posterior facet of the subtalar joint has been gaining popularity over the last 10 years. This technique allows better visualisation of the articular surface (21) and can be used to fine tune the reduction before internal fixation.

Primary subtalar fusion (Figure 18.8)

The goal of primary subtalar fusion is not only to achieve a solid arthrodesis, but also to restore the normal shape and alignment of the hindfoot. Reduction of the fracture is the initial step in the procedure in order to return to a more anatomical shape before the fusion is undertaken. The choice of reduction technique can be either open or minimally invasive; the articular cartilage is then removed using flexible osteotomes, nibblers and/or high speed burrs. The use of structural bone graft may be required if there are large defects created by the fracture pattern. Internal fixation is undertaken using screws alone or in combination with a plate to maintain fracture reduction and secure the fusion.

Surgical techniques for fractures not involving the posterior facet

Tuberosity fracture fixation

A displaced tuberosity fracture can result in pressure necrosis of the skin overlying the heel. Surgical treatment is therefore aimed at urgently reducing any tension on the soft tissues and restoring the function of the gastrocsoleus complex. As bone quality is often poor in patients with these injuries, percutaneous lag screw fixation alone may not be sufficient enough to counteract the pull of the Achilles tendon (13). Augmentation with bone anchors sutured onto the Achilles tendon has been described to prevent failure of the fixation. Tightness of the gastrocnemius muscle is often a feature and is thought to contribute to the pathogenesis of the injury. Surgical release prior to fixation has therefore been advocated to aid in reduction and prevent further sequelae in the future.

Sustentaculum tali fracture fixation (Figure 18.10)

The sustentaculum tali is an important support for the medial arch of the foot. Displaced fractures will disrupt the middle facet of the subtalar joint, can lead to hindfoot varus and may cause problems with the excursion of the flexor hallucis longus tendon inferiorly. Anatomic reduction and rigid fixation will help to prevent potential complications. A medial skin incision along the line of the tibialis posterior tendon over the sustentaculum tali will expose the sheath of the underlying tendon. A safe approach through the bed of the sheath will allow for dorsal retraction of the posterior tibial tendon and plantar retraction of the flexor digitorum longus and flexor hallucis longus tendons, protecting the neurovascular bundle inferiorly. This exposes the sustentacular process and the medial wall of the calcaneum allowing for anatomical reduction of the fracture and fixation with screws or with a small plate (8).

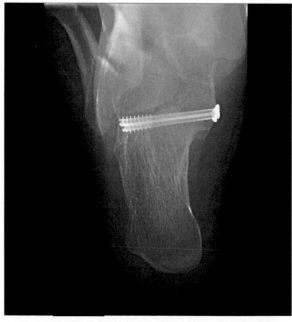

Figure 18.10 Postoperative imaging. Showing fixation of the sustentaculum tali with two cannulated screws.

Complications and how to manage them

Soft tissue necrosis

Soft tissue complications can occur acutely at the time of injury or later as a result of the further insult of surgery. The soft tissue envelope should be assessed at the time of injury, as any impending problems should be addressed urgently. Ice, elevation and careful monitoring should be implemented to ensure that swelling and subsequent tissue hypoxia is kept to a minimum.

After surgery, wound healing problems and skin breakdown are the most common complications (22). In the extended, lateral approach, breakdown usually originates from the tip of the flap created and extends along each limb of the incision thereafter. Avoidance of weight-bearing, rest, elevation and monitoring for signs of infection will allow the tissues a chance to recover. An early plastic surgical opinion should be sought.

Infection

Wound infections can be managed with antibiotics. However, the use of antibiotics for deep infections is controversial and should be guided by a microbiologist with a good knowledge of orthopaedic infections. If deep infection occurs then suppressive antibiotics may be used to control its progression until union of the fracture, followed by removal of the metalwork, thorough debridement of any contaminated tissues and achievement of soft tissue coverage. These procedures often require multiple areas of expertise and may be best managed in a tertiary setting.

Post-traumatic arthritis

Calcaneal fractures may result in post-traumatic arthritis of the subtalar or calcaneocuboid joints. The two factors that have been shown to correlate with the likelihood of developing arthritis are the severity of initial displacement and the accuracy of the reduction of the articular surfaces (22). Pain on walking on uneven surfaces and a stiff subtalar joint should alert to the presence of arthritis. There may also be evidence of a loss of joint space in the posterior facet of the subtalar joint on plain radiograph or CT scanning. MRI can help to confirm the diagnosis, but may be difficult to interpret if there is significant artefact created by the adjacent metalwork. Initial treatment should be through the use of anti-inflammatories, activity modification and the use of orthotics to support the foot shape and attempt to offload the subtalar joint. If this fails then a subtalar arthrodesis may be able to offer the patient relief of their symptoms.

Malunion

The alteration to the shape of the heel, especially in non-operative management, can lead to several problems.

The widened heel can make shoe fitting problematic, and therefore custom made orthotics may be required. Displacement of the lateral wall may lead to irritation of the peroneal tendons or, if extreme, may lead to abutment against the tip of the fibula leading to impingement pain. This may be further exacerbated if the calcaneum has united in a valgus alignment. Alternatively, a varus malunion may result in overload of the lateral border of the foot and ankle with lateral foot pain and callosities, fifth metatarsal stress fractures and weakening of the lateral ankle ligaments.

CT imaging can be useful in understanding the morphology of the calcaneus and for surgical planning. MRI imaging can be useful in assessing the peroneal tendons and showing bony oedema in fibula impingement.

Significant malunions with symptoms may require complex, multiplanar osteotomies to restore alignment and shape. Patients with symptoms from lateral wall impingement can be managed effectively through exostectomy of the lateral wall. Any co-existing issues with the peroneal tendons can also be dealt with using the same approach.

Take home messages

- Always check for other injuries associated with the mechanism.
- Assess the soft tissue envelope and protect it with rest, elevation and ice.
- CT imaging will help to understand the fracture and be able to guide both management and prognosis by using the Sanders Classification.
- The management plan should be tailored to both the patient and the fracture pattern.
- Postoperative complications are not uncommon and can cause significant morbidity.

Acknowledgement

The authors would like to thank Elise Sykes for her help and expertise in creating the graphics for this chapter.

References

1. Mitchell J, McKinley J, Robinson C. The epidemiology of calcaneal fractures. *The Foot.* 2009;19(4):197–200.
2. Haapasalo H, Laine H, Mäenpää H, Wretenberg P, Kannus P, Mattila V. Epidemiology of calcaneal fractures in Finland. *J Foot Ankle Surg.* 2017;23(4):321–4.
3. Netter F. *Atlas of Human Anatomy.* 5th ed. Philadelphia, PA: Saunders; 2011.
4. Essex-Lopresti P. The mechanism, reduction technique and results in fractures of the Os Calcis. *Brit J Surg.* 1952;39(157):395–419.
5. Daftary A, Haims A, Baumgaertner M. Fractures of the calcaneus: a review with emphasis on CT. *Radiographics.* 2005;25(5):1215–26.
6. Sanders R, Fortin P, DiPasquale T, Walling A. Operative treatment in 120 displaced intraarticular calcaneal fractures.

7. Results using a prognostic computed tomography scan classification. *Clin Orthop Relat Res.* 1993;(290):87–95.
7. Porter D, Schon L. *Baxter's The Foot & Ankle in Sport.* 2nd ed. Maryland Heights, MO: Mosby; 2008.
8. Della Rocca G, Nork S, Barei D, Taitsman L, Benirschke S. Fractures of the sustentaculum tali: injury characteristics and surgical technique for reduction. *Foot Ankle Int.* 2009;30(11):1037–41.
9. Lee S, Huh S, Chung J, Kim D, Kim Y, Rhee S. Avulsion fracture of the calcaneal tuberosity: classification and its characteristics. *Clin Orthop Surg.* 2012;4(2):134–8.
10. Wong-Chung J, Marley WD, Tucker A, O'Longain DS. Incidence and recognition of peroneal tendon dislocation associated with calcaneal fractures. *J Foot Ankle Surg.* 2015;21(4):254–9.
11. Myerson M, Manoli A. Compartment syndromes of the foot after calcaneal fractures. *Clin Orthop Relat Res.* 1993;290:142–50.
12. BOAST – Open Fractures [Internet]. *British Orthopaedic Assocaition.* London [updated 2017 Dec 1; cited 2020 May 11]. Available from: https://www.boa.ac.uk/resources/boast-4-pdf.html
13. Banerjee R, Chao J, Taylor R, Siddiqui A. Management of calcaneal tuberosity fractures. *J Am Acad Orthop Surg.* 2012;20(4):253–8.
14. Massen F, Baumbach S, Herterich V, Böcker W, Polzer H. Fractures of the anterior process of the calcaneus – clinical results following functional treatment. *Injury.* 2019;50(10):1781–6.
15. Buckley R, Tough S, McCormack R, Pate G, Leighton R, Petrie D, Galpin R. Operative compared with nonoperative treatment of displaced intra-articular calcaneal fractures: a prospective, randomized, controlled multicenter trial. *J Bone Joint Surg Am.* 2002;84(10):1733–44
16. Griffin D, Shaw E, Hutchinson C, Lamb, S. Operative versus non-operative treatment for closed, displaced, intra-articular fractures of the calcaneus: randomised controlled trial. *BMJ.* 2014;349:g4483.
17. Carr J. Surgical treatment of intra-articular calcaneal fractures: a review of small incision approaches. *J Orthop Trauma.* 2005;19(2):109–17.
18. Wallin K, Cozzetto D, Russell L, Hallare D, Lee D. Evidence-based rationale for percutaneous fixation technique of displaced intra-articular calcaneal fractures: a systematic review of clinical outcomes. *J Foot Ankle Surg.* 2014;53(6):740–3.
19. Buckley R, Leighton R, Sanders D, Poon J, Coles C, Stephen D, Paolucci E. Open reduction and internal fixation compared with ORIF and primary subtalar arthrodesis for treatment of sanders type IV calcaneal fractures: a randomized multicenter trial. *J Orthop Trauma.* 2014;28(10):577–83.
20. Zwipp H, Tscherne H, Wülker N. Osteosynthese dislozierter intraartikulärer calcaneusfrakturen. *Unfallchirurg.* 1988;91(11):507–15.
21. Pastides P, Milnes L, Rosenfeld P. Percutaneous arthroscopic calcaneal osteosynthesis: a minimally invasive technique for displaced intra-articular calcaneal fractures. *J Foot Ankle Surg.* 2015;54(5):798–804.
22. Lim E, Leung J. Complications of intraarticular calcaneal fractures. *Clin Orthop Relat Res.* 2001;391(1):7–16.

Venu Kavarthapu and Raju Ahluwalia

Introduction

Diabetic foot disease (DFD) is a common complication of diabetes carrying a high degree of morbidity and mortality. As its global prevalence rises, the burden of DFD on patients and healthcare systems is expected to increase further. A common presentation of DFD is diabetic foot ulceration (DFU) for which diabetic patients have a lifetime risk of 19–35% (1). DFU is estimated to proceed 85% of amputations. A major amputation is known to carry a 5-year mortality rate ranging from 40% to 90% (2).

Multidisciplinary care is a critical component of the management of such cohort of patients presenting with complex local pathology along with systemic manifestations of diabetes. In this chapter we explore the common clinical presentations of DFD in our foot and ankle practice and their multidisciplinary treatment with an emphasis on surgical component.

Risk factors for diabetic foot disease

The pathophysiology of DFD is complex and multifactorial. The risk factors for its development include peripheral neuropathy, peripheral vascular disease, infection and altered foot mechanics.

Peripheral neuropathy

Peripheral neuropathy develops due to a combination of occlusion of the vasa nervorum, endothelial dysfunction, alteration of myelin synthesis and glycosylation of nerve cell proteins. A combination of large and small fibre neuropathy leads to loss of protective touch and pain sensations – a risk factor for developing foot ulceration. Motor neuropathy is a late manifestation resulting in muscle weakness contributing to foot deformity and abnormal pressure distribution during weight-bearing.

The standard assessment tool for peripheral neuropathy is 10 gm Semmes-Weinstein monofilament – insensitivity to the 10 gm monofilament is associated with ×1.8 increased relative risk of DFU development (3). Characteristically, small fibre neuropathy develops first causing abnormalities of pain and temperature perception, followed by large fibre sensory neuropathy resulting in loss of vibration, touch, and proprioception and cutaneous autonomic neuropathy leading to abnormal sweating and dry skin. Motor neuropathy along with sensory neuropathy, may lead to the development of foot deformities, gait abnormalities and balance disorders. The presence of diabetic peripheral neuropathy is also key to the development of Charcot neuroarthropathy (CN).

Peripheral vascular disease

Diabetes significantly increases the risk of developing peripheral arterial disease (PAD), and it is estimated that PAD is present in nearly half of all DFU. Vascular event rates are higher in diabetic individuals with PAD than in non-diabetes population. PVD is a prognostic marker for slower healing of DFU infections, a higher risk of lower extremity amputation (both major and minor), unplanned hospital admissions, cardiovascular events and mortality (4).

Mechanical changes and deformities of the foot

Common deformities such as claw toes, hammer toes, bunions, hallux limitus or the foot contour changes secondary to CN induce significant biomechanical alterations during load-bearing (3) resulting ulcer formation. The classical sign of a motor neuropathy is cavovarus foot deformity resulting in prominent metatarsal heads and lesser toe clawing. The presence of associated sensory neuropathy will augment the risk of developing a DFU. One study noted that nearly 1/3rd of neuropathic feet with high pressure developed ulceration in contrary to 0% of rheumatoid feet with similar peak plantar pressure.

Systemic risk factors

In addition to neuropathy, the following factors are known to contribute to the development of a DFU: older age, longer duration of diabetes, suboptimal glycaemic control with HbA1c > 9%, male gender, nephropathy and higher body mass index (3). Factors such as cigarette smoking, elevated diastolic blood pressure, increased fasting triglycerides and presence of microalbuminuria are independently associated with diabetic neuropathy and DFU development (5). Medical comorbidities such as dialysis, previous cerebrovascular events and reduced mobility also confer additional risk.

Clinical manifestations of diabetic foot disease

DFD encompasses a spectrum of clinical manifestations contributed by a combination of local and systemic anomalies associated with diabetes. The common manifestations managed by a foot and ankle surgeon are outlined in Table 19.1.

Diabetic foot ulcer (DFU)

The critical differences between the neuropathic and neuroischaemic ulcers are outlined here. Repetitive load-bearing over peak plantar pressure areas callus build-up or blistering formation that progresses on to develop a DFU (6, 7).

1. Neuropathic ulceration occurs primarily on the plantar aspect, underneath the metatarsal heads, tips of toes or any other bony pressure points. Persistently increased pressure transmission through the bone prominences result in callus formation. If allowed to become too thick, the callus will press on the soft tissue underneath and cause ulceration. A layer of whitish, macerated, moist tissue found under the surface of the callus may indicate imminent ulceration. It is critical that the callus is removed to uncover the ulcer.

2. Neuroischaemic and ischaemic DFU are often seen on the margins of foot or in the tips of the toes (ischaemic infarction or gangrene).

A DFU can also be categorised as 'predominantly mechanical' or 'predominantly biological', based on the underlying abnormality contributing to ulceration. The 'mechanical' ulcers present with significant peak plantar pressures that result in ulceration in the background of underlying sensory neuropathy. These require predominantly 'mechanical' solutions that involve offloading of the pressure points ranging from orthosis and casting to surgical deformity correction. The 'biological' ulcers are due to associated vascular compromise or infection as the primary pathology.

Absence of pain is a common finding in most DFU presentations; indeed, even in pure vascular infarction, minimal pain is reported because of the underlying peripheral neuropathy. Infection, when present, will contribute additional elements such as skin erythema around the ulcer, thick exudate and malodour. The signs of infection may be subtle and should be carefully assessed clinically and radiographically. A DFU present for many months or recrudescing within a short period of epithelialisation may be indicative of underlying diabetic foot osteomyelitis (DFO). DFU warrants a detailed assessment, institution of appropriate care by a multidisciplinary foot team (MDfT) and regular monitoring

Table 19.1 Common diabetic foot conditions, their incidence and pathophysiology

Condition	Description	Incidence/ Prevalence	Pathology	Outcome
Diabetic foot ulceration	Defined as breach of epidermis, plantar or otherwise, and predicted by excessive callus formation	A worldwide DFU prevalence rate is 6.3% (9)	**Neuropathic** – where there is no significant vascular component **Neuroischaemic** – where both neuropathy and ischaemia co-contribute **Ischaemic** – where there is a predominant vascular compromise leading to tissue loss	Infection and tissue loss
Charcot neuroarthropathy	Bone fragmentation, disorganisation, deformity and instability along with impaired healing response	Global prevalence among patients with diabetes is estimated between 0.1% and 8%	Severe uncontrolled local inflammatory process, often in response to minor trauma, in the background of peripheral neuropathy resulting in osteolysis and bone fragmentation	Deformity and pressure ulceration

of the treatment response. Failure of reduction in ulcer size by more than 50% after 4 weeks of treatment results in a reduced likelihood of healing by 12 weeks. Recently, the concept of DFU in remission is gaining wider attention. Given the tendency of the diabetic foot to re-ulcerate, reactivate, recrudesce pain and require long-term surveillance, the concept has been widened to become the 'diabetic foot in remission' as a distinct clinical phenotype.

Charcot neuroarthropathy (CN)

CN is considered as one of the most devastating complications of diabetic peripheral neuropathy. CN was first described by Jean-Martin Charcot in 1868 in patients with tabes dorsalis, and its association with diabetes was later established by W Jordan in 1936. In CN, the combination of neuropathy and continued abnormal loading of the foot or an episode of minor trauma leads to abnormal and uncontrolled inflammatory response leading to bone and joints disorganisation, osteolysis, fractures, dislocations as well as skin and soft tissue changes in the foot and ankle region. This leads to deformity and/or instability of the foot, resulting in a 3.5-fold increased risk of ulcer development. CN is known to be associated with a decreased life expectancy of the affected individuals by about 14 years (8).

Active (Acute) CN

Acute CN typically presents as a painless, warm, swollen foot with visible erythema in lighter skinned individuals. There may be a poorly perceived history of minor trauma. Clinical examination often reveals a well-perfused foot with bounding pulses. The foot feels warm to touch and measurement reveals a higher local temperature by at least 2 degrees compared to the contralateral normal foot. There may be a deformity along with crepitus on palpation due to the underlying bone fragmentation, particularly in late presentations. Most common location of CN is the midfoot (50%), followed by hindfoot (30%). As the differential diagnosis includes cellulitis, deep venous thrombosis and even gout, many individuals experience a considerable delay in diagnosis.

Chronic or inactive CN

As the acute and uncontrolled inflammation settles, the CN affected foot progresses to the inactive phase, where the involved bones show a healing response. This results in foot deformity with or without instability. Chronic CN may present to the foot clinic with sequelae due to deformity, such as ulceration/osteomyelitis at the site of deformity or seeking reconstructive surgery for profound deformities such as 'rocker foot' from a midfoot collapse or varus hindfoot from ankle bones involvement. In such late presentations, usually months to years after the acute episode, one needs to remain vigilant for coexistent PAD.

Classically, staging of Charcot is done radiologically using the Eichenholtz classification (Stage 1 – destruction; Stage 2 – coalescence and Stage 3 – consolidation), with the recent addition of stage 0 to categorise clinical presentations of acute CN with normal appearance on plain radiographs, but MRI evidence of typical bone oedema and fragmentation.

Based on the location of these changes, CN has been classified anatomically by Sanders and Fryberg into 5 patterns – the metatarsal-phalangeal joints (pattern I), tarsometatarsal joints (pattern II), tarsal joints (pattern III), ankle joint (pattern IV) and body of calcaneum (pattern V). It is generally considered that the hindfoot Charcot has a significantly worse prognosis with a higher risk of major amputation.

General management of diabetic foot disease

Assessment of the diabetic foot

An adequate history to identify the risk factors is important, and a detailed general and local examination is vital during the assessment of a diabetic patient presenting with a foot problem. Many patients with diabetes present with neuropathy, vasculopathy, retinopathy, nephropathy and cardiac-related complications, and these require a systematic assessment on presentation. The main focus of foot examination should include on neuropathy, ischaemia and deformity. Thorough examination of all foot surfaces should be done for the presence of swelling, callus, skin breakdown, infection and tissue necrosis. Assessment of key pathologies of the diabetic foot is described in Table 19.2.

Early detection and treatment of ischaemia

Clinical assessment and common symptoms that should alert the clinician to possible vascular compromise are shown in Table 19.3. First-line assessment is usually noninvasive, but there is no single optimal modality present (9). An ankle brachial index (ABI) of >0.9, presence of triphasic pedal Doppler waveforms or a toe brachial index of ≥0.75 suggest the absence of PAD. ABI < 0.5 indicates severe ischaemia.

Measurement of transcutaneous cutaneous oxygen tension ($TcPO_2$, ≥25 mmHg) and toe blood pressure (≥30 mmHg increases pre-test probability of healing by 25%) may prognosticate the potential for healing. Some studies suggest that toe pressure is more sensitive than ankle pressure in the diagnosis of limb threatening ischaemia. Those with chronic limb-threatening ischaemia are likely to benefit from early revascularisation, either endovascular or, if suitable and medically fit, a surgical bypass, to help treat infection and ulceration.

Table 19.2 Assessment of the key pathologies of the diabetic foot and their investigations

Neuropathy Assessment & Investigations	The 10 gm Monofilament (10MF) is the most frequently used screening tool for assessment of the diabetic foot at risk. A neurothesiometer or 128 Hz tuning fork can be used for vibration thresholds. Pin prick test and temperature thresholds can help assess the small fibre function. Nerve conduction studies and skin biopsy tests can be performed if requited.
Diabetic foot ulcer Assessment & investigations	Clinical examination of the ulcer includes the determining the size, depth and the presence of infection. Any overlying callus needs to be completely excised to reveal the full extent of the ulcer. Positive probe-to-bone test indicates possible underlying osteomyelitis. A few classification systems are in practice to grade a DFU; the Texas classification is a commonly used one. Plain radiographs have low sensitivity and specificity in diagnosing osteomyelitis. MRI is currently considered as the gold standard with high sensitivity (88–100%) and specificity (40–90%) levels. Deep tissue and bone biopsies are essential to confirm the bacteriological diagnosis.
Charcot foot deformity Assessment & Investigations	In suspected active CN, W/B plain radiographs should be obtained immediately. Radiographic appearances of active CN include soft tissue swelling, bone fragmentation, bone destruction and joint dislocations. A normal x-ray does not exclude early CN and an MRI or nuclear medicine (CT SPECT) scan should be organised if required. Typical features of CN on MRI include soft tissue oedema, periarticular bone marrow oedema and microfractures. High update in all 3 phases of bone scan (early, blood pool and delayed phase) can be an indicative of CN. The clinical examination of a deformed inactive Charcot foot includes assessment of the fixed component of the deformity in the ankle, hindfoot, midfoot and forefoot regions, along with the degree of passive correction. The presence of fixed contracture of the tendons, particularly Achilles (equinus), tibialis posterior and tibialis anterior (hindfoot varus) is identified. Muscle weakness, particularly the peroneals and tibialis anterior, is a common occurrence. Any presence of bone prominence, particularly in the midfoot, is assessed. Plain weight-bearing AP and lateral radiographs of the foot and ankle help assess the bone deformities in detail. CT imaging with 3D reconstruction is extremely helpful for surgical planning. MRI or CT SPECRT imaging is helpful if there is any concern about chronic osteomyelitis.

Timely treatment of infection

A guide to the medical management of infected diabetic foot is provided in Table 19.4. In those with wound infection and suspected underlying osteomyelitis, attempts should be made to obtain a clean bone sample for microbiological culture and sensitivity (10). Antimicrobial therapy is then tailored to the appropriate cultured organism. A diabetic foot ulcer with no deep infection, significant deformity or marked vascular insufficiency usually responds well to bedside debridement and appropriate wound dressing, followed by culture specific oral antibiotic administration and offloading of the foot in a suitable brace until ulcer healing is achieved.

Appropriate wound management

Non-surgical management of diabetic foot ulcer includes cover with dressings to maintain the right degree of moisture on the wound bed, control exudate and avoid maceration of the surrounding skin. Little evidence is available from published literature to advocate one dressing or wound healing method over another (11). The benefit of sucrose-octasulfate dressing for the management of neuroischaemic ulceration with vascular indices that are above the threshold denoting critical limb ischaemia has been demonstrated in a multicentre randomised study (12). The use of Hyperbaric oxygen therapy has remained controversial but is offered as an adjuvant in some centres. There is evolving evidence for other adjuvant wound healing techniques such as LeucoPatch (13) and nitric-oxide systems (14). However, the cost-effectiveness of all three remains to

Table 19.3 Assessment of vascular pathology – clinical signs and symptoms indicative of significant vascular compromise

History of claudication with walking
Presence or history of a foot ulcer
Absent dorsalis pedis and posterior tibial arterial pulses
Advanced trophic skin changes, including decreased hair growth, abnormal toenails, discoloration or atrophy of the skin
Absent dorsalis pedis and posterior tibial arterial pulses
Venous insufficiency (especially in morbidly obese patients)
Non-traumatic partial or whole foot amputation

Table 19.4 A guide to the medical management of the diabetic foot infection

Assessment	Early recognition of infection by conducting a thorough clinical assessment, including the vascular examination. The blood investigations include serum C-reactive protein levels, as this is often elevated to greater than 100 mg/L in severe infections. Ultrasound examination can help assess the presence of soft tissue collections. MRI imaging can help determine presence of osteomyelitis and soft tissue collections.
Microbiological diagnosis	Requires collection of deep tissue specimens or bone biopsies for aerobic and anaerobic microbiological cultures prior to starting intravenous antibiotics. Alternatively, ultrasound guided aspiration can be performed.
Empirical antibiotic therapy	Appropriate empirical intravenous antibiotic therapy is commenced after obtaining deep tissue samples, as per the department protocol. Subsequently, antimicrobial therapy is guided by microbiological sensitivities.

be ascertained. Stem cell therapy holds promise in no-option ischaemia, but its clinical effectiveness remains unproven outside a few pioneering centres. Various growth factors are used to stimulate wound healing, but there is limited evidence to support their use in routine clinical practice. Indeed, the International Working Group on the Diabetic Foot (IWGDF) is yet to endorse any of these methods in their wound healing guidance (15).

Conservative management of CN and offloading

The medical management of active CN primarily is primarily offloading of the leg in a cast and protected weight-bearing. There is a strong scientific evidence to suggest the presence of abnormal osteoclastic activity in CN (16), and antiresorptive therapies were considered to correct this imbalance. The use of bisphosphonates (both oral and intravenous) in active CN has been investigated in small randomised controlled trials and as has the use of monoclonal antibody against receptor activator of nuclear factor-kappa B ligand (RANKL). However, none has reported a benefit in reducing the casting time, bone healing or resolution of the arthropathic process (17).

Immediate offloading of the leg in a total contact cast (TCC) and protected weight-bearing are considered as the gold standard in the management of acute CN. TCC facilitates even distribution of plantar pressure in the sole of the foot and transfers to the leg, along with reduction of oedema in the lower leg and ankle. Early initiation of casting minimises bone fragmentation and prevents progression to a major deformity. Despite this, the technical limitations of casting and non-acceptance by some patients has meant that TCC is underused. Removable fixed angled offloading devices are therefore increasingly used, but patient adherence to the offloading can be unpredictable and may result in delayed bone healing or treatment failures.

Key orthopaedic procedures in the management of diabetic foot disease

Surgical management has been a key component of care in the management of diabetic foot disorders for over the past 70 years (18). The initial focus of surgery was on infection control, but recently functional limb salvage/reconstruction procedures have successfully been added. It is critical that this service be delivered by an MDfT, which includes a diabetologist, podiatrist, orthotist, wound care specialist, orthopaedic surgeon, vascular surgeon, plastic surgeon, microbiologist and radiologist (Figure 19.1). The common conditions the foot and ankle surgeons are expected to deliver the service as part of an MDfT include the following.

Surgical management of infected diabetic foot

A guide to the surgical management of an infected diabetic foot is provided in Table 19.5. The commonest manifestation is an infected DFU, as over 50% of diabetic foot ulcers become infected, presenting as either acute or chronic infection complicated by osteomyelitis. Occasionally, infection presents with rapid progression along the tissue planes with spreading cellulitis, tissue necrosis and systemic inflammatory response. Such infections can be limb threatening without timely intervention and are labelled as 'diabetic foot attack' (19). The management of such infections is ideally delivered in an MDfT setting, using a structured approach. The management principles of diabetic foot attack include rapid diagnosis, identifying pathogens through microbiological culture of deep tissue specimens, targeted intravenous antibiotic therapy, emergent and radical surgical debridement.

An infected DFU requires resection of the infected and necrotic tissue to achieve eradication of infection

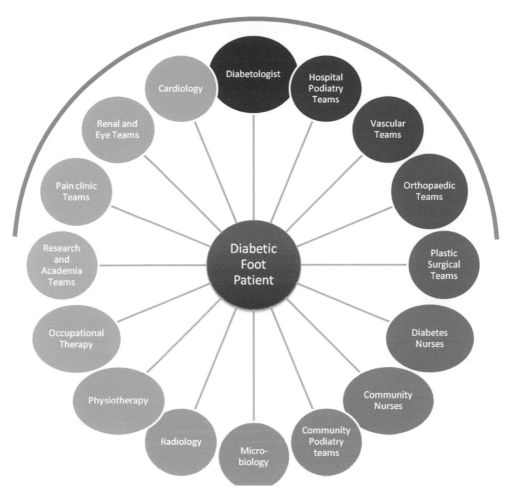

Figure 19.1 Multidisciplinary Foot Team (MDfT) – the constituent resources of a well-developed MDfT. Highlighted by the orange include the core team members.

and predictable ulcer healing. Non-healing/recurrence of a diabetic foot ulcer is often due to inadequate resection of the infected and non-viable tissues. The Red-Amber-Green (RAG) model provides a structured model of debridement of infected diabetic foot (20). The central part of the infected ulcer with necrotic portion is recognised as the 'red zone' (Figure 19.2). This tissue is normally included in the routine surgical debridement. However, the red zone is surrounded by relatively avascular and fibrous tissue that often harbours pockets of infection. This is considered as the 'amber zone'. This is surrounded by normal and healthy tissue – the 'green zone'. It is essential that the tissue in the red and amber zones be excised completely, down to the adjacent green zone, to excise all potentially infected tissue. This is applicable to bone debridement too. Deep tissue samples obtained from the red and amber zones are used for microbiological analysis. The tissue defect is managed with negative pressure wound therapy and serial change of dressings (Figure 19.3).

Chronic non-healing DFU or recurring ulcer with an underlying significant vascular compromise, chronic osteomyelitis or marked deformity often require a formal surgical debridement of the infected ulcer along with an exostectomy of the bone prominence, revascularisation or a deformity reconstructive procedure to achieve predictable ulcer healing and reduce the risk of recurrence.

Surgical management of acute CN

Most presentations with active CN respond favourably to immobilisation and offloading in a TCC until the inflammatory process is resolved, followed by gradual return to normal weight-bearing in a brace or custom-made shoes. However, the CN process can continue in some patients, despite adequate offloading, and this can lead to progression of deformity and foot instability resulting in ulceration and infection. The resulting 'fracture' haematoma during acute phase provides an

Table 19.5 A guide to the surgical management of diabetic foot infection	
Assessment of infected diabetic foot	Deep tissue specimens and bone biopsies can be done in the outpatient clinic and provide the most accurate microbiological diagnosis of diabetic foot infections.
Surgical debridement	Severe infection presentations (diabetic foot attack) require immediate and aggressive surgical debridement. 'Time is tissue' concept is applicable to this condition and unnecessary as delay in definitive surgical debridement may result in a limb loss. Repeat surgical debridement is mandatory if there is a suspicion of residual tissue necrosis or further deep collection. Any foot instability because of aggressive bone debridement can be managed with temporary stabilisation with threaded guide wires or an external fixator. Open wounds can be managed with negative pressure wound therapy (NPWT).
Adjuvant local antibiotic elusion and systemic antibiotics	Targeted intravenous antibiotic treatment is continued until the infection is completely cleared, as noted by improvement in the clinical parameters and serological markers. Local antibiotic eluding calcium sulphate preparations or similar products may be used at the time of surgical debridement to fill the bone voids or tissue defects and to provide high concentrations of antibiotic to the adjacent tissues.
Achieving skin cover	This may require a plastic surgical procedure for soft tissue cover of the wounds including split skin grafting for dorsal skin or local rotational flap for plantar skin.
Definitive stabilisation	Once the infection eradication is achieved, as noted clinically and serologically, a definitive reconstruction of the foot is performed as required. The aim is to achieve a normal shaped and stable foot so that the patient can mobilise without any risk of ulceration.

excellent medium for the pathogens aiding the progression of infection and tissue necrosis and potentially a major amputation. The lower extremity amputation rate in patients with CN has been reported to range from 3% to 9%. To achieve functional limb salvage, such presentations warrant immediate surgical stabilisation during Eichenholtz stage 1 of the disease. Such patients during active phase of CN should be admitted immediately and managed by an MDfT. The foot offloading in a TCC is continued and the leg is elevated to reduce swelling. Once the swelling and local warmth resolve, surgical stabilisation of the Charcot foot is undertaken using durable long-segment rigid internal fixation with optimal bone opposition principle that has been described in the following section. Recent studies with a small series have shown improved results of surgical reconstruction of active CN; most likely due to the recent improvements in the fixation methods and the access to multidisciplinary care (21).

Tendon balancing procedures for diabetic foot deformities

Tendon balancing procedures can be highly effective for some foot deformities. On the contrary, tendon transfer procedures are generally considered as ineffective in diabetic foot deformities as the associated motor neuropathy is a progressive condition and the muscle

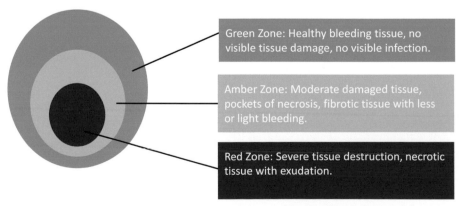

Green Zone: Healthy bleeding tissue, no visible tissue damage, no visible infection.

Amber Zone: Moderate damaged tissue, pockets of necrosis, fibrotic tissue with less or light bleeding.

Red Zone: Severe tissue destruction, necrotic tissue with exudation.

Figure 19.2 Principles of ulcer surgical debridement using RAG principle. The RAG model defines the area of debridement to create a healthy bed and wound margins. Elliptical incisions are preferred where possible to facilitate wound approximation and accommodate NPWT dressings.

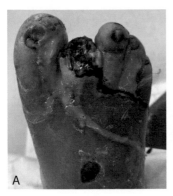
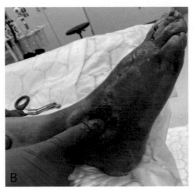
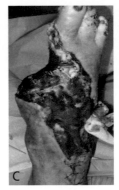
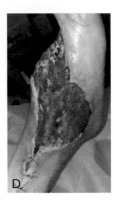

Figure 19.3 A case example of a diabetic foot attack. (A and B) Classical diabetic foot attack presentation with spreading infection with evidence of tissue necrosis. The infection started from a small ulcer at the tip of second toe and spread along the tissue planes and tendons. (C) Aggressive debridement is performed using RAG model. (D) After 2 cycles of NPWT, good granulation tissue response was noted. Transmetatarsal amputation along with wound coverage on the plantar side with local transposition flap and dorsally with split skin graft was later performed.

imbalance continues resulting in either recurrence or development of new deformities.

Tendon balancing procedures can be done on their own to correct flexible foot deformities or along with the bone correction procedures during reconstruction, to improve the deformity correction and muscle balance. The commonest procedure is percutaneous toe flexor tenotomy performed with a hypodermic needle to correct claw toe deformities with supple interphalangeal joints (Figure 19.4). These procedures can be safely performed in an outpatient or day surgery facility under local anaesthetic. Another common tendon balancing procedure is Achilles tendon release/lengthening. A tight Achilles is a common occurrence in DFD, causing increased plantar forefoot and midfoot pressure, leading to ulceration. Achilles tendon release is performed using Hoke's triple hemisection technique and this can be combined with metatarsal head resection, or joint arthroplasty to promote healing of associated plantar forefoot ulcer. Achilles tendon release requires bracing of ankle in neutral position for about 6 weeks.

Exostectomy

Exostectomy involves removal of underlying bone prominence to achieve direct pressure offloading of the ulcer without providing full deformity correction. Plantar ulcers associated with bone prominence, often seen in the midfoot that do not respond to debridement and offloading, should be considered for exostectomy. Current evidence suggests that medial midfoot exostectomy is a safe and reliable procedure, whereas the lateral column procedures involving the cuboid carry a higher risk of recurrence requiring a repeat procedure (22).

During exostectomy, the infected ulcer is excised and debrided thoroughly, and the underlying bone prominence is exposed. The area of exostosis is carefully

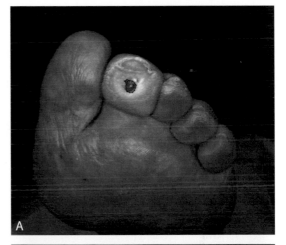
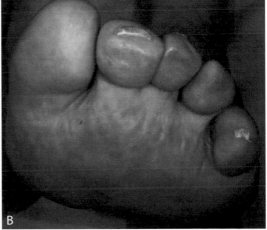

Figure 19.4 Flexor tenotomy. (A) Patient with a flexible IP joint contracture – released using a percutaneous flexor tenotomy technique, to prevent rubbing in the toe box. (B) The ulcer healed within 6 weeks.

mapped under fluoroscopy and by palpation. The exostosis is excised completely using an osteotome or an oscillating saw. Care is taken to make sure that any residual necrotic bone or residual bone prominence is resected. Occasionally, the foot becomes unstable due to the need for excessive bone resection, and this often requires a temporary stabilisation with threaded wires or an external fixator. Definitive fixation may be considered later, using the following techniques as discussed, after full infection clearance is achieved.

Forefoot procedures

The majority of forefoot procedures are related to deformity correction and offloading for ulceration. Hallux MTPJ resection arthroplasty (modified Keller's) is an effective surgical technique in the management of chronic plantar hallux ulcerations due to associated dorsiflexion deformity at the MTPJ. This allows complete removal of the infected part of the bones, increases the range of motion of the hallux and reduces plantar pressure. However, such procedures may induce transfer lesions affecting the lesser toes, particularly if they have fixed toe claw deformities. Other pressure relieving forefoot procedures involve osteotomies and metatarsal head resections to decrease the peak plantar pressure under the affected metatarsal heads. These techniques are considered for hard-to-heal plantar ulcers with failure of offloading measures and are often combined with Achilles tendon lengthening or gastrocnemius release to address the associated forefoot overload.

Surgical reconstruction of the before deformed Charcot foot

The reconstruction of a foot affected by CN is one of the most challenging surgical interventions. A deformed Charcot foot is often limb threatening, particularly in the presence of an ulcer. The amputation risk is 7 times higher for diabetes patients with an ulcer and 12 times higher with Charcot and an ulcer(23). The surgical aim of Charcot foot reconstruction is to achieve a normal shaped, plantigrade and stable foot that allows full weight-bearing using routine or modified shoes. Long-term stability of the reconstructed foot requires full deformity correction and solid bone fusion of all bones that are intended for fusion. Vascular assessment prior to the deformity correction, and revascularisation if required, is critical for predictable bone union. Detailed clinical and radiological assessment of the bone and soft tissue components of the deformity is essential for a successful outcome.

The surgical approach is planned according to the location of deformity and is often done on the convex side of the foot and ankle. The deformity correction is achieved by performing soft tissue releases, and bone osteotomies and wedge resections on the convex side of the deformity. It is critical that all joints intended for

fusion are thoroughly prepared. The choice of surgical fixation can be either with external fixation (circular frame) or internal fixation, as per the preference of the surgeon (24). However, many diabetic foot patients find it difficult to tolerate keeping the circular frame on for the full duration of treatment. The internal fixation techniques have become more popular recently with the introduction of Charcot specific devices and more published data is now available with good outcomes.

Infection around the internal fixation devices is a major concern in this group of patients; however, most published literatures indicate low or acceptable infection rates (24–29). The generally accepted principle of internal fixation during Charcot foot reconstruction is the 'Super-construct' technique described by Sammarco et al., 2010, about a decade ago, which recommended a 'long-segment fixation' that involved extension of the bone fusion to beyond the zone of injury. This is achieved by extending the fixation to the adjacent joints that are not affected by CN (30). Since then, this principle has been refined further as 'durable long-segment rigid fixation with optimal bone opposition' as non-rigid fixation was found to have higher failure rates (27–29, 31, 32).

Actively infected deformed Charcot requires two-stage reconstruction (28, 32). The first stage consists of aggressive surgical debridement of the ulcer and infected bone using the principles described earlier, and removal of all bone prominences, along with osteotomy at the deformity to provisionally restore the normal foot shape. Local antibiotic eluding calcium preparations are used to fill the bone voids and for local antibiotic delivery. Temporary stabilisation of the osteotomised bones is achieved with judicious use of threaded guide wires or an external fixator. Administration of targeted and culture specific IV antibiotics is continued until there is clinical and serological evidence of infection eradication. negative pressure wound therapy (NPWT) is used to manage the soft tissue defects. After a period of 6–10 weeks of treatment, the infection eradication is usually achieved, and the second stage of definitive fixation is performed.

Metal work failure is a well-recognised complication following Charcot foot reconstruction using the internal fixation method (32). The incidence is higher among patients with high BMI and in those that require a two-stage reconstruction. However, the surgical revision rate is not higher among the patients with hardware failure and their ambulatory status is similar to those without hardware failure.

Principles of hindfoot deformity correction

Ankle and subtalar joint reconstruction is achieved by performing bone wedge resections on the convex side of the deformity and applying long-segment rigid internal fixation construct applied along the lines of the weight-bearing forces (27, 28). An intramedullary (IM) hindfoot fusion nail (tibio-talar-calcaneal nail) is a load sharing device and provides better mechanical environment compared to staples, screws, standard plates and angled plates (Figure 19.5A–C). It has a higher bending and torsional stiffness compared to plates or other devices and can provide intraoperative compression and optimal bone apposition, and thereby better bone fusion rates.

Where there is significant bone loss in the hindfoot region, the following principles may be considered:

1. Locking screws are normally inserted into talus and calcaneus through the IM nail, but in the presence of significant bone loss or osteopenia, optimal rigid fixation may not be achieved and the locking screw may be subjected to excessive load at its bone interphase. This can potentially result in screw migration or breakage. Hydroxyapatite (HA) coating to the locking screws has been shown to reduce screw migration (27). In addition, screw bone on-growth may increase the self-loosening threshold of these locking screws.

2. If the degree of bone loss is marked in the hindfoot, the IM nail alone may not provide enough rigid fixation, as there is often some rotational instability. In such situations, an additional screw fixation inserted retrograde from calcaneus into distal tibia (Figure 19.5D) or a plate fixation from distal tibia to medial column (Figure 19.5E) increases the rotational stability of the construct significantly.

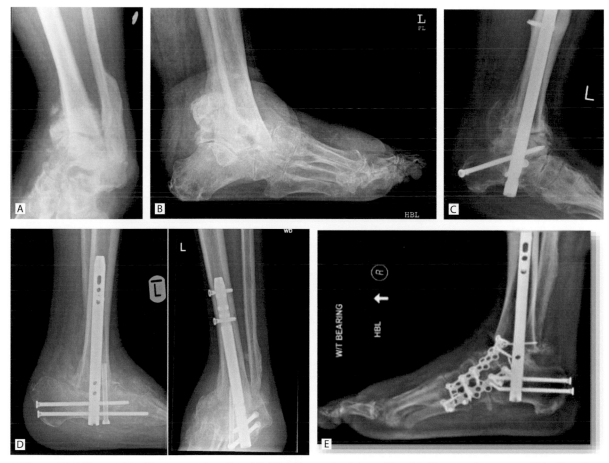

Figure 19.5 Charcot hindfoot reconstruction. (A) AP radiograph of the ankle with Charcot changes and hindfoot in varus alignment. (B) Lateral radiograph of foot and ankle with Charcot changes in the ankle and relative preservation of the midfoot. (C) The Charcot hindfoot deformity is managed with a hindfoot nail. (D) In this case example with talectomy, further rotational stability of the hindfoot nail construct was achieved with an additional calcaneotibial screw. (E) In this case example, additional rotational stability of the hindfoot nail construct was achieved with extension of the medial column plate to distal tibia.

Table 19.6 Charcot midfoot deformity patterns

1	**Rocker bottom forefoot abduction:** The Rocker bottom forefoot abduction pattern is the commonest and results in collapse of the medial column (rocker bottom) causing relative lengthening and forcing the forefoot into abduction. This leads to dissociation of the Meary's angle and talar-1st metatarsal angle in the dorsoplantar plane, along with reduction of calcaneal pitch and contracture of Achilles tendon in severe deformities. Depending on the location of midfoot CN changes, the rocker bottom may affect only on the medial or both medial and lateral columns.
2	**Dorsal subluxation/dislocation:** Dorsal subluxation or dislocation of the forefoot from the midfoot/hindfoot due to destruction of midfoot articulation resulting in shortening of the foot due to overlapping these segments.
3	**Forefoot adduction:** The forefoot adduction pattern is the least common and may be associated with fracture of bases of lateral metatarsals and/or peroneus brevis muscle/tendon dysfunction.

Principles of midfoot reconstruction

The midfoot is the most commonly affected region in CN of the foot and ankle. This often results in midfoot collapse, leading to rocker bottom deformity and forcing the forefoot into abduction. The deformities fall into one of three surgical patterns as shown in Table 19.6 (29).

Reconstruction requires correction and stabilisation of the medial column usually using an extended medial approach exposing the medial column. After adequate

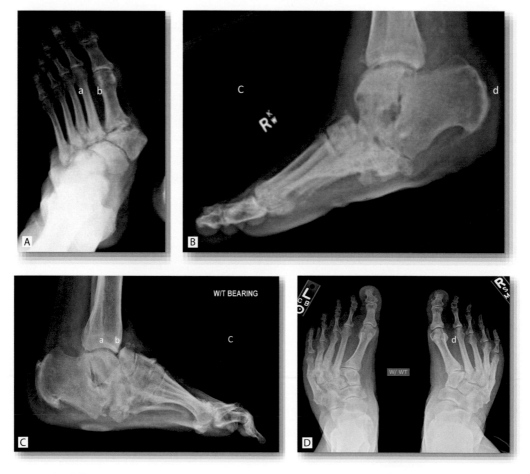

Figure 19.6 The different patterns of midfoot Charcot deformity. (A and B) Dorsoplantar and lateral views of foot showing rocker bottom forefoot abduction midfoot Charcot pattern. (C) Lateral view of foot showing dorsal subluxation/dislocation pattern. (D) Dorsoplantar views of both feet showing forefoot adduction pattern.

surgical exposure, creating thick soft tissue flaps, an appropriate medial/plantar-based wedge osteotomy is performed under fluoroscopy guidance (Figure 19.7A and b). The apex of the wedge aimed at within the cuboid bone leaving its lateral cortex intact. The planter prominence is included in the resection mass.

Compressive fixation of the osteotomy is undertaken with 1 or 2 cannulated lag screws across the osteotomy and/or a locking plate using long-segment rigid fixation principle (Figure 19.7C,D). Alternatively, an IM medial column beam is inserted either retrograde through the metatarsal head into talus or antegrade through the posterior body of talus in to 1st metatarsal shaft. The rotational stability of the beam fixation is enhanced with a medial or dorsomedial neutralisation plate if required (Figure 19.7E).

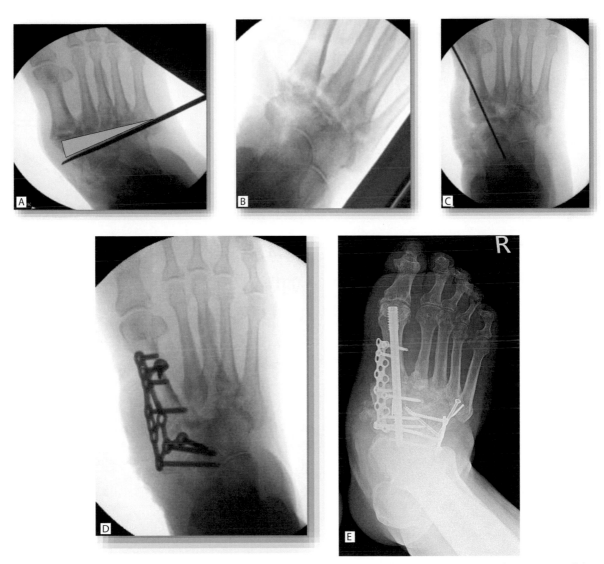

Figure 19.7 Principles of midfoot deformity correction by performing wedge resection. (A) Distal osteotomy of the wedge resection (blue shaded) passes through the base of the 1st–3rd metatarsals and the proximal osteotomy commonly goes through the cuneiform/navicularis/talar head parts medially depending on the degree and location of the deformity. (B) The apex of the osteotomy is aimed within the cuboid bone near the lateral cortex so that this is preserved and used a hinge to stabilise the osteotomy. In this case example, the apex is close to the distal part of cuboid bone. (C) This intact lateral cortex of the cuboid acts as a strong hinge allowing plastic deformation of the lateral cortex during correction of forefoot abduction deformity. The correction is provisionally held in place with a Kirschner wire. (D) The osteotomy is stabilised with a locking plate. (E) An example of beam and plate construct in midfoot Charcot correction.

In certain complex deformities, e.g., a previous divergent dissociation of the Lisfranc joint, an additional plate fixation is required to bridge the base of 2nd or 3rd metatarsal to the tarsal bones. Dorsal subluxation pattern deformity and rocker bottom deformities with significant involvement of the lateral column require additional lateral column fixation using a separate lateral approach. This is achieved by using a smaller diameter beam inserted through the 4th metatarsal retrograde or calcaneum in an antegrade direction. Alternatively, a low-profile locking plate spanning the base of 4th metatarsal to the anterior part of calcaneum can be used.

Management of foot and ankle trauma

The management of foot and ankle trauma in patients with diabetes is similar to other diabetic foot conditions and warrants a detailed foot assessment and access to MDfT. This is especially true if there is no history of significant trauma, as this may represent an acute CN in the presence of peripheral neuropathy. Diabetes control, degree of neuropathy and the vascular status are key elements for risk stratification and the development of complications. These presentations can be broadly categorised and managed as the following two groups:

1. In compliant patients with well-controlled diabetes (HbA1c < 6.5), and without peripheral neuropathy, angiopathy or nephropathy (uncomplicated diabetes); displaced fractures are managed with standard open reduction and internal fixation. Undisplaced fractures can be managed by standard cast treatment. Extended non–weight-bearing mobilisation is recommended for all these patients as the bone healing response is known to be slow. The patients need to be clinically and radiologically monitored for extended periods to ensure that the fracture healing is complete and there is no late fracture displacement.

2. In patients with poorly controlled diabetes (HbA1c > 6.5), poor or non-compliance, along with manifest complications of neuropathy, angiopathy or nephropathy (complicated diabetes); and with a history of no or minimal trauma, the fracture can be managed as an acute CN. It is recommended that the fixation principles used in Charcot reconstruction are considered in such presentations, with an emphasis on using a long-segment rigid fixation technique (Figure 19.8). Table 19.7 outlines the surgical risks of lower leg and ankle fractures management in these groups.

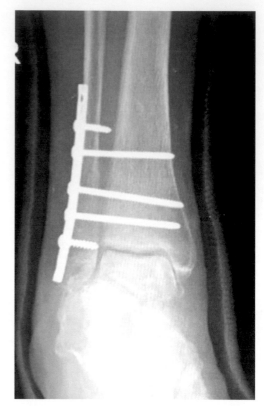

Figure 19.8 AP view of ankle showing lateral malleolar fracture fixation using the principle of long-segment rigid plate fixation.

Amputations in diabetic foot disease

Severe diabetic foot infection with critical ischaemia and associated marked tissue loss may not be amenable for limb preservation or reconstruction. An amputation is often the only option available in such conditions.

Risk factors associated with amputation include the duration of ulcer longer than 1 month, PAD, higher Wagner grade, wound infection, proteinuria and osteomyelitis. Fifteen per cent of foot ulcers result in amputations (33). All patients require multidisciplinary work-up with the relevant amputation team including a prosthetist. The level of amputation is judged by the level of infection and vascular supply. This is often performed as a two-stage procedure in combination with NPWT for the wound management, to address any residual infection. A definitive resection level and stump closure is undertaken at 5–7 days.

Postoperative management includes daily change of soft stump dressings until complete wound healing before the initial prosthesis fitting. An alternative is fitting an immediate postoperative prosthesis (IPOP), a rigid dressing typically made of fibreglass applied

Table 19.7 Outcomes after tibial and foot ankle fractures

Lower limb injuries	Outcomes and risks compared to non-diabetic patients
Tibial fracture	Closed fractures of the tibia in diabetics have an increased risk of delayed union, requirement for exchange nailing and an increased rate of surgical site infection compared to patients without diabetes.
Pilon fracture	There is a 10.7-fold increase in complications among those undergoing surgical management with routine fixation. The rate of non-union/delayed union is increased by 3.95-fold with surgical management.
Ankle fracture	Diabetes is a known risk factor for complications after ankle fracture. Classifying outcomes by stratifying the type of diabetes into complicated vs. uncomplicated, complicated diabetes has a: 3.8 times higher risk of overall complication 3.4 times higher risk for malunion, non-union or CN 5 times higher risk of requiring revision surgery

in the operating room. While maintaining the knee in extension, IPOP maintains shape of the stump and reduces oedema. Recent studies show it reduces the rate of surgical revision and achieves early ambulation and rehabilitation, resulting in psychological benefits and decreased complications from prolonged bed rest (34). The common amputation levels considered in DFD are:

1. Transmetatarsal, midfoot and Chopart
2. Pirogoff amputation or ankle disarticulation (Syme's amputation)
3. Below-knee
4. Through knee or above knee

The clinical outcomes following a major amputation are poor and associated with significant morbidity, in comparison to patients without diabetes. The complication rates in these procedures can be high, as one study revealed 33% rated their result as fair or poor at a mean follow-up of 44.9 months. The 5-year survival rate following a major amputation is low at 30–60% and such decision should only be considered if functional limb salvage is not possible.

Take home messages

- DFD develops due to 3 main pathologies – infection, ischaemia and neuropathy, contributing to the commonest complications – neuropathic and ischaemic ulceration.
- Foot and ankle surgeons have an increasingly important role in an MDfT, with surgical procedures offered for treatment of DFD ranging from simple tendon balancing procedures to major two-stage Charcot foot reconstructions.
- A painless, swollen, red and warm foot with no history of significant trauma in a patient with diabetic neuropathy is an acute CN until proved

otherwise. Immediate offloading of the foot and referral to an MDfT is essential.
- Diabetic foot ulcer with features of rapid spread of infection, such as tissue necrosis, spreading erythema and systemic response, may represent a diabetic foot attack. The concept of 'time is tissue' is applicable to this potentially limb threatening condition.
- Foot and ankle fractures in patients with complicated diabetes, particularly with history of no significant trauma, warrant a multidisciplinary approach and may require long-segment rigid fixation and extended period of immobilisation for satisfactory outcomes.

References

1. Armstrong DG, Boulton AJM, Bus SA. Diabetic foot ulcers and their recurrence. N Engl J Med. 2017; 376(24):2367–75.
2. Thorud JC, Plemmons B, Buckley CJ, et al. Mortality after nontraumatic major amputation among patients with diabetes and peripheral vascular disease: A systematic review. J Foot Ankle Surg. 2016; 55:591–9.
3. Abbott CA, Carrington AL, Ashe H, Bath S, Every LC, Griffiths J, et al. The North-West Diabetes Foot Care Study: Incidence of, and risk factors for, new diabetic foot ulceration in a community-based patient cohort. Diabet Med. 2002; 19(5):377–84.
4. Hinchliffe RJ, Brownrigg JR, Apelqvist J, Boyko EJ, Fitridge R, Mills JL, et al. IWGDF guidance on the diagnosis, prognosis and management of peripheral artery disease in patients with foot ulcers in diabetes. Diabetes Metab Res Rev. 2016; 32(Suppl 1):37–44.
5. Tesfaye S, Selvarajah D. The Eurodiab study: What has this taught us about diabetic peripheral neuropathy? Curr Diab Rep. 2009; 9(6):432–4.
6. Edmonds ME, Foster AV. Diabetic foot ulcers. BMJ. 2006; 332(7538):407–10.
7. Game FL, Attinger C, Hartemann A, Hinchliffe RJ, Londahl M, Price PE, et al. IWGDF guidance on use of interventions to

enhance the healing of chronic ulcers of the foot in diabetes. Diabetes Metab Res Rev. 2016; 32(Suppl 1):75–83.

8. van Baal J, Hubbard R, Game F, et al. Mortality associated with acute Charcot foot and neuropathic foot ulceration. Diabetes Care. 2010; 33:1086–9.

9. Hingorani A, LaMuraglia GM, Henke P, Meissner MH, Loretz L, Zinszer KM, et al. The management of diabetic foot: A clinical practice guideline by the Society for Vascular Surgery in collaboration with the American Podiatric Medical Association and the Society for Vascular Medicine. J Vasc Surg. 2016; 63(2 Suppl):3S–21S.

10. O'meara S, Nelson E, Golder S, Dalton J, Craig D, Iglesias C. Systematic review of methods to diagnose infection in foot ulcers in diabetes. Diabet Med. 2006; 23(4):341–7.

11. Lázaro Martínez JL, Álvaro-Afonso FJ, Ahluwalia R, Baker N, Ríos-Ruh JM, Rivera-San Martin G, Van Acker, K. Debridement and the Diabetic Foot (2019) D-Foot International https://d-foot.org/images/Debridement.pdf

12. Edmonds M, Lazaro-Martinez JL, Alfayate-Garcia JM, Martini J, Petit JM, Rayman G, et al. Sucrose octasulfate dressing versus control dressing in patients with neuroischaemic diabetic foot ulcers (Explorer): An international, multicentre, double-blind, randomised, controlled trial. Lancet Diabetes Endocrinol. 2018; 6(3):186–96.

13. Game F, Jeffcoate W, Tarnow L, Jacobsen JL, Whitham DJ, Harrison EF, et al. LeucoPatch system for the management of hard-to-heal diabetic foot ulcers in the UK, Denmark, and Sweden: An observer-masked, randomised controlled trial. Lancet Diabetes Endocrinol. 2018; 6(11):870–8.

14. Edmonds ME, Bodansky HJ, Boulton AJ, Chadwick PJ, Dang CN, D'Costa R, et al. Multicenter, randomized controlled, observer-blinded study of a nitric oxide generating treatment in foot ulcers of patients with diabetes – ProNOx1 study. Wound Repair Regen. 2018.

15. Game FL, Attinger C, Hartemann A, Hinchliffe RJ, Londahl M, Price PE, et al. IWGDF guidance on use of interventions to enhance the healing of chronic ulcers of the foot in diabetes. Diabetes Metab Res Rev. 2016; 32(Suppl 1):75–83.

16. Mabilleau G, Petrova NL, Edmonds ME, Sabokbar A. Increased osteoclastic activity in acute Charcot's osteoarthropathy: The role of receptor activator of nuclear factor-kappaB ligand. Diabetologia. 2008; 51(6):1035–40.

17. Petrova NL, Edmonds ME. Conservative and pharmacologic treatments for the diabetic charcot foot. Clin Podiatr Med Surg. 2017; 34(1):15–24.

18. Frykberg R, Wukich D, Kavarthapu V, Zgonis T, Dalla Paola L. Surgery for the diabetic foot: A key component of care. Diabetes Metab Res Rev. 2019; 36(Suppl 1):e3251.

19. Vas PRJ, Edmonds M, Kavarthapu V, et al. The diabetic foot attack: "'Tis Too Late to Retreat!". Int J Low Extrem Wounds. 2018; 17(1):7–13.

20. Ahluwalia R, Vainieri E, Iam J, et al. Surgical diabetic foot debridement: Improving training and practice utilizing the traffic light principle. Int J Low Extrem Wounds. 2019; 18(3):279–86.

21. Simon SR, Tejwani SG, Wilson DL, Santner TJ, Denniston NL. Arthrodesis as an early alternative to nonoperative management of Charcot arthropathy of the diabetic foot. J Bone Joint Surg Am. 2000; 82-A(7):939–50.

22. Laurinaviciene R, Kirketerp-Moeller K, Holstein PE. Exostectomy for chronic midfoot plantar ulcer in Charcot deformity. J Wound Care. 2008; 17:53–5.

23. Chantelau E. The perils of procrastination: Effects of early vs. delayed detection and treatment of incipient Charcot fracture. Diabetes Med. 2005; 22:1707–12.

24. Ha J, Hester T, Foley R, et al. Charcot foot reconstruction outcomes: A systematic review. J Clin Orthop Trauma. 2020; 11(3):357–68.

25. Dayton P, Feilmeier M, Thompson M, Whitehouse P, Reimer RA. Comparison of complications for internal and external fixation for Charcot reconstruction: A systematic review. Foot Ankle Surg. 2015; 54(6):1072–5.

26. Shazadeh Safavi P, Jupiter DC, Panchbhavi V. A systematic review of current surgical interventions for Charcot neuroarthropathy of the midfoot. J Foot Ankle Surg. 2017; 56(6):1249–52.

27. Siebachmeyer M, Boddu K, Bilal A, Hester TW, Hardwick T, Fox TP, et al. Outcome of one-stage correction of deformities of the ankle and hindfoot and fusion in Charcot neuroarthropathy using a retrograde intramedullary hindfoot arthrodesis nail. Bone Joint J. 2015; 97-B(1):76–82.

28. Vasukutty N, Jawalkar H, Anugraha A, et al. Correction of ankle and hind foot deformity in Charcot neuroarthropathy using a retrograde hind foot nail – The Kings' experience. Foot Ankle Surg. 2018; 24(5):406–10.

29. Kavarthapu V, Vris A. Charcot midfoot reconstruction—surgical technique based on three deformity patterns. Ann Joint. 2020; 5:28.

30. Sammarco VJ, Chevillet J. The role of internal fixation in surgery of the Charcot foot and the evolution of "superconstruct" techniques. Current Orthopaedic Practice. 2010; 21(3):233–9.

31. Butt DA, Hester T, Bilal A, Edmonds M, Kavarthapu V. The medial column synthes midfoot fusion bolt is associated with unacceptable rates of failure in corrective fusion for Charcot deformity: Results from a consecutive case series. BJJ. 2015; 97-B(6):809–13.

32. Kummen I, Phyo N, Kavarthapu V. Charcot foot reconstruction—how do hardware failure and non-union affect the clinical outcomes? Ann Joint. 2020; 5:25.

33. Ugwul E, Adeleye O, Gezawa I. Predictors of lower extremity amputation in patients with diabetic foot ulcer: Findings from MEDFUN, a multi-center observational study. J Foot Ankle Res. 2019; 12:34.

34. Sumpio B, Shine SR, Mahler D, Sumpio BE. A comparison of immediate postoperative rigid and soft dressings for below-knee amputations. Ann Vasc Surg. 2013; 27(6):774–80. https://doi.org/10.1016/j.avsg.2013.03.007.

Further resources

1. Michael E. Edmonds, Bauer E. Sumpio. 'Limb Salvage of the Diabetic Foot – An Interdisciplinary Approach'. ISBN 978-3-319-17917-9, ISBN 978-3-319-17918-6 (eBook), https://doi.org/10.1007/978-3-319-17918-6 (Springer 2019)

2. You Tube – Acute Charcot Foot Reconstruction – https://youtu.be/5y-W15FF0rE

3. You Tube – Diabetic Foot Ulcer Debridement – https://youtu.be/LSrrvYqM854

4. You Tube – Charcot Hindfoot Reconstruction – https://youtu.be/4RICN-dzsAE

5. You Tube – Two-stage Charcot Hindfoot and Midfoot Reconstruction – https://www.youtube.com/watch?v=DrGSqiQgAak&t=66s

20 Surgical principles of amputations

Arul Ramasamy, Aabid Sanaullah, and Donatas Chlebinskas

Introduction

The most common cause for foot amputation is due to vascular insufficiency or as a sequelae of diabetic foot complications, and these are discussed in more detail in Chapter 19. Other causes include trauma, congenital deformities, tumours and chronic infection. The decision to amputate, particularly in the traumatic setting, can often be difficult. Whilst it is the instinct of the surgeon to favour limb salvage over amputation, the overriding aim must be to improve the quality of life of the patient.

Amputation in a trauma setting

The treatment of severe, leg-threatening injuries often necessitates an immediate or early decision between limb reconstruction and amputation. The initial decision requires a prediction of treatment outcomes based on the patient and injury characteristics. Factors that may lead to amputation include (1):

- Irreparable vascular injury
- Warm ischaemia time greater than 8 hours
- Severe crush with minimal remaining viable tissue
- A severely damaged limb which may constitute a threat to the patient's life

Given the advances in modern limb salvage techniques, anatomical indications for amputation, such as 'unreconstructable', should not be used, unless the case has been discussed with a specialist centre. In addition, no limb should be amputated on the basis that the patient would be better off without it, unless it has been fully discussed with the patient. In practice, this is rarely possible at the first operation, and so limb salvage should normally be attempted if possible (2).

The presence of a numb sole of foot has traditionally been quoted as an indication for amputation. However, recovery of protective sensation has been reported in 50% of civilian trauma patients and has also been noted in 90% of the UK military patients (3, 4). Therefore, an insensate foot should not be considered an indication for amputation.

Several scoring systems have been developed to guide the decision to amputate after severe lower limb trauma. Although they may be helpful as a retrospective governance tool, the relatively low sensitivity and specificity of these scores makes them unreliable as decision-making tools. This is particularly well illustrated in the prospective study of the Lower Extremity Assessment Project in the United States, which documented relatively low sensitivities and some inconsistencies when five of the more commonly used scoring systems were applied to 556 lower limb injuries and it was felt that clinical utility was not provided (5). In addition, they are not predictive of the shorter or longer term functional outcome.

The decision to amputate in the trauma setting should be made by the most senior surgeon available and should ideally be made by two surgeons and documented clearly in the medical notes. The UK military produced guidelines for performing amputations in the combat setting and those guidelines are equally applicable in civilian trauma practice and are summarised in Table 20.1 (6).

It must be remembered that in the acute trauma setting, the aim of the initial procedure is to perform an adequate debridement of devitalised soft tissue and non-viable bone. This is an evolving state, dependent upon the level of tissue contamination and the patient's physiology. It may require serial debridement of tissue to remove all non-viable tissue, and only at that stage can formal creation of an amputation stump occur.

General considerations

One of the main aims of foot amputation surgery is to salvage as much of the functioning foot as possible. Partial foot amputations have the advantage that they allow the use of relatively normal footwear with the need for only minor modification. In addition, they are likely to lead to better function, greater mobility, lower energy consumption, increased sensory input and less distortion of body image compared to transtibial amputation.

Table 20.1 Guidelines for performing amputations
Pre-operative guidelines
The examination findings, together with the indications to amputate the limb should be documented
Existing limb salvage scores should not be used
Where possible, the decision to amputate should be confirmed with a second surgeon
All wounds to be photographed. Radiographs should be obtained prior to amputation
Neurological dysfunction should not be part of the limb salvage algorithm
Operative technique
The site of the amputation should be the lowest level possible
Guillotine amputations should not be performed
No fashioning of flaps at initial debridement
Bones should be cut at the most distal soft tissue level
Amputation should not be carried at the level of any fracture unless this is the appropriate skin/soft tissue level
No part of the wound to be closed at initial surgery
No attempt to be made to prevent skin retraction

However, this must be tempered by the principles that the salvaged foot must achieve good healing with a stable soft tissue envelope, and the foot must be plantigrade to remain functional. Whilst a more distal amputation is preferable, the surgeon must be aware, that potentially longer healing times and soft tissue complications can result in significant morbidity in the patient. In these cases, a more proximal amputation that results in a well-healed stump that allows early ambulation may be in the patient's best interests. This decision needs to be made on a case-by-case basis, involving the patient, prosthetist and other members of the multidisciplinary team.

Determination of amputation level

The prime determinant of the amputation level is the need for a viable, healthy soft tissue envelope to support the amputated limb. Failure to debride the soft tissue and infected bone fully will lead to flap failure and persistent infection. Thus, the surgeon must be aggressive in the debridement of infected and necrotic soft tissue and bone. Whilst the flaps suggested in the following sections are in optimal tissue, the surgeon must not be afraid to make irregular flaps and then to re-evaluate closure once only healthy tissue remains.

The use of tourniquets in amputation surgery has previously been proscribed. However, Biehl et al. demonstrated that wound healing rates in diabetic and vascular patients undergoing amputation was similar in tourniquet and non-tourniquet groups (7). If a tourniquet is used, then it should be released once the amputated part is removed to check for haemostasis and flap viability prior to wound closure. Secondly, the presence of vascular bypass grafts should be identified as it is inadvisable to apply a tourniquet over such grafts.

When the final skin flaps are created, there should be visible bleeding from the skin edges. If it is not present, then a more proximal amputation may need to be considered. In cases of peripheral vascular disease, joint decision-making with a vascular surgeon is important to identify the correct level of amputation. It may be possible that, with appropriate vascular intervention, a more distal amputation level can be achieved.

Several factors, both local and systemic, influence wound healing and should be addressed in the pre-operative period where possible. Local factors include having adequate blood supply and arterial Doppler ultrasound has value in assessing this. A toe pressure of 40 mm Hg or greater is associated with improved wound healing (8). Transcutaneous oxygen measurements ($TcPO_2$) have also been advocated to predict wound healing. Pinzur et al., noted that a $TcPO_2$ greater than 30 mm Hg was associated with higher rates of wound healing (9). Other local factors include, reducing oedema of tissues by ensuring the limb remains elevated in the postoperative period, as well as preventing infection by adequate surgical debridement and administering culture specific antibiotics.

Systemic factors include optimisation of glycaemic control in diabetics and improving nutritional indices prior to surgery. Wound healing is likely to be improved when (10):

- Total lymphocyte count >1500/μL
- Serum albumin >3.5 g/dL
- Total protein >6.2 g/dL
- Haemoglobin >11 g/dL

Specific amputation levels

Foot amputations range from terminalisation of the distal phalanx to below knee amputation (BKA) (Figure 20.1). Each has their indication, surgical technique and complications and they are discussed here.

Hallux amputation

Amputation of the hallux can be performed either through the proximal phalanx base or through a metatarsophalangeal disarticulation. Although the disarticulation is technically easier, the amputation through the phalangeal base maybe preferable because it preserves the function of the flexor hallucis brevis tendon and the plantar fascia. This helps maintain some of the weight-bearing function of the first ray, and thereby reduce transfer loading to the second and third metatarsal heads.

A racket handle incision is made around the hallux enabling excision of all non-viable tissue. It is important that at *least 1 cm* of the proximal phalanx is preserved. At least one of the sesamoids must be retained because the sesamoidal-phalangeal attachment complex is key to maintaining the weight-bearing function of the first ray.

If the soft tissues or underlying osteomyelitis do not allow preservation of the proximal phalanx, then disarticulation through the metatarsal phalangeal joint (MTPJ) is acceptable. When considering amputation through this level, the soft tissue flaps should be equal to at least half of the proximal phalanx. The cartilage of the metatarsal head can be retained, and sesamoid complex should be inspected. Often the sesamoids retract after disarticulation, but on occasions they do not and can create plantar pressure under the metatarsal head. This could potentially increase the risk of ulceration in the neuropathic patient. In these cases, or if the sesamoids are enlarged or arthritic, then a concomitant sesamoidectomy should be considered. Once the amputation has healed, the patient can be fitted with custom-moulded shoe insert to help balance the weight-bearing pressure over the forefoot and to reduce sliding inside the shoe.

The most common complications of this amputation level are related to inadequate perfusion of the stump leading to flap necrosis. This may necessitate a more proximal amputation. Secondary effects of the amputation include a varus and hyperextension deformity of the second toe, which can lead to ulceration at the DIPJ or PIPJ, as well as the base of the metatarsal head.

Toe amputations

Amputations of the lesser toes are the most common amputation performed in the foot. They can be done either as a disarticulation through the MTPJ or through the proximal phalanx. The advantage of the partial amputation is that the residual stump acts to maintain the toe space and prevents the migration of the two adjacent toes towards each other into the gap created by the removed digit. Much like the hallux amputation, the incision can be made using either a racket -type, fish mouth or dorsal and plantar flaps (Figure 20.2).

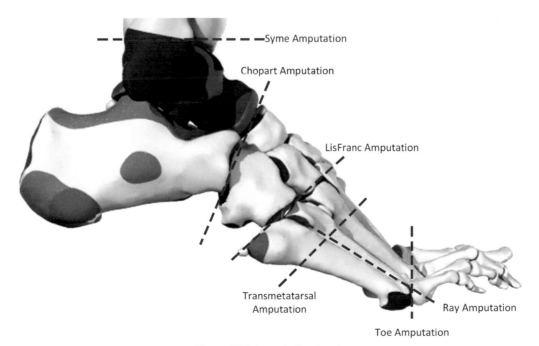

Figure 20.1 Amputation levels.

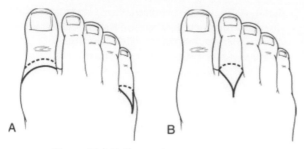

Figure 20.2 Hallux and toe amputations.

Complications from digit amputations include wound problems from haematoma formation or poor balancing of the soft tissues resulting in uneven tension of the sutures. Late complications include drifting of the adjacent toes to fill in the space. Where a partial amputation is performed, occasionally the stump can become dorsally elevated caused by a hyperextension contracture of the MTPJ. This may necessitate an MTPJ disarticulation, or release of the extensor tendons and MTPJ capsule.

Ray amputations

This is defined as an amputation involving the toe with part or all of its corresponding metatarsal. It is indicated in trauma in healthy patients and for infection and gangrene in diabetic patients. It has the advantage that it maintains the overall length of the foot, allowing the patient to mobilise in their own footwear. In addition, by maintaining the skin of the sole of the foot, it provides a durable soft tissue envelope to mobilise on. A consequence of a ray amputation is that it narrows the foot and causes the foot to slide within the shoe. It also increases the pressure exerted on the remaining metatarsals. Both these issues can be managed by a suitable orthotic placed in the shoe. When considering ray amputations, they can be categorised as border ray amputations (first and fifth metatarsals), central ray resections (second to fourth metatarsals) and multiple ray amputations.

Border ray amputations

The first and fifth metatarsal amputations can usually be achieved with either a medial or lateral incision, respectively. The toe and the metatarsal are then removed based on the level of the osteomyelitis and soft tissue envelope. The bases of both metatarsals are retained where possible to maintain the tibialis anterior and peroneus brevis tendon attachment intact. When creating the flaps, a longer plantar flap consisting of the weight-bearing skin is preferable to provide a durable base. It is important to keep as big as a soft tissue flap as possible to allow to a tension-free closure. Excessive trimming of the flaps can lead to tension at the suture line, leading to dehiscence or wound necrosis.

Central ray amputations

Amputation of the second, third or fourth metatarsal is often less common than the border ray amputations. The incisions are made from dorsal to plantar in the webspace and the intermetatarsal space. The metatarsal and toe is removed. The base of the metatarsal should be preserved where possible to prevent destabilising the midfoot and the defect is closed. It is important to note that over-excessive skin debridement can make closure of the wound difficult and care should be taken to ensure that the soft tissue envelope is sufficient. If this is not the case, then a more proximal amputation of the metatarsal may be required. Once the amputation has occurred, the void created by loss of the toe is often filled by the adjacent toes drifting into that space.

Multiple ray amputations

Amputation of more than two rays is possible, but it is vitally important that the patient is provided with a custom fitted insole in the shoe to prevent the severely narrowed foot to slide within the footwear. Medial based partial amputations can lead to imbalance when walking and force extra pressure on the lesser metatarsals, leading to further ulcerations. If more than three ray amputations are considered, then a transmetatarsal amputation (TMA) should be performed due to the excessive loading on the remaining metatarsals.

Transmetatarsal amputation

The TMA was first described by McKittrick in 1949 and is a well-recognised foot salvage procedure in the treatment of severe gangrene, infection or tissue loss in the forefoot. It has the advantage over more proximal amputations in that it preserves the attachment to tibialis anterior and peroneus brevis. This maintains active dorsiflexion, as well as counteracts the pull of the triceps surae that can lead to an equinus contraction. In addition, it allows patient to ambulate in their footwear with a custom total contact insole. The prerequisites for a TMA include absence of infection proximal to the level of amputation, no significant deformity of the midfoot or hindfoot, ability to create healthy skin flaps and a patent pedal arterial arch.

Full thickness dorsal and plantar skin flaps are developed, superficial to the long flexor and extensor tendons, retaining as much skin as possible. The proximal metatarsals are divided parallel to the floor with an oscillating saw in non-infected bone. Any sharp edges are smoothed. The second tarsometatarsal (TMT) joint's integrity is maintained and the Lisfranc ligament is left intact. Thus, the first and second metatarsals are cut at the same level. The third to fifth metatarsals are cut as a cascade to the lateral border of the foot. The base of the fifth metatarsal is preserved, as it is the attachment of peroneus brevis. Similarly, the insertion of the tibialis anterior is preserved on the first metatarsal base. Once the amputation is completed, the skin flaps are trimmed, leaving plantar skin in preference to dorsal skin, to allow easy closure (Figure 20.3). If 5 degrees of ankle dorsiflexion cannot be achieved, then a concomitant Tendo-Achilles procedure is performed (11).

The main risk associated with this procedure is the development of recurrent ulceration on the stump. This can be caused by either a plantar projection of one of the residual metatarsal stumps or by new bone formation at the distal metatarsal. This can be treated by surgical excision. At the same time, increased loading of the metatarsal stumps can arise from an equinus deformity. This may necessitate an Achilles lengthening or capsular release of the ankle and subtalar joints.

The Lisfranc amputation, which is the disarticulation at the TMT joints, is similar to a TMA in technique, but requires reimplantation of the tibilias anterior and

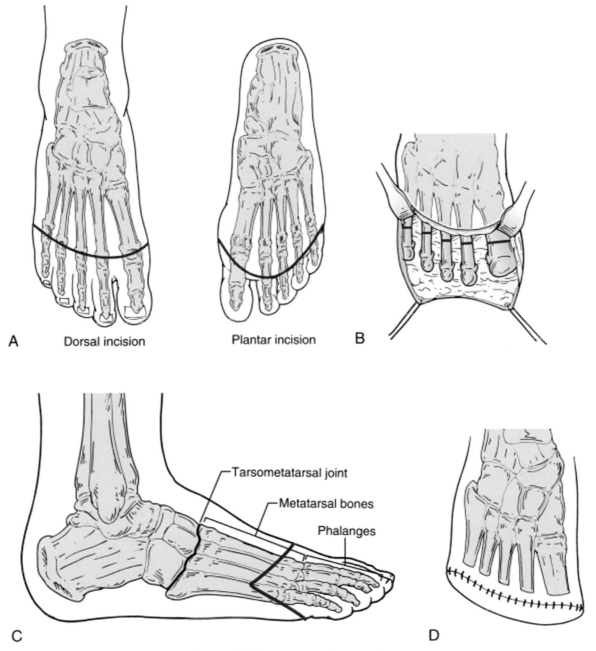

A   Dorsal incision   Plantar incision   B

Tarsometatarsal joint

Metatarsal bones

Phalanges

C   D

Figure 20.3 Transmetatarsal amputation.

peroneus brevis tendons in order to achieve a balanced foot. An Achilles lengthening should be considered in all cases.

Chopart amputation

The Chopart amputation involves the disarticulation of the foot at the level of the talonavicular and calcaneo-cuboid joint. This amputation level has some advantages compared to more proximal amputations:

- It does not provide much shortening of the limb.
- Postoperatively the patient can be fitted with an Ankle-Foot-Orthosis (AFO), allowing normal shoe wear.
- By maintaining the heel, distal weight-bearing is through tough weight-bearing skin.

Like the TMA, a long plantar flap is developed to provide soft tissue coverage. In order to balance the foot appropriately, the tibialis anterior tendon is transferred to the talar neck, extensor hallucis longus and peroneus brevis are transferred to the anterior process of the calcaneus to prevent an equinovarus deformity. Extensor digitorum longus can also be sutured to the distal end of the plantar fascia to prevent proximal migration of the plantar structures. An Achilles tenectomy (removal of 2–3 cm of the tendon) is performed concurrently through a separate posterior medial incision to prevent an equinovarus deformity. Following surgery, the ankle should be splinted in slight dorsiflexion for 6 weeks.

Whilst theoretically the Chopart amputation offers many advantages, the opportunity to utilise it is often very seldom. The major limiting factor is the need for adequate, healthy soft tissue coverage. This tissue envelope is similar to that required for a TMA. When this is not present, a more proximal amputation level should be considered. As such, it has been used as the last opportunity to avoid major amputation for diabetic patients. Faglia et al. (2016) reported a relatively high complication rate within this cohort of patients with a 31.9% ulcer recurrence and 27.7% major re-amputation rate (12).

Syme amputation

The Syme amputation involves disarticulation of the foot at the level of the ankle, removal of the malleoli and anchoring of the heel pad to the weight-bearing surface. The long-lever arm afforded by the distal amputation, the ability to bear weight on the end of the limb on robust heel pad skin and a self-suspending prosthetic fit would suggest that this would offer a good functional outcome and has been shown to be more energy efficient than a midfoot amputation (13). It is indicated in trauma, gangrene and infection. As it does not interfere with the distal tibial growth plate, it has also been used in the management of paediatric congenital deformities

such as fibular hemimelia, proximal focal femoral deficiency and congenital pseudoarthrosis of the tibia.

The surgical approach involves forming an anterior flap by an incision 1.5 cm below the lateral malleolus that is continued over the front of the ankle to point 1.5 cm below the medial malleolus. The plantar incision is then continued down to bone and then traverses the sole of the foot and vertically up to the lateral malleolar incision. Care must be taken to avoid damaging the neurovascular bundle on the medial side. The bundle lies between flexor hallucis longus and flexor digitorum longus and if damaged can lead to necrosis of the heel pad flap. The anterior tendons are then cut and retracted and the anterior tibial vessels tied and cut. Once bone is seen, careful blunt and sharp dissection of the calcaneus and talus is performed to separate it from the soft tissue envelope. At this stage the Achilles tendon is carefully dissected off the calcaneus, and the skin must not be breached as this will form the heel weight-bearing surface.

Once the calcaneus and talus are removed, the prominence of the medial malleolus and lateral malleolus are cut so that they are flush with the tibial plafond. The soft tissue pad is then stabilised by suturing the plantar fascia to the anterior tibia (Figure 20.4).

The most common complication of the Syme amputation is the failure of healing. The soft tissue flap is reliant on the blood supply to remain uninjured during surgery. Any injury to the vessels during dissection can lead to necrosis of the flap. Furthermore, excessive trimming of the lateral and medial skin flaps to prevent dogears can lead to reduced perfusion to the heel flap. The second complication is failure to stabilise the soft tissue stump securely. This can lead to a mobile and displaced heel pad that interferes with direct weight-bearing.

Pinzur et al. demonstrated 88% success rate in a retrospective review in diabetic patients with Syme amputation. They emphasised the importance of appropriate patient selection, made on the basis of clinical examination and an assessment of the wound-healing parameters, i.e., vascular inflow (ultrasound Doppler ischemic index of 0.5 or transcutaneous partial pressure of oxygen between 20 and 30 mm Hg), tissue nutrition (serum albumin of 2.5 g/dL) and immunocompetence (14).

Below knee amputation

The BKA is necessary when foot salvage amputations have failed or not deemed appropriate due to the level of infection, vascular dysfunction or soft tissue damage. Traditionally, the ideal below knee stump should be 15 cm below the level of the knee joint. However, advances in prosthetics have resulted in successful prosthetic fitting with much smaller residual stumps. Whilst a longer below knee stump provides a longer lever

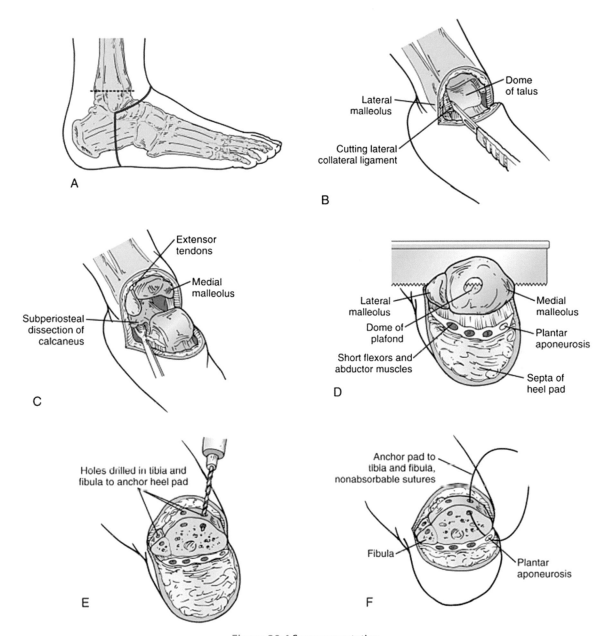

Figure 20.4 Syme amputation.

to generate power, an overly long stump may preclude fitting of more advanced micro-processor controlled motorised prosthesis. This highlights the importance of discussing amputation level with the prosthetic team prior to surgery.

The classic Romano-Burgess amputation involves fashioning a long posterior flap. This has the advantage of providing distal padding under the weight-bearing portion of the tibia. However, it is important to fashion the stump appropriately to prevent large dog-ears on both sides of the stump, which can make fitting a temporary prosthetic difficult. For this reason, some surgeons prefer using a skew flap technique, which allows for more consistent shaping of the stump (15).

One of the controversies in BKA has been the use of bone-bridging procedures. Theoretically, by creating a synostosis between the tibia and fibula, this may reduce pain within the residual stump. This may be more important in more proximal transtibial amputations, where the interosseous membrane is relatively absent leading to abduction of the fibula on weight-bearing. First described by Ertl in 1949, it involves implanting a corticoperiosteal block between the bones. Later, screw fixation or a suture button technique has also been employed. Despite showing promising results in single surgeon case series, a randomised controlled trial in the US military casualties demonstrated a higher complication rate with no significant improvement in functional outcome (16).

Complications following BKA include infection, wound problems and painful neuroma formation in the short term. In the longer term, phantom limb pain may be disabling. It is important to realise that as the stump matures and the patient starts their prosthetic journey, issues with excess soft tissue or prominent bone may lead to ulceration or rubbing. This may necessitate the need for stump refashioning in the future.

Following BKA, it should be recognised that functional outcomes are significantly reduced compared to non-amputees in both physical and mental health domains. This is irrespective of whether the amputation is performed for vascular insufficiency or trauma. BKA results in an increase of baseline energy expenditure of 25–40% based on the level of amputation and prosthetic use diminishes with increasing age and time after amputation.

Take home messages

- Amputations in trauma should be a two-surgeon decision and where possible limb salvage should be considered unless it is to the detriment to the patient.
- An insensate sole of the foot is not an indication for amputation.
- The key to a successful amputation is the complete excision of infected and non-viable tissue, leaving a healthy soft tissue envelope that will heal.
- When performing a TMA, care must be taken to preserve the base of the first and fifth metatarsals to maintain the attachment of the tibialis anterior and peroneus brevis tendon.
- Ertl bridging procedures in BKAs are not associated with better outcomes but may have a higher complication rate.

References

1. Ramasamy A, Hill AM, Clasper JC. "Improvised explosive devices: pathophysiology, injury profiles and current medical management," *BMJ Military Health* 155(4) (2009): 265–72.
2. Clasper J, Ramasamy A. "Traumatic amputations," *Br J Pain* 7(2) (2013): 67–73.
3. Bosse MJ, McCarthy ML, Jones AL, Webb LX, Sims SH, Sanders RW, MacKenzie EJ, Lower Extremity Assessment Project (LEAP) Study Group. "The insensate foot following severe lower extremity trauma: an indication for amputation?" *J Bone Joint Surg Am* 87-A (2005): 2601–8.
4. Birch R, Misra P, Stewart MP, Eardley WG, Ramasamy A, Brown K, Shenoy R, Anand P, Clasper J, Dunn R, Etherington J. "Nerve injuries sustained during warfare: part II: outcomes," *J Bone Joint Surg Br* 94(4) (2012):529–35.
5. Bosse MJ, MacKenzie EJ, Kellam JF, et al. "A prospective evaluation of the clinical utility of the lower-extremity injury-severity scores," *J Bone Joint Surg Am* 83-A (2001): 3–14.
6. Clasper JC. "Amputations of the lower limb: a multidisciplinary consensus," *J R Army Med Corps* 153(3) (2007): 172–4.
7. Biehl III WC, Morgan JM, Wagner Jr FW, Gabriel RA. "The safety of the Esmarch tourniquet," *Foot Ankle* 14(5) (1993): 278–83.
8. Apelqvist J, Castenfors J, Larsson J, Stenström A, Agardh CD. "Prognostic value of systolic ankle and toe blood pressure levels in outcome of diabetic foot ulcer," *Diabetes Care* 12(6) (1989): 373–8.
9. Pinzur MS, Sage R, Stuck R, Ketner L, Osterman H. "Transcutaneous oxygen as a predictor of wound healing in amputations of the foot and ankle," *Foot Ankle* 13(5) (1992): 271–2.
10. Dickhaut SC, DeLee JC, Page CP. "Nutritional status: importance in predicting wound-healing after amputation," *J Bone Joint Surg Am* 66(1) (1984): 71–5.
11. Humphrey JA, Kanthasamy S, Coughlin P, Coll AP, Robinson AAH. "Outcome of trans-metatarsal amputations in patients with diabetes mellitus," *Foot (Edinb)* 40 (2019): 22–6.
12. Faglia E, Clerici G. "Outcomes of Chopart amputation in a tertiary referral diabetic foot clinic: data from a consecutive series of 83 hospitalized patients," *J Foot Ankle Surg* 55(2) (2016): 230–4.
13. Pinzur MS, Gold J. "Energy demand for walking in dysvascular amputees as related to the level of amputation," *Orthopedics* 15(9) (1992): 1033–7.
14. Pinzur MS, Stuck R, Sage R. "Syme ankle disarticulation in patients with diabetes," *J Bone J Surg Am* 85(9) (2003): 1667–72.
15. Robinson KP. "Skew-flap below-knee amputation," *Ann R Coll Surg Engl* 73(3) (1991): 155–7.
16. Tintle SM, Keeling JJ, Forsberg JA, Shawen SB, Andersen RC, Potter BK. "Operative complications of combat-related trans-tibial amputations: a comparison of the modified burgess and modified Ertl tibiofibular synostosis techniques," *J Bone J Surg Am* 93(11) (2011): 1016–21.

21 Principles of lower limb prosthetics and rehabilitation

Rajiv S Hanspal and John Sullivan

Introduction

Limb amputation surgery and prosthetic replacement is one of the earliest recorded surgical operations dating back to 5th century BC. Historian Herodotus relates the story of a Persian soldier and prisoner who cut off his foot in order to secure his freedom and replaced it with a wooden foot. The common cause of amputation has generally been traumatic and as a life-saving procedure. Most of the developments in amputation and prosthetics have generally been associated with war, as is evident even today. However, in the western world, the cause of amputation is increasingly due to vascular disease. Amputation becomes a necessary surgical procedure to remove a limb that has otherwise become useless and life threatening.

Nevertheless, it should be viewed as a positive reconstructive procedure to 'fashion' a residual limb (stump) that will facilitate optimal biomechanical function and locomotion. With technical advances in prosthetics and a wider acceptance of disability in current western society, amputation is increasingly considered a 'treatment option' as opposed to a 'necessity'. In these circumstances, a pre-amputation consultation with a specialist prosthetic rehabilitation team is strongly recommended. This helps with goal planning, managing expectations and the preparation of an effective rehabilitation programme with a view to achieving the best possible outcome.

Indications

Essentially, the indications for a lower limb amputation (Box 21.1) are to remove a non-viable limb (gangrene), to reduce pain (ischaemic), to preserve life (malignancy,

---

Box 21.1 Indications for amputation
- Remove non-viable limb – gangrene
- Relieve symptoms – ischaemic limb
- Preserve life – malignancy
- Improve function – limb deformity, neuropathic limb, congenital deficiency

---

gangrene) or to improve function (congenital deficiency, neuropathic, late complications of trauma). In the UK, the commonest cause remains vascular (65%). Other causes are trauma (early or late complications), infection including failed joint replacement, tumours, neuropathies or congenital limb deficiency (1). Recently, there has been an increase in amputation as an optional treatment with the aim of improving mobility and function with the use of advanced prostheses.

Stages of rehabilitation

Pre-amputation consultation

The stages of rehabilitation are set out in detail in the British Society of Rehabilitation Medicine Standards (2). A pre-amputation consultation is particularly useful when amputation is elective and planned as a treatment option. It facilitates appropriate advice and discussion of all treatment options. A meeting with the specialist prosthetic rehabilitation team facilitates further clinical opinion and advice about the amputation with discussions of realistic goals, prosthetic options and projected outcome. It provides an opportunity to advise the operating surgeon regarding the optimum level of amputation and ideal length of stump. Specialist therapy advice for potential adaptive equipment and environmental changes, including return to employment or leisure activities, can also be considered (3). It may be appropriate to start a therapy program preoperatively. Pain management may also need to be addressed preoperatively. It has been shown that pain control (epidural or patient control analgesia) started preoperatively and continued in the same form post-amputation reduces the incidence of phantom and amputation related pain.

Amputation

The aim of amputation, especially for those who are likely to mobilise with a prosthesis, is to fashion a new end organ for locomotion. A surgeon with experience in appropriate techniques should perform the amputation. The amputation should be timely and be given

---

Box 21.2 Principles of amputation surgery

- Skin: Healthy, sensate and tension free repair
- Muscle: Debulked to reduce stump size and optimise shape
- Nerves: Gentle traction before division proximally with a sharp knife
- Blood vessels: Double ligation
- Bone: Adequate length with chamfered edges and avoid periosteal stripping

---

Box 21.3 Selection of amputation levels

- Most distal level that achieves healing
- Preserve knee joint if possible
- Avoid proximal joint contracture
- Ensure adequate clearance distance to allow space for prosthetic joints
- Bone: Adequate length with chamfered edges and avoid periosteal stripping

Specific

- Transfemoral: 15 cm proximal to knee joint to allow space for soft tissue cover and prosthetic knee unit
- Transtibial: 8 cm per metre of patient height
- Syme's amputation: Ensure good end-bearing stump. Prosthetic results better than Boyd, Chopart or Lisfranc

---

appropriate priority on the surgical list. Recognised surgical techniques should be used. Tourniquet should be used in all cases except in those with vascular disease. Meticulous handling of soft tissues is essential to ensure good healing.

The stump should have healthy skin cover though this may not always be possible due to the nature of the original trauma and tissue injury (Box 21.2). Rarely, special techniques may be used to provide skin cover with the aim of ensuring adequate length (skin grafting or fillet of sole technique), i.e., to allow a possible transtibial level instead of a transfemoral amputation (4). Scars in weight-bearing areas of the stump and adherence to underlying bone should be avoided.

Muscles should be cut a few centimetres longer than the level of bone section. Adequate myoplasty with appropriate debulking of muscle should ensure a good stump shape for prosthetic socket use. For myodesis, adequate muscle is required to ensure repair of opposing muscles without tension.

Over traction of nerves should be avoided. The nerves should be divided with a sharp knife after applying gentle traction and then allowed to retract. This should help minimise neuroma formation. Recently, Targeted Muscle Reinnervation (TMR) surgery (5) is being considered at the time of an elective amputation as studies have shown this to be therapeutic for stump and phantom pain.

Blood vessels are ligated with double ligatures considered for major arteries. Tourniquet should be released before muscle repair. Meticulous haemostasis avoids haematoma formation, not an uncommon complication. Appropriate drain should be used.

Length of amputation stump

The level of bone section depends on the level of amputation planned (Box 21.3). The optimum level for a transtibial amputation is 8 cm per metre of the patient's height. For transfemoral amputation, the level of bone section is generally considered to be 15 cm proximal to the knee joint when the distal muscle cover will effectively reduce the distance of knee clearance (distance from the end of the stump to the level of the knee joint) to about 12 cm.

This is adequate space to accommodate most prosthetic knee units. Excessive periosteal stripping should be avoided to limit secondary changes at the stump end. The cut ends should be gently shaped to avoid spikes or sharp edges. The end result should be a gently tapered and contoured stump appropriate for socket fitting.

The characteristics of the amputation stump have a significant influence on the ability to tolerate and control a prosthesis (Figure 21.1). The stump is a mechanical

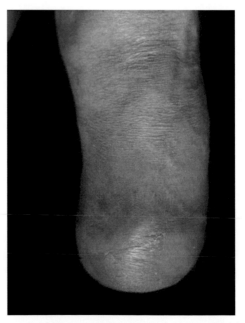

Figure 21.1 Mature conical transtibial stump suitable for prosthetic use.

lever and a short stump reduces the mechanical advantage. A correlation exists between the length of stump and quality of gait. A short transfemoral stump and the associated loss of adductor mass magnify the Trendelenburg effect, a common characteristic of transfemoral gait (6).

Other considerations

When considering the optimum level of amputation, joints should be preserved and fixed deformities avoided. Retention of the knee provides a better functional outcome than a transfemoral amputation. Ideally, a unit performing amputations should have a 2.5 to 1.0 ratio of transtibial to transfemoral amputations. Amputations through the joint may be functionally beneficial, but there are associated cosmetic limitations. If a patient is unlikely to mobilise with prostheses or if there is a possibility of becoming a bilateral amputee, a knee disarticulation should be considered as this facilitates improved bed mobility due to the end bearing and leverage properties of the stump. The authors have never seen through hip or pelvic amputation for a foot and ankle pathology in their career spanning over 30 years.

Disarticulation through a joint

Good end bearing properties are essential for knee disarticulation, Gritti-Stokes or Syme's amputations to achieve the designed benefits of this level of amputation. While these levels have functional advantages, the cosmetic appearance of the prostheses may be disappointing for some. The length of the prosthetic socket needs to accommodate the bulbous end of the amputation stump and choice of prosthetic knee and prosthetic foot may be restricted. At the foot and ankle level, the Syme's amputation gives better results than the Boyd, Chopart or Lisfranc amputations. The Chopart and Boyd amputations do not provide adequate space distally for the prosthetic foot. The Lisfranc and some other midfoot amputations present problems at the end of the stump due to high forces during gait. Amputation through a metatarsal bone is unlikely to require prosthetic assistance apart from a space filler.

Paediatric amputation

In children (1), an amputation through the diaphysis is avoided in preference to a disarticulation (e.g., Syme's). This is because the growing upper end of the tibia is retained in the stump and as the child grows, it presents through the skin often requiring surgical trimming every 2–4 years until skeletal maturity. The Syme's stump in a child does not have the same disadvantages as in adults and functionally ends up as a 'below knee' amputation for prosthetic replacement.

Postoperative management

This period should ensure good pain control. If a preoperative epidural or Patient Controlled Analgesia (PCA) is started, it should ideally continue for 3 days. Physical measures like elevation of the limb should be accompanied. It is still generally recommended that rigid plaster dressings are used for transtibial amputees to control swelling, pain and fixed contractures. The authors however warn against the use of rigid dressings in teams or on wards that are not used to regular use of plaster of Paris. This is because it may be necessary to remove the plaster urgently if there are symptoms or signs of swelling. A Cochrane systematic review (7) identified uncertainty with regard to the efficacy of rigid dressings over soft dressings though they have been routinely advised in various guidelines.

Alternatives are available although graduated compression socks (e.g., Juzo™) are the commonest measure used in the UK. The compression sock is first applied a few days post-amputation when signs of healing are evident and the surgeon approves. This helps control postoperative oedema and pain. Wheelchairs should have stump-elevating boards.

Complications

Early complications directly related to the amputation are wound healing and pain. Wound problems may require revision surgery especially if the chances of healing remain in doubt and early mobilisation and prosthetic use is desired.

Both may also be late complications – as discussed in section 'Later consequences or sequelae after lower limb amputations'.

Early prosthetic rehabilitation

Prosthetic rehabilitation should ideally be undertaken under the supervision of a team specialised in this field to achieve the best holistic results and outcomes (2). The use of an early walking aid such as the Pneumatic Post Amputation Mobility Aid (PPAM Aid) with a maximum pressure of 40 mmHg or Femurette, are an essential part of early rehabilitation in the physiotherapy gym (Figure 21.2). Early walking aids facilitate early standing, posture control, early mobilisation, stump oedema control as well as improving morale. Early walking aids also assist as an assessment tool for predicting achievable outcomes and goals (Box 21.4).

The amputee's general medical condition, physical fitness and cognitive status will influence the outcome in terms of prosthetic rehabilitation and mobility. Many amputees who are systemically unwell will not have the required level of fitness to follow a prosthetic rehabilitation pathway. It has been shown that there is a positive linear relationship between cognitive ability and level of mobility achievable with a prosthesis (8).

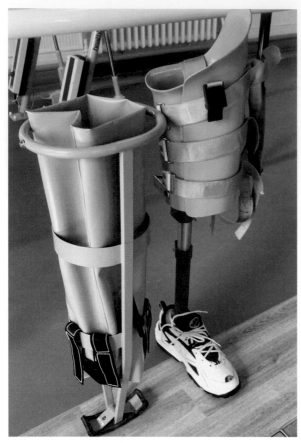

Figure 21.2 Early walking aids. Pneumatic Post Amputation Mobility Aid (PPAM Aid) and Femuette.

Sensory impairment, especially visual impairment and neglect, may be additional problems to overcome. Cardiorespiratory fitness is important because of the additional energy required for walking with a prosthesis (9). Musculoskeletal impairment including motor weakness and joint contractures especially in the lower

limbs will impair mobility. Upper limb problems like weak grasp or lack of dexterity make independent donning and doffing difficult. Coexisting medical problems such as heart failure or renal impairment can affect the socket fit due to associated peripheral oedema and fluctuating stump volume. All these factors need to be considered when assessing the amputee and setting expectations and realistic goals. The aim however should be a return to maximum independence and participation in society.

Principles of prostheses

Access to prosthetic rehabilitation services remains variable across the globe. The provision of technologically advanced prosthetics is prevalent in countries with advanced healthcare systems. The WHO and the International Society for Prosthetics and Orthotics (ISPO) have published international standards (10) for global use, including an implementation manual. The use of local resources is strongly recommended.

Successful outcomes following amputation surgery are not dependent upon sophisticated levels of prosthetic provision. Adherence to sound principles in rehabilitation and good quality technical support can achieve excellent results within the boundaries of regional, social and economic constraints.

Good practice in amputation surgery can have a profound impact upon outcomes and quality of life for prosthetic users (11). The amputation marks the beginning of the rehabilitation journey and re-integration into society.

Prosthetic socket

The linkage between the amputation stump and prosthesis is termed the socket (Box 21.5). The socket is a bespoke component designed to accommodate the amputation stump and facilitate the comfortable transmission of forces during gait.

The level of socket comfort (12) experienced by amputees varies over time. During the course of a day the stump volume can change due to factors including, activity level, temperature and fluid retention. Amputees manage the fit of their socket by using additional socks to accommodate changes in volume or by moderating activity to remain within parameters of comfort.

The socket needs to be adjusted from time to time and replaced periodically as the stump matures or the body mass alters (13). The shape of the stump is captured using traditional plaster of Paris techniques or, as is increasingly the case, digital scanning. The positive plaster or digital model requires modification to produce a 'biomechanical' interface.

Cotton socks have been the traditional interface between the stump and socket. Liners are now widely

---

Box 21.4 Common outcome measures used in the UK for the rehabilitation of lower limb amputees with prostheses

- SIGAM Mobility Grade
- Harold Wood Stanmore Mobility Grade
- Locomotor Capability Index
- Timed Walking Test
- Socket Comfort Score
- Barthel Index for activities of daily living
- Hospital Anxiety & Depression Scale (HADS)
- Numerical Rating Score (NRS) for pain
- EQoL 5D

Box 21.5 Summary of prosthetic prescription

Socket
- Accommodate amputation stump
- Transmission of stump interface forces during gait
- End-bearing with joint disarticulation
- Often designed in combination with liners – PUR, Silicone, TPE

Suspension
- Means of attaching the prosthesis and minimising instability
- External – waist belt, external hip joint
- Supracondylar self suspending to capture anatomical shape
- Use of liners – locking pin, vacuum suspension
- Skin suction
- Osseointegration

Knee joints
- Simple joint for locked knee gait, voluntary unlock for sitting
- Mechanical joint for free knee gait – swing and stance phase control
- Accurate alignment to facilitate safe and efficient gait
- Single axis or polycentric, geometric, hydraulic, pneumatic control
- Microprocessor knee control, high level of safety and control

Prosthetic foot modules
- Simple design SACH foot, material deformation
- Multiaxial foot modules incorporating mechanical ankle joint
- Energy storing – carbon fibre or composite used for high impact
- Microprocessor ankle units
- Powered ankle joints
- Selection based on activity, goals and body weight

Additional
- Torsion adapter to absorb rotational forces during gait
- Telescopic shock absorbers to absorb axial impact forces
- Cosmetic fairing – foam cover or high definition silicone
- Now more acceptable to wear prosthesis without cosmetic covering

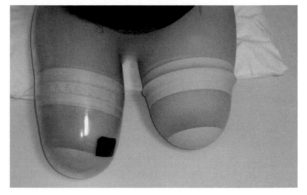

Figure 21.3 Transfemoral silicone liners on a bilateral amputee. Clear diagnostic/test socket *in situ* on the right side. Note the circumferential sealing rings designed to facilitate vacuum suspension of the prosthesis.

(PUR) and silicone are the three materials predominantly used to manufacture liners. The materials have different mechanical properties and selection is based upon individual requirements. Liners serve a range of functions including soft tissue containment, reduction in shear forces, cushioning, suspension (Figure 21.3) and protection of vulnerable tissue (14).

Prosthetic alignment

This refers to the dimensional relationship between the ground reaction force vector and anatomical/prosthetic landmarks such as the socket, hip, knee and ankle joints. Poor alignment results in discomfort, instability and inefficiency of gait. Characteristics of the amputation stump that affect alignment include, muscle imbalance, length of stump and contractures.

Transtibial prostheses

Transtibial socket design

Socket comfort is the primary priority for most amputees. An uncomfortable socket can restrict or completely prevent mobility. The Patella Tendon Bearing (PTB) design of socket has been prevalent since the mid 1960s. This socket design captures and applies load to pressure tolerant areas namely the patella tendon, paratibial areas and popliteal region. Space is introduced over pressure sensitive areas in particular the head of fibula, cut end of tibia and tibial crest. This requires a method of rectification that adds material to a positive model to introduce space and removes material over pressure tolerant areas to apply increased load. Latterly, the same techniques can be applied to digital models.

The introduction of liners has facilitated alternative methods of designing the transtibial socket and transmitting weight through the stump. PUR liners can be

used worn directly over the stump prior to donning the socket. Thermoplastic elastomer (TPE), polyurethane

used to achieve loading across the whole surface area of a well-fashioned stump. The flow characteristic of polyurethane redistributes material away from areas of peak pressure until equal pressure distribution is achieved. This concept is referred to as total surface bearing. The choice of socket design and interface material is considered in combination depending upon the features of the stump. A TPE liner may be more appropriate to provide cushioning over a bony stump. TPE is an inert material useful to protect sensitive scar tissue for example. Silicone liners are particularly effective when stabilisation of excess soft tissue is required.

Transtibial suspension

The method of securely attaching the prosthesis to the body is referred to as the suspension system. Effective suspension eliminates movement between the socket and stump during gait (15). Inadequate suspension allows movement of the socket causing instability of the prosthesis, abrasions, reduced proprioception and increased risk of falls.

Supracondylar suspension is inherent in the socket design encompassing the curve of the femoral condyles and providing a self-suspending socket. Cuff straps are less commonly used. The strap is secured circumferentially proximal to the femoral condyles with down-straps attached to the socket.

Some liners incorporate suspension systems within their design. For example, the use of a distal locking pin that engages with a ratchet mechanism inside the socket to provide mechanical fixation. Vacuum systems are employed using a circumferential airtight sealing ring around the liner. Air is expelled from the socket via a one-way expulsion valve situated distal to the seal creating a vacuum suspension.

Knee suspension sleeves are commonly used. These attach to the proximal brim of the socket extending over the knee onto the lower thigh. The sleeve can be used in combination with an expulsion valve to provide a vacuum effect.

Prosthetic foot module

The simplest design of prosthetic foot is termed solid-ankle cushion heel (SACH). Deformation of the foot during gait facilitates shock absorption and forward progression.

Energy storing feet mainly consist of carbon fibre or composite materials. Energy storing feet do not incorporate ankle joints. Energy is stored as the material deforms during the loading cycle and released at toe off. These designs can be seen at their most effective in the Paralympic running events.

Multi-axial feet with ankle joints range from mechanical and hydraulic designs to units incorporating microprocessor technology and powered plantar flexion. Evidence indicates that the incorporation of an ankle joint, with plantar and dorsi flexion facilitates forward progression, greater symmetry during gait and a reduction in forces acting around the stump.

Foot module selection is based upon factors including patient goals, body weight and activity levels. Manufacturers provide guidance to assist appropriate product selection.

Additional components can be introduced into the prosthetic system such as torsion adapters and shock absorbers to reduce the effect of rotational and impact forces particularly with high activity amputees.

Transfemoral prostheses

The absence of the knee joint presents additional challenges compared to transtibial level. Walking with an above knee prosthesis demands additional energy expenditure over and above non-amputee, or transtibial amputee gait (9). Transfemoral prostheses incorporate a prosthetic knee unit, in addition to the other routine components (Figure 21.4). Forces generated during gait are predominantly transmitted through the socket in the pelvic region, in particular the ischial tuberosity.

Transfemoral socket, liners and suspension

Sockets can be designed as ischial bearing, ischial containment, total contact or suction sockets. Liners are also widely used and the benefits of liners are as previously discussed.

Secure suspension of the transfemoral prosthesis can be difficult to achieve particularly with short stumps. Inadequate suspension causes movement of the socket around the stump, discomfort, insecurity and an increased risk of falls. The simplest form of suspension is a soft elastic belt extending from the prosthesis around the waist. This can also be the least effective design of suspension particularly for obese amputees with a diffuse body shape.

A waist belt with an external hinged hip joint can be used in conjunction with weak hip musculature. The belt suspends the prosthesis and the pendulum effect of the hip joint reduces the effort to walk.

Liners incorporating distal locking pins or rubber sealing rings in combination with vacuum systems are commonly used to suspend transfemoral prostheses These systems negate the requirement for a belt around the waist, which can be bulky and restrictive.

Skin suction sockets, less commonly used since the introduction of liners, offer effective suspension on a well-fashioned stump. The stump is drawn into the socket using a nylon sheath or bandage. Once fully into the socket a one-way expulsion valve maintains a negative pressure providing direct suction suspension.

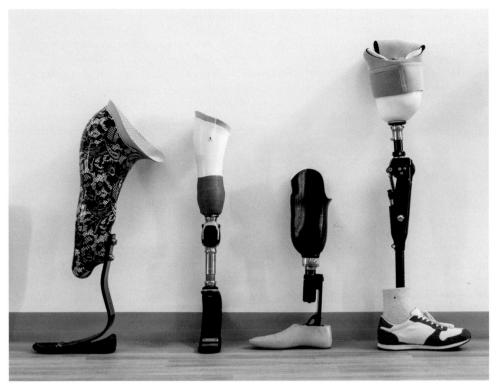

Figure 21.4 Range of prostheses, left to right: Congenital deformity with carbon foot, child above knee prosthesis with hydraulic knee, transtibial prosthesis with locking pin suspension and above knee prosthesis with waist belt and mechanical knee joint.

Prosthetic knee units

Prosthetic knee joints range considerably in complexity; the simplest remain locked during gait and can be voluntary unlocked for sitting. Amputees capable of a free-knee gait utilise knees incorporating swing and stance phase control mechanisms.

Stance phase control facilitates a recovery time in the event of a stumble or misplacement of the foot. The mechanism used can be a simple friction brake or a more complex yielding hydraulic design. The geometry of the knee influences stability with particular regard to polyaxial joints as opposed to single axis joints. Biomechanical alignment is critical during stance phase and the ground reaction force vector should be anterior to the knee centre when the joint is straight generating an extension moment.

Microprocessor knees are widely used inferring an increased level of safety and intuitive gait (16). Various designs are available incorporating hydraulic, pneumatic and magnetorheological fluid to facilitate stance and swing phase control. Sensors measure real time spatial, temporal and angular parameters as well as forces generated during gait. The knee responds and adjusts in real time to changing situations such as an increase in walking speed, unintended stumbles or negotiation of steps and slopes.

Foot module

Prosthetic feet and additional components are as described under transtibial considerations. Suffice to say that the transfemoral prosthesis should be viewed as a biomechanical system with the various components working harmoniously to optimise gait, safety and socket comfort. Recent additional developments in prosthetic systems utilise biomimetic principles and microprocessor technology to facilitate communication and synchronisation between the prosthetic knee and foot module. For example, as the knee flexes, the ankle joint dorsi flexes to assist with ground clearance.

Joint disarticulation considerations

Knee disarticulation

Disarticulation through the joint, either ankle or knee, can provide a durable and functional amputation stump with full end bearing properties. This avoids the requirement to transmit weight through more proximal structures.

Advantages of a knee disarticulation include a long lever arm providing effective control of the prosthesis and improved proprioception. The muscle complex acting around the hip remains intact with minimal lateral deviation of the trunk during gait. The bulbous shape of the femoral condyles can be utilised to suspend the prosthesis via a self-suspending socket.

The long stump can be considered a disadvantage cosmetically. There is insufficient space available to accommodate the dimensions of a prosthetic knee. This results in disproportionality with regard to the knee centres particularly noticeable in sitting. Knee units are available with low build heights incorporating a stable polyaxial design that can to some extent mitigate dimensional inequality.

Amputations through the distal femur such as the Gritti-Stokes strive to address the disadvantages of the knee disarticulation amputation. In the event that end bearing properties are unsatisfactory following amputation the result is a long tranfemoral stump without the distal weight-bearing properties considered an advantage following a knee disarticulation.

A knee disarticulation can facilitate excellent outcomes for a cohort of amputees whose main goal is functionality over and above cosmetic appearance (17).

Ankle disarticulation

The Syme's ankle disarticulation can produce a functional end bearing stump. It is now unusual to come across a Syme's amputation and prosthetic manufacture needs to be bespoke to achieve a good prosthetic outcome. Disadvantages include the bulbous shape, poor cosmesis around the ankle and limited options for components. An advantage of a Syme's is the ability to mobilise on the stump without a prosthesis. It remains an excellent operation in growing children and is effectively treated as a 'below-knee' amputation in terms of prosthetic provision.

Partial foot amputation

Prosthetic solutions for partial foot amputations such as the Lisfranc remain limited. Provision falls between orthotic and prosthetic services. Although the degree of loss is relatively small compared to higher level amputations, the outcome can be just as, if not more, debilitating. Provision of a silicone foot prosthesis or insole with toe filler is the most common intervention.

Special prostheses

Dedicated activity prostheses

Designed to facilitate specific activities that cannot be achieved using a general day-to-day limb. Dedicated activity prostheses are usually prescribed for leisure and sports including swimming, running, cycling, skiing and climbing. Prosthetic foot modules are available designed to accommodate a variety of activities ranging between day-to-day walking and function as well as leisure activities such as the gym. For example, a carbon fibre foot module with a shock absorber can be used for daily use and higher impact sports. It is often the case that a specific design of prosthesis is only required for individuals participating in an activity at club or competitive level. Examples here include running blades for use on the track or a bespoke cycling prosthesis for competitive cycling. A water activity prosthesis (18) may be required for occupational reasons or to access a swimming pool. Standard foot modules that are also waterproof can be used to access water-based environments. A more specific device with an adjustable ankle and flipper attachment may be required for diving. It should be noted that the majority of amputees who swim do so without a prosthesis.

Direct skeletal fixation

Also termed osseointegration, this technique refers to the attachment of a prosthesis to a metal implant originating inside the residual long bone extending through an aperture in the soft tissue (Figure 21.5). The component that extends through the soft tissue is referred to as the abutment and this is the point of attachment for the prosthesis. Osseointegration, originally developed in Sweden, became established in the field of dental implants. Its application to attach prostheses to long bones was first applied in 1990. Latterly a number of skeletal prosthetic attachment systems have been developed and teams are working to refine the procedure (19). Techniques require one or two surgical procedures and a lengthy rehabilitation programme. The rehabilitation protocol varies depending upon the adopted system. Osseointegration negates the requirement for a socket and is most commonly applied to transfemoral amputees who are unable to fulfil their functional potential using a socket system. Osseointegration overcomes some of the problems associated with a conventional socket such as soft tissue irritation and discomfort. Prosthetic attachment is achieved by mechanical fixation to the abutment using an Allen key or rotary chuck device. Improvements in mobility and quality of life are reported (20, 21). The absence of a socket extending proximally allows unrestricted movement of the hip. Problems can be encountered including superficial infection, deep infection and mechanical trauma resulting in deformation or loosening of the intraosseous implant. These events may require removal of the system and a return to conventional socket use. Osseointegration and subsequent rehabilitation should be undertaken under the supervision of a multidisciplinary team experienced in the technique.

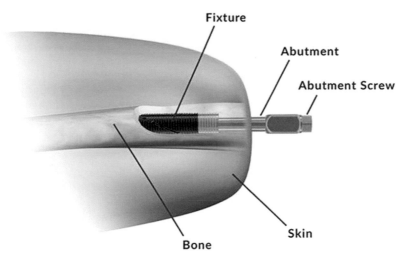

Figure 21.5 Image of components used for direct skeletal fixation. The external prosthesis attaches to the abutment. (Courtesy of Integrum, Molndal, Sweden.)

Targeted muscle reinnervation (TMR)

Initially developed at the Rehabilitation Institute of Chicago as a method of intuitively controlling myo-electric upper limb prostheses using electromyographic signals (EMG). The residual nerves that served the amputated arm are transferred into chest or upper arm muscles. Once reinnervated these muscles deliver appropriate and intuitive commands to control components such as the prosthetic hand, wrist or elbow. The technique has been found useful in the management of amputation-related pain including neuroma and phantom pain (5) for lower as well as upper extremity amputees. Peripheral nerve endings following amputation are transferred into redundant target muscles. Indications are that the target muscle provides feedback to the peripheral nerve reducing neuroma sensitivity and phantom limb pain.

Amputee review and rehabilitation

Established amputees need lifelong review and follow-up (2). This is to respond to changes in the amputation stump requiring adjustment the prosthetic fit, mechanical repair or changes required for different functional need and provision of replacement prosthesis. It is generally accepted that a lower limb prosthesis may require replacement every 5 years, dependent on its use (14).

Later consequences or sequelae after lower limb amputations

Pain and gait deviations are the commonest problems in people with lower limb amputations (Box 21.6).

The pain may be in the stump or in the phantom limb. Stump pain is generally due to socket fit problems, impaired gait or specific local pathology like sores and neuromas. The incidence of phantom pain has generally reduced due to improved peri-amputation multidisciplinary management but remains between 10–20%. A long pre-amputation history predisposes to post-amputation and phantom pain. Treatment modalities currently used are wide ranging from pharmacological

---

Box 21.6 Problems after amputation

Early (specific postoperative)
- Haematoma
- Delayed healing secondary to ischaemia
- Skin necrosis
- Infection
- Pain, including phantom symptoms
- Joint contractures

Later (during rehabilitation)
- Pain: Stump pain and phantom pain
- Impaired mobility
- Prosthetic fitting unsatisfactory
- Anxiety and depression

Long term
- Pain: Stump pain and phantom pain
- Diminished mobility
- Impaired gait
- Increased energy required for walking
- Back pain
- Other muscular joint pains, e.g., hips and knees
- Anxiety and depression
- Personal relationship problems
- Occupational and leisure consequences

drugs including anti-epileptic medication used for neuropathic pain, physical treatment like massage, acupuncture, use of magnet incorporated socks or liners, cognitive behaviour therapy like distraction techniques, relaxation techniques, hypnotherapy, eye movement desensitising and reprocessing (EMDR), mirror therapy, use of visual reality and rarely surgical intervention including spinal stimulator implants and TMR.

Impaired gait may require socket adjustment or realignment of the prostheses supported by physiotherapy gait re-education.

There is an increased energy required to walk with a prosthesis. This is generally quoted as an additional 10% energy for unilateral transtibial amputees and 60% for unilateral transfemoral amputees increasing to 200% for bilateral transfemoral amputees.

There is an increased incidence for some degenerative changes in major proximal joints (22). However, this is not significant enough to require joint replacement surgery, the incidence of which remains low. It is expected that the amputees 'titrate' their walking proportionately and symptoms are treated with medication or physiotherapy. There is also an increased incidence of low back pain that is generally due to the altered mechanics of gait.

Psychological problems should not be underestimated. This is more prevalent following amputations related to trauma and in upper limb amputees. Presentation is generally 12–18 months after the amputation when the reality of day-to-day problems become apparent upon return to the community and social life or employment (23).

Appropriate adaptations and environmental changes at home and work should not be overlooked.

Studies have shown that two-thirds of amputees under the age of 65 years return to work (24, 25). Support at work is recommended for successful return to employment.

Lifelong follow-up or access to a specialist prosthetic rehabilitation unit is recommended.

Take home messages

- A lower limb amputation should be viewed as a positive reconstructive procedure to 'fashion' a residual limb (stump) that will facilitate optimal biomechanical function and locomotion using a prosthesis.
- The ideal amputation stump should be of optimum length, well healed with healthy and sensate skin cover, gently tapered in shape with chamfered bone ends, absence of proximal fixed deformities.
- Good mobility does not necessarily require the most advanced technology but a prosthesis, however simple, that is appropriate to the individual's needs and supported with dedicated therapy should ensure successful rehabilitation.

- Common complications are socket fit problems, stump and phantom limb pain, impaired gait and increased energy requirement, back pain, hip and knee pain, psychological problems, difficulties at work and leisure.
- Lifelong follow-up is advised for prosthetic maintenance and appropriate repair, renewal or adaptation to changes in the stump.

References

1. Calder P, Hanspal RS. *Management of the Limb Deficient Child.* Oxford Text Book of Orthopaedics and Trauma Chapter 13–14, *edC Bulstrode* (Oxford University Press, 2011).
2. British Society of Rehabilitation Medicine *"Amputee and Prosthetic Rehabilitation – Standards and Guidelines* (3rd Edition). Report of a Working Party. Co-Chairs: Hanspal RS, Sedki I. British Society of Rehabilitation Medicine, London 2018. ISBN: 978-0-9927275-1-2
3. College of Occupational Therapists, *"Occupational therapy with people who have had lower limb amputations. Evidence-based guidelines".* Edited by Anita Atwal, Jane McLaughlin, Georgia Spiliotopoulou. (Lavenham Press, 2011).
4. Ghali S, Harris P, Khan U, Pearce M, Nanchahal J. Leg Length Preservation with Pedicled Fillet of Foot Flaps following Traumatic Amputations; *Plast Reconstr Surg.* Feb 2005; 115(2): 498–505.
5. Dumanian GA, Potter BK, Mioton LM, et al. Targeted Muscle Reinnervation Treats Neuroma and Phantom Pain in Major Limb Amputees: A Randomized Clinical Trial. *Annals of surgery.* 2019; 270(2): 238–246.
6. Gottschalk FA, Stills M. The Biomechanics of Trans Femoral Amputation. *Prosthet Orthot Int.* 1994; 18: 12–17.
7. Kwah LK, Webb MT, Goh L, Harvey LA. Rigid Dressings versus Soft Dressings for Transtibial Amputations (Review). *Cochrane Database of Systematic Reviews.* 2019; (6). Art. No: CD012427.
8. Hanspal RS, Fisher K. Assessment of Cognitive and Psychomotor Function and Rehabilitation of Elderly People with Prostheses. *BMJ.* 1991; 302: 94.
9. Goktepe AS, Cakir B, Yilmaz B, Yazicioglu K. Energy Expenditure of Walking with Prostheses: Comparison of Three Amputation Levels. *Prosthet Orhot Int.* 2010; 34(1): 31–36.
10. WHO Standards for Prosthetics and Orthotics. Geneva: World Health Organization; 2017. Licence: CCBY-NC-SA 3.0IG0. ISBN 978-92-4-151248-0.
11. Sooriakumaran S, Uden M, Mulroy S, Ewins D. The Impact a Surgeon Has on Primary Amputee Prosthetic Rehabilitation: A Survey of Residual Lower Limb Quality. *Prosthet Orthot Int.* 2018; 42(4): 428–436.
12. Hanspal RS, Fisher K, Nieveen R. Prosthetic Socket Comfort Score. *Disabil Rehabil.* 2003; 25(22): 1278–1280.
13. Nair A, Hanspal RS, Zahedi MS, Saif M, Fisher K. Analyses of Prosthetic Episodes in Lower Limb Amputees. *Prosthet Orthot Int.* 2008; 32(1): 42–49.
14. Richardson A, Dillon MP. User Experience of Transtibial Prosthetic Liners: A Systematic Review. *Prosthet Orthot Int.* Feb 2017; 41(1): 6–18.
15. Al Shuaili N, Aslani N, Duff L, McGarry A. Transtibial Prosthetic Socket Design and Suspension Mechanism: A Literature Review. *Prosthet Orthot Int.* 2019; 31(4): 224–245.

16. NHS England Specialised Commissioning Agency. Clinical Commissioning Policy: Microprocessor Controlled Prosthetic Knees. NHS England: 2016; 16061/P. Prepared by NHS England Specialised Services Clinical Reference Group for Complex Disability Equipment-Prosthetics.

17. Hagberg E, Berlin OK, Renstrom P. Function after through Knee Compared with below knee and above Knee Amputation. *Prosthet Orthot Int*. 1992; 16: 168–173.

18. Hanspal RS, Nieveen R. Water Activity Limbs. *Prosthet Orthot Int*. 2002; 26: 218–225.

19. Herbert JS, Rehani M, Stiegelmer R. Osseointegration for Lower Limb Amputation: A Systematic Review of Clinical Outcomes. *JBJS Rev*. 2017; 5(10): e10.

20. Matthews DJ, Arastu M, Uden M, Sullivan JP, Bolsakova K, Robinson K, Sooriakumaran S, Ward D. UK Trial of the Osseointegrated Prosthesis for the Rehabilitation for Amputees: 1995-2018. *Prosthet Orthot Int*. 2018; 43(1): 112–122.

21. Hagberg K, Ghassemi Jahani SA, Kulbacka-Ortiz K, Thomsen P, Malchau H, Reinholdt C. A 15 Year Follow-up of Transfemoral Amputees with Bone-anchored Transcutaneous Prostheses. *Bone Joint J*. 2020; 102-B(1): 55–63.

22. Jingsheng W, Siqun W, Yibing W, Jianguo W, Chen F, Huang G, Chen J, Wei L, Jiang J, Xia J. Lower Limb Amputation and Rehabilitation in Total Joint Arthroplasties in the Ipsilateral Limb. *Prosthet Orthot Int*. 2014; 38(3): 185–192.

23. Fisher K, Price EM. The Use of Standard Measure of Emotional Distress to Evaluate Early Counseling Intervention in Patients with Amputations. *J Prosthet Orthot Int*. 2003; 15(1); 31–34.

24. Fisher K, Hanspal RS, Marks L. Return to Employment after Major Lower Limb Amputation. *Int J Rehabil Res*. 2003; 26(1): 51–54.

25. Burger H, Marincek C. Return to Work after Lower Limb Amputation. *Disabil Rehabil*. 2007; 29(17): 1323–1329.

Further resources

WHO Standards for Prosthetics and Orthotics. Geneva: World Health Organisation: 2017. Licence: CC BY-NC-SA 3.0.IGO ISBN 978-92-4-151248-0

ISO International Standards Organisation (1993). Prosthetics and orthotics – limb deficiencies – Part 2: method of describing lower limb amputation stumps. ISO 8548-2

ISO International Standards Organisation (1993). Prosthetics and orthotics – limb deficiencies – Part 3: method of describing upper limb amputation stumps. ISO 8548-3

Sangoh Lee and Raj Bhatt

Introduction

Foot and ankle pain are common presenting symptoms that can have a significant impact on the quality and activity of daily living. Up to 1 in 5 people in a given population has been found to have foot pain, which increases with age, female sex and obesity (1). It is often difficult to obtain a firm diagnosis on clinical examinations alone and imaging has therefore become an integral part of the diagnostic workup. We discuss the image findings of pathologies related to the foot and ankle.

Imaging modalities

Plain radiographs/computed tomography (CT)

Plain radiograph is the 1st line imaging modality for the assessment of the foot and ankle. It allows clear delineation of the osseous anatomy and is useful in the diagnosis of osteoarthritis, fractures and bone tumours. It is also widely used for postoperative surveillance of prosthesis and assesses bone union after a fracture. CT gives greater information regarding the anatomy and the surrounding soft tissue structures. Thin slice (<1 mm) bone window images are obtained, which can be manipulated via multiplanar or 3D reconstructions to visualise the area of interest to a greater detail.

Ultrasound (US)

US is an easily accessible and relatively cheap imaging modality that allows assessment of the soft tissue structures. It is especially useful in the assessment of the tendon, ligament, joint effusion and synovitis. Dynamic imaging can be performed at the time of the scan to assess the functional status of the examined structure, which is a significant advantage over other imaging modalities. However, this technique is user dependant and achieving the correct diagnosis will invariably depend on the skill and experience of the operator.

Magnetic resonance imaging (MRI) protocol

MRI provides exquisite details of tendons, ligaments, bones, joints and surrounding soft tissue structures. The foot and ankle should be imaged separately with dedicated surface coils using a small field of view. Imaging the foot and ankle together in a large field of view results in images with poor spatial resolution. This will limit the assessment of small structures, and subtle pathologies around the foot and ankle can be missed leading to erroneous diagnoses.

The ankle should be imaged in three orthogonal planes: coronal, sagittal and axial. The coronal images are obtained with the medial and lateral malleoli in the same plane. The sagittal images are obtained perpendicular to the coronal plane and the axial images are obtained covering the distal syndesmosis to the calcaneal heel pad (2).

The foot is imaged in an oblique axial plane through the long axis of the metatarsal bone. The coronal plane is imaged perpendicular to the oblique axial images and the sagittal plane is obtained to cover the medial and the lateral malleoli (Figure 22.1). Obtaining a mixture of T1- and T2-weighted images in at least two orthogonal planes are useful to evaluate the anatomy of the foot and ankle. Proton Density (PD) fat saturated sequences are useful for the assessment of the articular cartilage. The Short Tau Inversion Recovery (STIR) and T2-weighted fat saturated sequences accentuate fluid, which is seen in most pathologies such as oedema, tenosynovitis and joint effusion (Figure 22.1).

Image findings

Developmental/congenital

Tarsal coalition is defined as partial or complete union of two or more bones of the midfoot and hindfoot and is a frequent cause of hindfoot pain (Figure 22.2). Coalition can be osseous, fibrous or cartilaginous. Approximately 90% of tarsal coalition involves talocalcaneal or

Coronal	Sagittal	Axial	T1/T2/PD FSE
Coronal	**Sagittal**	**Axial**	PD/T2 FS FSE

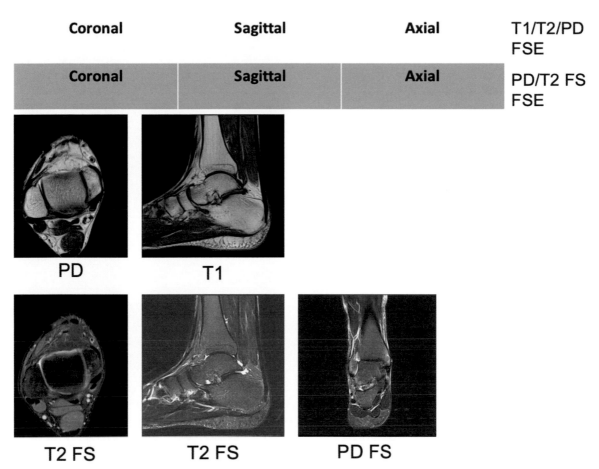

PD   T1

T2 FS   T2 FS   PD FS

Figure 22.1 A combination of spin echo and fat suppressed sequences are used in the assessment of the foot and ankle joints. It is important to image the foot and ankle separately in order to have adequate spatial resolution for subtle diagnoses.

calcaneonavicular joints. The initial investigation is with plain radiograph.

Calcaneonavicular coalition demonstrates elongation of the anterior calcaneal process mimicking 'an anteater's nose' on lateral radiograph (Figure 22.3).

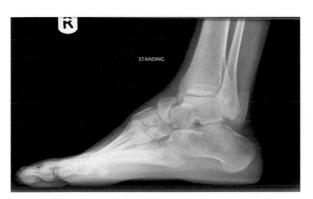

Figure 22.2 Lateral plain radiograph shows calcaneocuboid coalition.

Coalition of the talocalcaneal joint at the middle facet is common at the level of the sustentaculum tali. A lateral view of talocalcaneal coalition simulates a letter 'C', known as the 'C sign' (Figure 22.4).

CT allows detailed anatomy of the various coalitions and is an important assessment tool for surgical planning. MRI is used to investigate whether the coalition is cartilaginous, fibrous or osseous and can identify bone marrow oedema (BMO) in an unsuspected yet symptomatic coalition. Treatment is usually conservative with non-steroidal anti-inflammatory drugs (NSAIDs), steroid injections and physiotherapy. Failure of conservative therapy results in surgery with local resection or arthrodesis.

Osteochondral lesion of the talus (OLT)

OLT occurs due to trauma or repetitive microtrauma to a focal area of the talar dome. A combination of ankle inversion and axial loading are the main mechanisms of injury. This causes chondral shearing with injury to

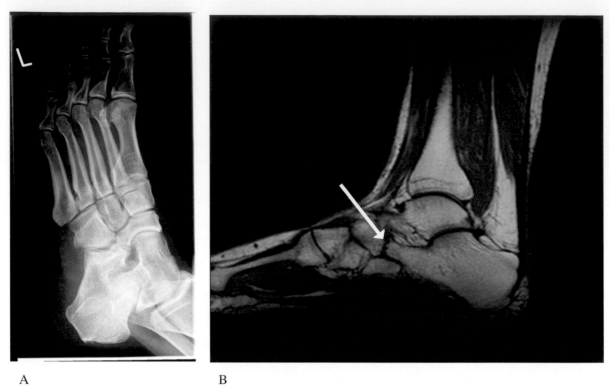

A   B

Figure 22.3 Calcaneonavicular coalition (A) medial oblique plain radiograph of the left foot showing the calcaneo-navicular collation. (B) Sagittal T1-weighted MRI shows fibrous calcaneonavicular coalition with elongated anterior process of the calcaneus.

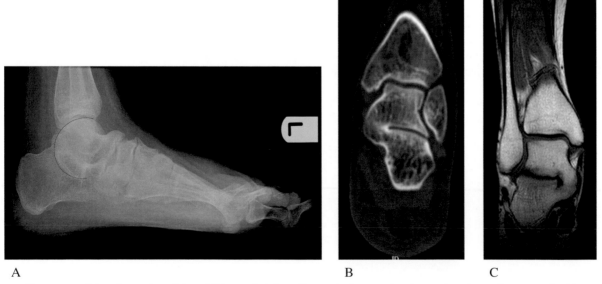

A   B   C

Figure 22.4 Talocalcaneal coalition. (A) Lateral plain radiograph shows talocalcaneal coalition depicting the 'C sign'. (B) Coronal CT multiplanar reconstruction demonstrates osseous talocalcaneal coalition at the middle facets. (C) Coronal T1-weighted MRI showing osseous talocalcaneal coalition.

Table 22.1 Hepple classification of OLT based on MRI (4)

Stage	MRI findings
I	Articular cartilage oedema only
IIA	Chondral injury with underlying fracture and surrounding BMO (acute)
IIB	Stage IIA without surrounding BMO (chronic)
III	Detached but non-displaced bone fragment
IV	Displaced bone fragment
V	Subchondral cyst formation

the subchondral bone plate and it is often associated with ankle fracture and/or ligamentous sprain injury. The most symptomatic, therefore surgical treated lesion, was found to be within the central third of the lateral talar dome, followed by the central third of the medial talar dome. This is contrary to the belief that these lesions occur along the anterolateral and posteromedial margins of the talar dome. The medial lesions were also shown to be larger in surface area although the depth remained similar (3). The Hepple staging system is used to grade the degree of OLT on MRI (Table 22.1) (4). Stages 1 and 2 demonstrate chondral injury only, commonly involving the medial margin of the talar dome, while lateral lesions are almost always associated with a history of trauma. Stages 3 and 4 demonstrate detached fragment with varying degree of displacement. The lateral lesions are more likely to be displaced and is therefore often more symptomatic. Stage 5 demonstrates subchondral cyst formation (Figure 22.5).

A weight-bearing plain radiograph is the 1st line imaging modality of choice. The sensitivity of picking up OLT on a plain radiograph is low. However, it is able to assess the presence of a concurrent fracture and other anatomical variants. CT is useful to assess the size of the subchondral cyst and the displaced fragment, although it cannot confidently assess the degree of chondral injury and identify the subchondral BMO. MRI can demonstrate subchondral BMO and a high signal fluid cleft around the fragment can identify a stage 3 lesion that is detached but remains undisplaced.

Ankle impingements

Imaging is useful in identifying the aetiology of the ankle impingement, which can occur circumferentially around the ankle joint. By far the commonest types of impingements are posterior, anterior and anterolateral impingements. The image findings of ankle impingements can often be non-specific. Therefore imaging should be interpreted in the context of appropriate clinical history and examination.

Posterior ankle impingement occurs due to repetitive plantar flexion of the ankle leading to compression and injury of the bone and adjacent soft tissue in the posterior ankle (5). There are several predisposing factors, which include the presence of os trigonum, Stieda process, downward sloping of the posterior tibia, fracture of the lateral tubercle of the posterior process of talus and Haglund deformity. Pain and tenderness of the posterior ankle exacerbated by plantar flexion occurs due to impingement, tenosynovitis of the flexor hallucis longus and injury to the posterior talofibular ligament (PTFL) (5). MRI can demonstrate posterior capsular thickening and tenosynovitis. BMO of the lateral tubercle of the posterior talar process is also a feature of posterior ankle impingement (Figure 22.6).

Anterior ankle impingement occurs as a result of chronic repetitive trauma. This results in enthesophyte

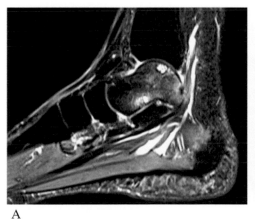
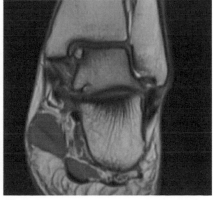

A   B

Figure 22.5 Osteochondral lesion of the talus (OLT). (A) MR sagittal STIR MRI showing a prominent subchondral cyst of the talar dome with associated bone marrow oedema commonly seen in OLT. There is also a concurrent subchondral cyst of the subtalar joint. (B) MR coronal T1-weighted MRI showing OLT at the medial margin of the talar dome.

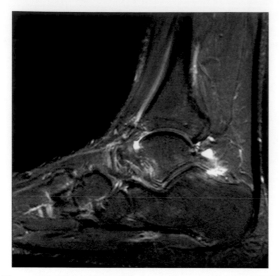

Figure 22.6 Posterior ankle impingement. Sagittal STIR MRI showing synovitis within the posterior recesses of the ankle and subtalar joints. There is associated BMO around the elongated lateral tubercle of the posterior talar process compatible with posterior ankle impingement.

formation along the anterior margin of the tibial plafond and the talar neck, leading to restricted dorsiflexion of the ankle joint. MRI demonstrates joint effusion with localised synovitis within the anterior recess of the ankle joint. There is usually associated capsular thickening/scarring demonstrated by thickened synovial lining of the anterior ankle joint.

The anterolateral recess of the ankle is a pyramidal shaped space between the tibia medially and fibula laterally. Although small amounts of fluid can be present in an asymptomatic individual, fibrosis and localised synovitis of this recess can cause symptoms upon internal and external rotations with restricted dorsiflexion of the ankle joint. The commonest cause of anterolateral impingement is sprain injury of the ATFL. Ganglion cyst, osteophyte, avulsed osseous fragment and osteochondral injury have also been reported as contributory aetiology. MRI is the imaging modality of choice, which demonstrates localised synovitis on a fluid sensitive sequence, as shown by fluid in the recess in the presence of an appropriate clinical history and relevant predisposing aetiologies. Low SI on T1- and T2-weighted images can also be present in the presence of fibrosis that can elicit the symptoms (Figure 22.7).

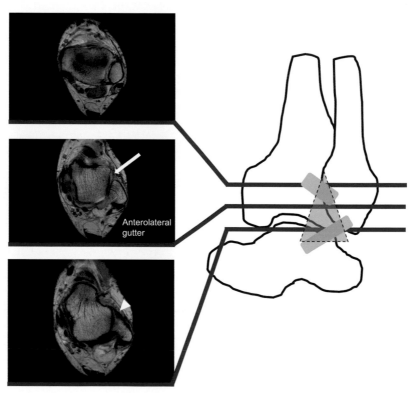

Figure 22.7 Anterolateral ankle impingement. Axial T1-weighted MRIs showing the anatomy of the ankle anterolateral gutter between the AITFL and ATFL. The ATFL is thickened here in keeping with a chronic sprain injury (arrow head). There is isointense fluid SI on these T1-weighted images suggestive of synovitis (arrow). With appropriate clinical history, this is compatible with anterolateral ankle impingement.

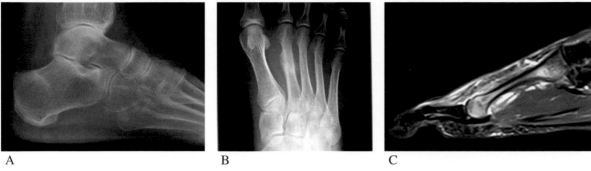

Figure 22.8 Stress fracture. (A) Lateral plain radiograph, which shows a thin sclerotic line in the superior aspect of the posterior calcaneum in keeping with bone healing. (B) DP radiograph of the forefoot, which shows callus formation at the shaft of the 2nd metatarsal bone in keeping with a stress fracture. (C) Sagittal T2-weighted fat saturated MRI showing florid BMO of the 2nd metatarsal bone with adjacent soft tissue oedema in keeping with a stress response.

Stress fracture

Stress fracture occurs as a consequence of mismatch between the bone strength and the mechanical stress exerted on the bone. Chronic repetitive mechanical stress exerted on a normal bone is a fatigue fracture whereas a normal stress exerted on a pathological bone is an insufficiency fracture. Stress fracture has insidious onset, which presents as chronic, worsening pain with little or no history of trauma.

Calcaneus is the most commonly affected tarsal bone and is usually due to excessive physical activity. The 2nd and 3rd metatarsal bones are commonly affected in the forefoot. Early stress fractures are difficult to appreciate on a plain radiograph and it may take several days for the bone healing to occur that manifests as sclerosis and periosteal reaction (Figure 22.8). Bone scan will show increased radioisotope uptake as there is increased bone turnover. MRI is highly sensitive in identifying radiographically occult stress fractures. It demonstrates low SI fracture line on T1- and T2-weighted imaging with bone marrow, periosteal and soft tissue oedema (Figure 22.9). Isolated BMO without fracture can be present which is indicative of an early stress response. Treatment is usually conservative with rest and pain management.

Plantar fasciitis

Plantar fasciitis is the most common cause of inferior heel pain. Classically present as plantar heel pain, it is exacerbated by passive dorsiflexion and weight-bearing

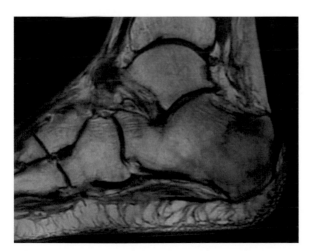
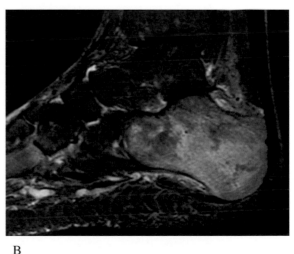

Figure 22.9 Calcaneal stress fracture. (A) T1-weighted MRI showing a low-SI lines in keeping with calcaneal stress fractures. (B) T2-weighted fat saturated MRI, which again delineates the fractures. There is associated bone marrow oedema throughout the calcaneum with surrounding soft tissue oedema, deep to the plantar fascia and within the Kager's fat pad.

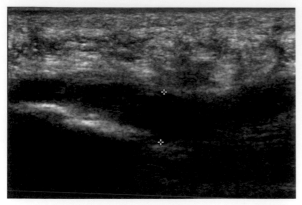

Figure 22.10 Plantar fasciitis. Longitudinal US image of the plantar fascia. There is marked thickening of the plantar fascia measured between the two cross-hairs. Plantar fascia is diagnosed when the thickness is measured greater than 3 mm.

after a period of prolonged rest. The cause of the pain is multifactorial and includes degeneration, microtears and low-grade inflammation of the fascial and perifascial soft tissue (6). Commonly affected groups include obese patients and athletes who perform excessive running. Seronegative spondyloarthropathies, such as ankylosing spondylitis, Reiter syndrome and psoriatic arthritis associated enthesopathy are also known causes of plantar fasciitis (7). The calcaneal spur is best demonstrated on a lateral plain radiograph; however, it is a non-specific finding that is also seen in asymptomatic individuals. US shows hypoechoic fascia with fusiform thickening, defined as being greater than 3 mm in thickness (Figure 22.10).

MRI shows intra-fascial intermediate SI on T1- and PD-weighted images with high SI on fluid sensitive and T2-weighted images. There is also high SI within the perifascial soft tissue and fat pad. Seronegative spondyloarthropathy related plantar fasciitis is usually bilateral and associated with retrocalcaneal bursitis and Achilles tendinitis (Figure 22.11) (7).

Plantar fibromatosis

Plantar fibromatosis is a benign yet locally invasive neoplasm involving the plantar fascia. There is abnormal proliferation of the fibrous tissue, which replaces the plantar aponeurosis and can slowly invade adjacent skin and deep musculature (8). It is associated with other fibroproliferative conditions such as Dupuytren and Peyronie diseases, although flexion deformity is not a

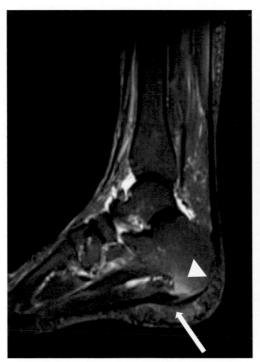

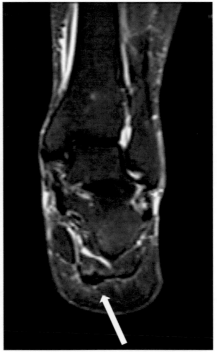

A   B

Figure 22.11 Plantar fasciitis. (A) Sagittal and (B) Coronal T2-weighted fat saturated MRIs, which demonstrate marked thickening of the central band of the plantar fascia with intrinsic high signal suggestive of a partial tear (arrows). There is also reactive bone marrow oedema at its calcaneal insertion in keeping with enthesitis (arrow head).

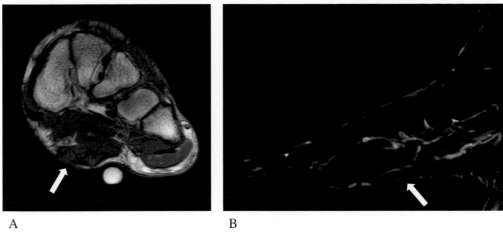

A   B

Figure 22.12 Plantar fibroma. (A) Coronal T1-weighted and (B) sagittal T2-weighted fat saturated MRIs showing isointense SI on T1 and low SI on T2-weighted imaging with fusiform thickening of the plantar fascia. Findings are in keeping with a plantar fibroma.

common finding (9). On US, plantar fibromatosis demonstrates low or mixed echogenic discrete, nodular thickening along the plantar fascia. MRI is the modality of choice in assessing plantar fibromatosis. As with US, there is nodular thickening along the plantar fascia, which is low or intermediate SI on T1- and T2-weighted images due to the acellular, fibrous nature of the lesions (Figure 22.12).

Achilles tendinosis

The Achilles tendon is formed by the medial and lateral heads of the gastrocnemius and soleus muscles and inserts to the posterior aspect of the calcaneus. It is surrounded by loose connective tissue known as the paratenon, which consists of visceral and parietal layers (10). There is a relatively poor vascular supply between 2–6 cm of the Achilles tendon, proximal to the calcaneal insertion. This area is known as the 'watershed zone' and directly correlates with slow tendon repair and thus is the site of most Achilles tendon pathologies (10).

Normal Achilles tendon has uniformly low SI on MRI and is flattened or slightly concave anteriorly and measures approximately 6 mm in thickness. Insertional Achilles tendinosis occurs at its calcaneal insertion in the presence of inflammatory arthropathy, manifested by thickening of the tendon with associated retrocalcaneal bursitis (Figure 22.13).

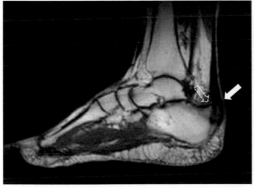
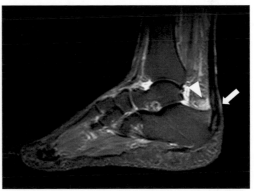

A   B

Figure 22.13 Insertional Achilles tendinosis. (A) Sagittal T1-weighted MRI, which demonstrates marked thickening of the Achilles tendon at its calcaneal insertion (arrow). There is associated Haglund deformity (dotted arrow) and synovitis within the posterior recess of the ankle joint compatible with posterior ankle impingement. (B) Sagittal T2-weighted fat saturated MRI of the same patient. There is associated intrinsic high signal within the tendon substance consistent with tendinosis. There is retrocalcaneal bursitis (arrow head) and subtle fluid posterior to the Achilles tendon in keeping with paratenonitis (arrow).

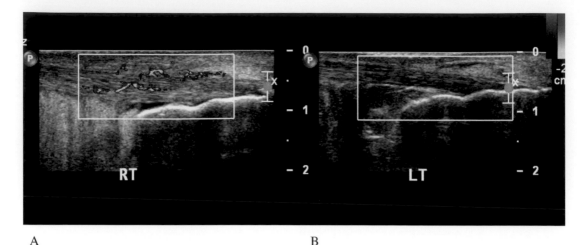

A   B

Figure 22.14 Insertional Achilles tendinosis. (A) Longitudinal US image of the Achilles tendon as it inserted onto the calcaneus. There is subtle expansion of the Achilles tendon with notable intrinsic neovascularity. There is associated small volume of fluid within the retrocalcaneal bursa. (B) Longitudinal US image of the normal contralateral Achilles tendon, which shows uniform morphology with absent vascularity.

Achilles tendinosis is best assessed by US and MRI. US can identify fusiform expansion of the Achilles tendon with neovascularity, which is predominantly seen along its ventral surface at its interface with the Kager's fat pad (Figure 22.14). On MR, Achilles tendinosis demonstrates expansion with intrinsic high SI on T2-weighted images. Subtle findings include small intra-substance or ventral surface high signals consistent with microtears (Figure 22.15).

Tendon dysfunction

Tibialis posterior tendon (TPT) dysfunction is a spectrum of pathologies that include tenosynovitis, tendinosis, partial intra-substance tear and complete tendon rupture.

The normal TPT appears hypointense in all sequences. A small amount of fluid can be present around the tendon in this location; however, this should

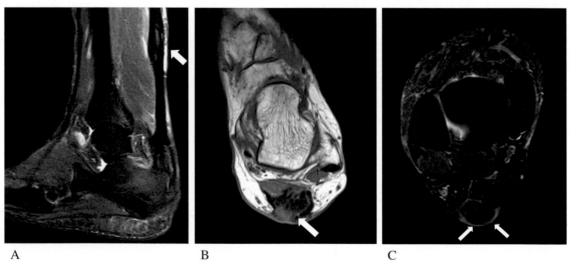

A   B   C

Figure 22.15 Achilles tendinosis. (A) Sagittal STIR MRI, which demonstrates marked thickening of the Achilles tendon at its 'watershed zone' away from its calcaneal insertion (arrow). There is intrinsic fluid signal suggestive of interstitial tear. (B) Axial T1-weighted MRI showing marked expansion of the Achilles tendon with intrinsic intermediate SI that extends towards its ventral and dorsal surfaces suggestive of high-grade partial tears (arrow). (C) Axial T2-fat saturated MRI showing hemi-circumferential oedema around the paratenon, present along the dorsal surface of the Achilles tendon. Findings are in keeping with Achilles paratenonitis (arrow).

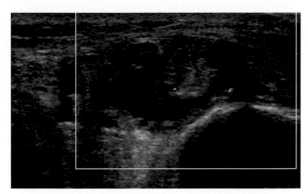

Figure 22.16 Tibialis posterior tendon (TPT) dysfunction. Transverse US image showing concentric fluid around the TPT measuring greater than 2 mm in depth. There is associated Doppler signal within the tendon sheath in keeping with neovascularity. Appearances are consistent with tenosynovitis of the TPT.

be less than 2 mm in depth (11). The distal 1–2 cm of the tendon can also appear slightly expanded with mildly high SI. The tendon sheath terminates 1–2 cm from the main TPT insertion to the navicular tuberosity. It has previously been suggested that no fluid should be present in this distal portion of the tendon (11). However, a more recent study found that a small volume of fluid here can be normal, seen in 65% of MRIs performed regardless of the clinical history (12)

The commonest cause of adult acquired hindfoot valgus deformity is TPT dysfunction. TPT maintains the longitudinal arch of the foot in conjunction with the spring ligamentous complex. TPT dysfunction or spring ligament rupture can exert exaggerated stress on the other, which will eventually fail, causing hindfoot valgus (also known as flatfoot deformity). Unrecognised malalignment can progress to a fixed deformity with secondary subtalar and tibiotalar osteoarthritis.

Tenosynovitis is inflammation of the tendon sheath, which is a synovial membrane that surrounds a tendon. Tenosynovitis manifests as excessive (>2 mm) fluid surrounding a morphologically normal tendon. US demonstrates hypoechoic fluid accumulation within the tendon sheath with increased vascularity (Figure 22.16). On MR, there is circumferential fluid collection around the tendon, which shows high SI on T2-weighted imaging, low to intermediate SI on T1-weighted imaging (Figure 22.17).

Tendinosis appears as tendon enlargement with or without increased intra-substance SI. Partial tear appears as linear high intra-tendinous SI, and complete rupture as an empty tendon sheath with a full-thickness disruption of the tendon substance. The tendon may become stretched prior to a complete rupture, in which case it will appear attenuated and of smaller calibre to the adjacent flexor digitorum longus tendon (Figure 22.17) (11).

A longitudinal split tear of the peroneus brevis tendon (PBT) commonly occurs as it traverses around the retromalleolar groove. This manifests as a C-shaped PBT that is seen on either side of the intact peroneus longus tendon (PLT). There is often concurrent tenosynovitis, peroneal tendon subluxation/dislocation, osteophytosis and reactive BMO of the adjacent fibula (Figure 22.18).

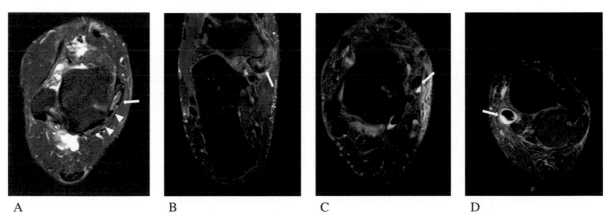

A   B   C   D

Figure 22.17 Tibialis posterior tendon (TPT) dysfunction. Axial T2-weighted fat saturated MRIs showing: (A) Significantly attenuated TPT (arrow) when compared to the adjacent flexor digitorum longus and flexor hallucis longus tendons (arrow heads). (B) Marked expansion of the TPT with intrinsic increased SI at its insertion to the navicular tuberosity (arrow). There is associated bone marrow oedema at the enthesis in keeping with enthesitis. There is also oedema around the distal 2 cm of the TPT in keeping with paratendinitis. (C) Fluid around the TPT in keeping with tenosynovitis. There is a linear fluid SI through the substance of the TPT in keeping with a longitudinal split tear (arrow). (D) Concentric fluid around the TPT in keeping with tenosynovitis (arrow). The tendon appears expanded with a fluid signal extending into the tendon substance in keeping with a partial tear.

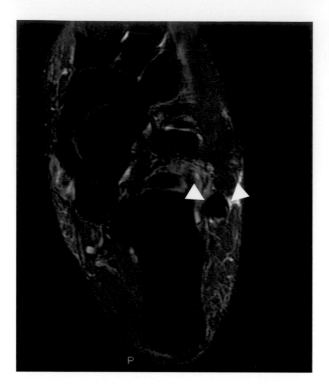

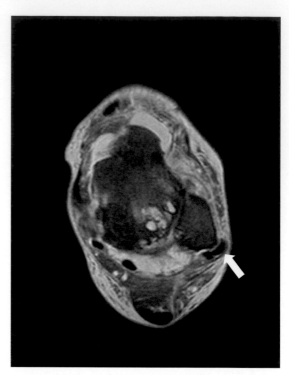

A

B

Figure 22.18 Peroneal tendon pathology. (A) Axial T2-weighted fat saturated MRI showing a C-shaped PBT around the PLT in this inframalleolar position (arrow heads). This is consistent with longitudinal split tear of the PBT. (B) Axial PD-weighted fat saturated MRI showing subluxation of the PBT with periosteal stripping of the superior peroneal retinaculum at its fibular insertion. Appearances are in keeping with Oden type 1 injury.

In order to truly understand the degree of hindfoot deformity, a weight-bearing imaging needs to be performed to replicate the physiological stress exerted on the foot. Weight-bearing radiograph and CT are therefore used to evaluate the degree of hindfoot deformity for preoperative planning.

Ligament injuries

There are three groups of ligaments that support the ankle joints: the syndesmotic ligaments, the medial deltoid ligaments and the lateral collateral ligaments. The syndesmotic ligaments are comprised of anterior inferior tibiofibular ligament (AITFL) and posterior inferior tibiofibular ligament (PITFL). The deltoid ligamentous complex comprises of deep and superficial layers. The deep layer is made up of anterior tibiotalar ligament (ATTL) and posterior tibiotalar ligament (PTTL) and the superficial layer is a fan-shaped, sheet like structure that consists of tibiospring, tibionavicular, tibiotalar and tibiocalcaneal ligaments, named depending on where they insert distally. The lateral collateral ligaments are comprised of anterior talofibular ligament (ATFL), calcaneofibular ligament (CFL) and posterior talofibular ligament (PTFL).

Appearance of the ligament depends on the severity of the injury, which can be broadly divided into interstitial, partial or complete tears. Low-grade sprain or interstitial injury can demonstrate only mild peri-ligamentous oedema with or without morphological changes to the ligament, which can be thickened with ill-defined margins. There can also be associated soft tissue or BMO and localised synovitis as seen in the anterolateral ankle impingement. This is often accompanied by altered signal characteristics of the ligament, which demonstrates high SI on PD and T2-weighted images as a result of oedema and haemorrhage. This causes the loss of the normal striated pattern that is often seen in AITFL, deep deltoid ligaments and PTFL (Figure 22.19). Partial tears consist of thinning of the ligament with partial discontinuity of the ligament. Complete tear represents full thickness disruption of the ligament, which is often retracted with a fluid-filled defect in its place. There is often accompanying joint effusion which can leak into the extra-capsular soft tissues due to the disruption of these capsular ligaments.

ATFL is the most commonly injured ligament, which occurs due to ankle inversion with or without plantar flexion (Figure 22.20). As the weakest ligament within

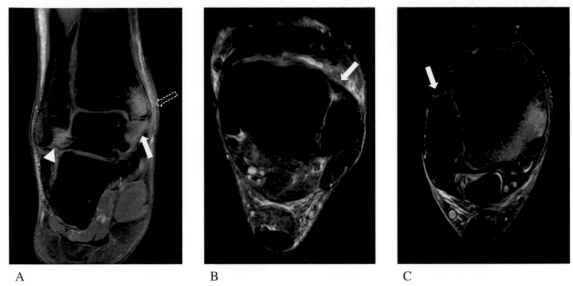

A   B   C

Figure 22.19 Ankle ligament injuries. (A) Coronal PD-weighted fat saturated MRI showing high signal and loss of the normal striated pattern of the deep deltoid ligaments (arrow) and the PTFL (arrow head) in keeping with high-grade sprain injuries. There is associated periosteal and BMO of the medial malleolus in keeping with periosteal stripping injury of the superficial deltoid ligaments (dotted arrow). (B) Axial T2-weighted fat saturated MRI showing thickening of the AITFL with periligamentous oedema in keeping with a sprain injury (arrow). (C) Axial T2-weighted fat saturated MRI showing thickening of the AITFL, which is torn and retracted from its fibular attachment in keeping with a full thickness tear (arrow).

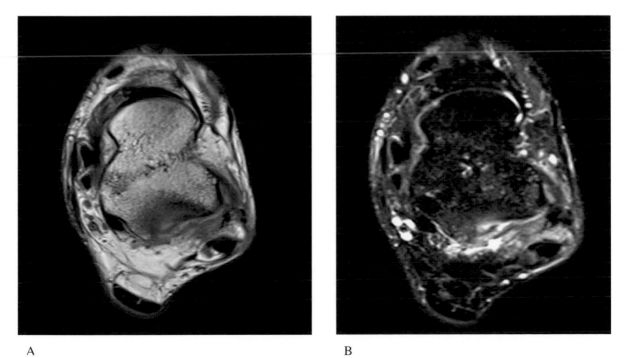

A   B

Figure 22.20 ATFL high-grade sprain injury. (A) Axial PD-weighted MRI showing thickening of the ATFL, which is mildly lax. (B) Axial T2-weighted fat saturated MRI of the same patient also showing thickening of the ATFL with associated periligamentous oedema.

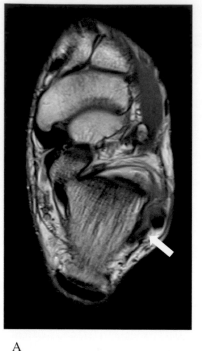
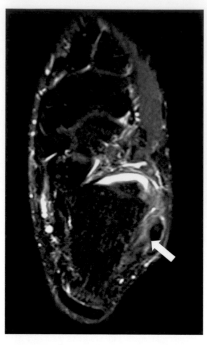

A   B

Figure 22.21 CFL high-grade sprain injury. (A) Axial PD-weighted MRI showing thickening of the CFL (arrow). (B) Axial T2-weighted fat saturated MRI of the same patient also showing thickening of the CFL with intrinsic high SI with associated periligamentous oedema (arrow). There is leakage of subtalar joint effusion to the peroneal tendon sheath suggestive of CFL tear.

the lateral ligamentous complex, ATFL is injured in isolation in up to two-thirds of cases. In the remaining cases, the injury can propagate posteriorly affecting the CFL, then the PTFL (Figure 22.21). Avulsion injury related to the ATFL is also thought to occur more commonly at its fibular attachment.

Hypertrophic and accessory muscles

Hypertrophic and accessory muscles, although common anatomical variants, are frequently overlooked during evaluation of images. Although most are incidental findings and typically asymptomatic, occasionally accessory muscles can cause pain, compartment syndrome and compressive neuropathy. The advent of cross-sectional imaging has allowed accurate assessment of these accessory muscles.

Peroneus quartus tendon is located within the peroneal retinaculum. It commonly originates from the peroneus brevis muscle and has various different insertions along the lateral margin of calcaneus, although it is commonly seen inserting onto the retrotrochlear eminence of the calcaneus. It has been associated with lateral ankle pain and/or instability and the presence of an extra tendon within the peroneal retinaculum can cause crowding, leading to anterior subluxation, degeneration and longitudinal split tear of the PBT (13).

Flexor digitorum accessorius longus (FDAL) tendon can arise from any structure in the posterior compartment of the leg. FDAL tendon traverses through the flexor retinaculum into the tarsal tunnel where it is closely related to the posterior tibial artery and the tibial nerve. Due to its intimate relationship with the neurovascular bundle in the tarsal tunnel, it is predisposed to tarsal tunnel syndrome and tenosynovitis of the FDL tendon (Figure 22.22).

Accessory soleus arises deep to the soleus muscle and descends anterior to the Achilles tendon. It presents as a soft tissue mass in the posteromedial aspect of the ankle, which can clinically mimic sarcoma (Figure 22.22). It can also cause significant pain and this is thought to be secondary to increased intra-fascial pressure, leading to insufficient blood supply and compartment syndrome (14). It has been successfully treated with fasciotomy, tendon release and excision. Accessory soleus appears as a soft tissue density that obliterates the normal Kager fat pad anterior to the Achilles tendon on plain radiography.

Sinus tarsi syndrome

The sinus tarsi is a cavity that courses posteromedial to anterolateral direction. It is found laterally between the talus and the calcaneus and continues medially to

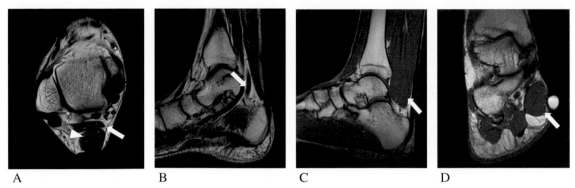

A B C D

Figure 22.22 Accessory muscles. (A) Axial T2-weighted MRI showing a muscular structure posterior to the FHL tendon in keeping with the FDAL accessory muscle (arrow). There is also a low-lying accessory soleus muscle (arrow head). (B) Sagittal T1-weighted image of the same patient showing the FDAL muscle (arrow) seen posterior to the FHL tendon. (C) Sagittal T1-weighted MRI of a different patient showing the low-lying accessory soleus muscle deep to the Achilles tendon (arrow). (D) Coronal T1-weighted MRI showing the hypertrophic abductor hallucis muscle where the patient was symptomatic (arrow).

form a canal. It contains the cervical and talocrural interosseous ligaments and these ligaments stabilise the calcaneus in relation to the talus. Sinus tarsi syndrome usually occurs as a consequence of an ankle sprain. Patients present with persistent lateral foot pain after a history of trauma with ankle inversion. The main cause is due to fibrosis or tear of the cervical and talocrural interosseous ligaments, synovial herniation and bleeding into the sinus tarsi. Although up to 70% of cases are due to trauma, it can be caused by ganglion cyst, gout, rheumatoid arthritis, seronegative spondyloarthropathies and pigmented villonodular synovitis (PVNS) (15).

Conventional radiography is not a useful imaging modality in the assessment of sinus tarsi syndrome. MRI is useful in the assessment of ligamentous disruption, especially in T1-weighted coronal and sagittal planes. A very sensitive but not specific feature of sinus tarsi syndrome is a loss of normal fat within the sinus tarsi, which manifests as the loss of high SI on T1-weighted imaging. This represents pathology, which includes fibrosis, inflammation and fluid accumulation (Figure 22.23).

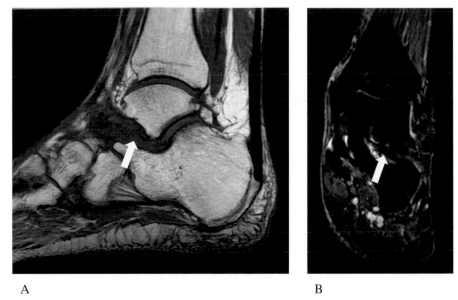

A B

Figure 22.23 Sinus tarsi syndrome. (A) Sagittal T1-weighted MRI showing the obliteration of fat within the sinus tarsi suggestive of synovitis or fibrosis (arrow). This is depicted by the loss of normal high SI within the sinus tarsi. (B) Coronal T2-weighted fat saturated MRI of the same patient showing thickening of the talocalcaneal interosseous ligament (arrow) in keeping with a chronic sprain injury of the sinus tarsi ligaments.

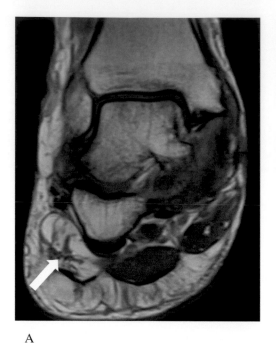 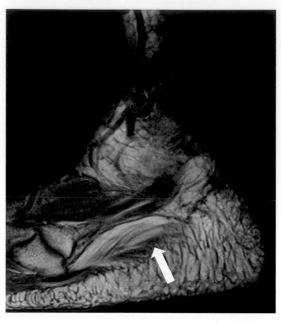

A   B

Figure 22.24 Baxter neuropathy. (A) Coronal T1-weighted MRI showing fatty infiltration of the abductor digiti minimi muscle depicted by high SI on this image (arrow). Notice the difference when compared to the other intrinsic muscles of the foot. (B) Sagittal T1-weighted image of the same patient showing fatty infiltration of the abductor digiti minimi muscle (arrow).

Baxter neuropathy

Baxter neuropathy is caused by compression of the inferior calcaneal nerve (Baxter nerve), which is the first branch of the lateral plantar nerve. It supplies the abductor digiti minimi, lateral one-third of the quadratus plantae, flexor digitorum brevis, long plantar ligament and the adjacent vessels. Predisposing factors include hypertrophy of the abductor hallucis muscle, which is often seen in long distance runners, hindfoot valgus deformity, calcaneal spur, plantar fasciitis and seronegative spondyloarthropathies. Patients present with sensory changes in the lateral one-third of the plantar surface of the foot as well as motor weakness of the abductor digiti minimi. Patients can also present with chronic heel pain, which is often difficult to distinguish from plantar fasciitis on clinical examination alone. Compression of the Baxter nerve can occur at three sites: adjacent to the hypertrophied abductor hallucis muscle, the medial edge of the quadratus plantae as the nerve takes a sharp turn from vertical to horizontal plane and, most commonly, adjacent to the medial calcaneal tuberosity (16).

MRI is the investigation of choice for Baxter neuropathy. T1-weighted imaging will show atrophy and fatty infiltration of the abductor digiti minimi. This is often accompanied by neurogenic oedema, which manifests as high SI on T2-weighted imaging of the abductor digiti

minimi and less commonly the flexor digitorum brevis and quadratus plantae muscles (Figure 22.24).

Tarsal tunnel syndrome

Tarsal tunnel syndrome is caused by entrapment of the tibial nerve within the tarsal tunnel that is found in the medial aspect of the ankle formed by the flexor retinaculum. The tunnel content consists of tibialis posterior, flexor digitorum longus, flexor hallucis longus tendons and the neurovascular bundle. Although up to 50% of cases are idiopathic, pathology of any of these contents can cause compression of the posterior tibial nerve resulting in pain and paraesthesia of the toes and heel (17). Causes include varicosities, neurogenic tumours, ganglion cyst, tenosynovitis, accessory or hypertrophied muscles, bone deformities and os trigonum (Figure 22.25).

Charcot neuropathic osteoarthropathy vs osteomyelitis

Charcot neuropathic osteoarthropathy (CNO) is a progressive disease affecting bones, joints and the surrounding soft tissue in patients with peripheral neuropathy, occurring among 0.1–29% of the diabetic population. Early identification and treatment of CNO is key as delayed diagnosis can lead to foot and

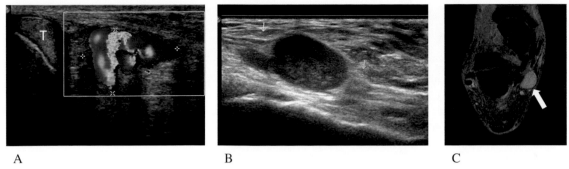

Figure 22.25 Tarsal tunnel syndrome. (A) Transverse US image of the tarsal tunnel showing distended varicosity adjacent to the TPT (T) depicted by vascularity on this colour Doppler image. (B) Transverse US image of the tarsal tunnel showing a well-defined ovoid mass, which can be seen along the course of the tibial nerve. This is in keeping with a peripheral nerve sheath tumour. (C) Axial PD-weighted fat saturated MRI showing a large well-defined fluid SI structure within the tarsal tunnel. This is in keeping with a ganglion cyst.

ankle deformity, foot ulceration, osteomyelitis and amputation (18).

Imaging is key in the diagnosis of CNO. It is often difficult to differentiate osteomyelitis with joint destruction seen in CNO. Ahmadi et al. found that osteomyelitis and CNO could be differentiated most effectively on MRI (19). The presence of sinus tract from a skin ulcer, replacement of the soft tissue-fat interface, extensive BMO, diffuse or thick rim enhancement of the joint fluid and bone erosion near the sinus tract support the diagnosis of osteomyelitis. Subluxed or dislocated abnormal midfoot joints with preservation of the subcutaneous fat, absence of enhancing soft tissue collection and presence of intra-articular loose bodies are more in keeping with CNO (Figure 22.26) (19). Since osteomyelitis occurs adjacent to a skin ulcer, it is usually found in weight-bearing surfaces of the forefoot (metatarsophalangeal joint [MTPJ]) and hindfoot (posterior calcaneus) (Figure 22.27). CNO on the other hand is predominantly a joint-based disease that preferentially affects the midfoot (tarsal and tarsometatarsal joints).

Inflammatory arthritis

Inflammatory arthritis is a multi-systemic disorder with predominant musculoskeletal features. It is an immune mediated inflammatory response that causes bilateral inflammatory synovitis, commonly affecting the peripheral appendicular joints. MTPJs are preferentially affected. The talonavicular joint is the most frequently affected joint amongst the tarsal joints. Like other joints, there is marginal erosion caused by pannus formation

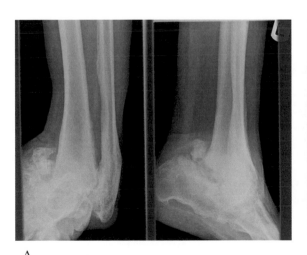

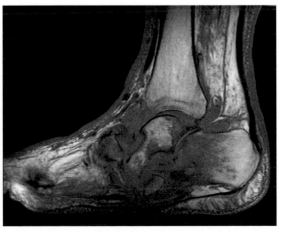

Figure 22.26 Charcot neuropathic osteoarthropathy. (A) AP and lateral plain radiographs showing marked disorganisation, destruction and bone debris involving the ankle and subtalar joints. (B) Sagittal T1-weighted MRI showing destruction and disorganisation centred on the midfoot joints.

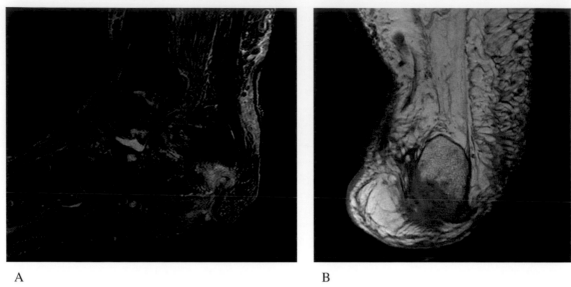

A   B

Figure 22.27 Calcaneal osteomyelitis. (A) Sagittal T2-weighted fat saturated MRI showing a clear sinus tract extending from the skin surface to the weight-bearing surface of the calcaneus where there is florid BMO. (B) Coronal T1-weighted MRI of the same patient showing corresponding low SI within the region of the BMO in keeping with bone marrow infiltration that is seen in osteomyelitis.

with periarticular osteopaenia due to a combination of disuse and hyperaemia. This causes symmetrical, deforming arthritis with uniform joint space loss, which may eventually lead to ankylosis.

Plain radiograph has low sensitivity for structural damage and cannot assess soft tissue inflammation. US is useful in the diagnosis of joint effusion, synovitis, erosion and image-guided corticosteroid injection for symptom relief. MRI can be utilised when US findings are equivocal and is highly sensitive in the diagnosis of synovitis, tenosynovitis and BMO, which is thought to be a precursor of marginal erosions (Figure 22.28) (20).

Intermetatarsal (Morton's) neuroma

Morton's neuroma is benign fibrosis of the plantar interdigital nerve with a reported prevalence of up to 33% (21). It is thought to be due to chronic ischaemia and compression of the nerve by the transverse intermetatarsal ligament. It causes pain or paraesthesia that radiates commonly between the 2nd and 3rd webspaces to the toes.

US is the imaging modality of choice in identifying Morton's neuroma, which has an equal sensitivity to MRI (22). Morton's neuroma appears as a hypoechoic

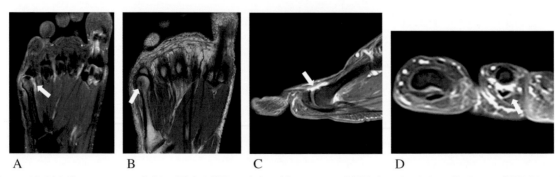

A   B   C   D

Figure 22.28 Inflammatory arthritis. (A) Axial T2-weighted fat saturated MRI showing joint effusion and BMO involving the 5th MTPJ (arrow). (B) Axial T1-weighted MRI of the same patient showing a small erosion (arrow) at the 5th metatarsal head where there was BMO. (C) Sagittal contrast enhanced T1-weighted fat saturated MRI showing joint effusion of the 2nd MTPJ (arrow), which enhances with contrast in keeping with synovitis. (D) Coronal contrast enhanced T1-weighted fat saturated MRI showing enhancing flexor tendon sheath effusion of the 2nd toe in keeping with tenosynovitis (arrow).

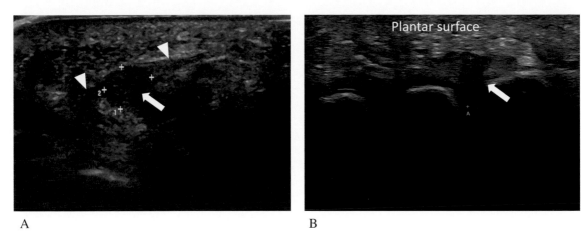

A   B

Figure 22.29 Morton's neuroma. (A) Longitudinal US image between the 3rd webspace. This demonstrates a well-defined, hypoechoic thickening (arrow) of the plantar interdigital nerve (arrow heads). (B) Transverse US image showing a hypoechoic lesion bulging towards the US probe, which is positioned along the plantar surface of the forefoot.

well-defined lesion that is seen along the expected course of the plantar interdigitial nerve. Sonographic Mulder sign can be elicited by compressing the metatarsal heads whilst the US probe is placed along the plantar surface of the symptomatic webspace (Figure 22.29). When metatarsal heads are compressed, Morton's neuroma is displaced towards the US probe with the characteristic click and this may reproduce the symptoms.

Historically it was thought that Morton's neuroma became symptomatic when measured larger than 5 mm in transverse dimension on MRI (21). Cohen et al. however found a discrepancy between the size of the Morton's neuroma on excision and the measurement performed during the US. This was found to be due to overestimation in US due to the surrounding bursal thickening and fluid, which often co-exist, as well as neural fibrosis and degeneration (23). It is therefore

commonly called a Morton's neuroma-bursal complex. This highlights the importance of clinical history and examination when determining the management, rather than relying on its size alone. MRI is reserved for equivocal US findings with atypical presentation. It is both low on T1- and T2-weighted imaging and there is often associated intermetatarsal bursitis (Figure 22.30). Treatment options include image guided steroid injection, radiofrequency ablation and surgical excision.

Plantar plate Injury

Plantar plate tears occur due to hyperextension and axial loading, most commonly on the 2nd MTPJ. There is controversy as to which imaging modality is superior in diagnostic accuracy. Meta-analyses have shown that the sensitivity and specificity of US is reported

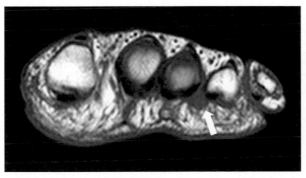
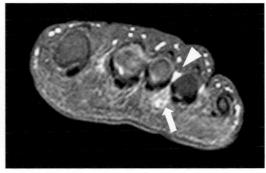

A   B

Figure 22.30 Morton's neuroma. (A) Coronal T1-weighted MRI showing a low-SI lesion bulging towards the plantar surface of the forefoot between the 3rd webspace in keeping with a Morton's neuroma (arrow). (B) Coronal T2-weighted fat saturated MRI of the same patient showing the high SI Morton's neuroma at the plantar margin of the 3rd webspace (arrow). There is associated intermetatarsal bursitis, which can be seen more centrally (arrow head).

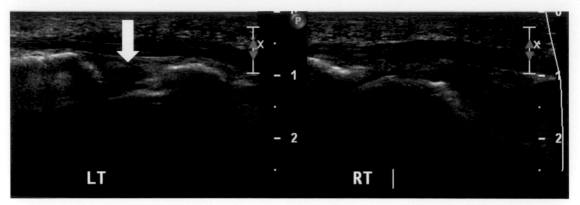

Figure 22.31 Plantar plate tear. Longitudinal US image of the 2nd MTPJ, which shows an area of hypoechoic defect within the plantar plate of the left foot. Note the normal appearance of the plantar plate of the right foot.

as 93% and 33%, whereas MRI is reported as 95% and 54%, respectively (24). The benefits of US are its availability, cost-effectiveness and ability to perform a dynamic investigation. On US, plantar plate is a relatively hypoechoic, homogenous and striated structure that envelopes the plantar surface of the MTPJ with the flexor tendon traversing superficially. It is closely related to the accessory collateral ligaments, which blend in with the plantar plate on either side from the metatarsal head. There is loss of this homogenous echotexture of the plantar plate with a fluid-filled gap when it is torn (Figure 22.31). This can be accentuated on dynamic testing, which will demonstrate joint subluxation.

There are direct and indirect signs of a plantar plate tear on MRI. The direct sign includes discontinuity of the plantar plate from its osseous attachments or at its attachments to the accessory collateral ligaments. Joint effusion or intra-articular contrast can be seen to decompress through the defect to the surrounding soft tissue or into the flexor tendon sheath. Indirect signs of plantar plate tear include a pseudoneuroma sign, where it mimics the presence of a Morton's neuroma (Figure 22.32). This occurs secondary to pericapsular

fibrosis from the plantar plate tear and has a strong sensitivity (91%) and specificity (90.9%) (25). Morton's neuroma is usually centrally located within the webspace, whereas the pericapsular fibrosis is eccentric in its location.

Take home messages

- Imaging is an integral part of the diagnosis and management of the foot and ankle disorders.
- Correlation of findings on imaging with clinical signs and symptoms is key to achieving a correct diagnosis.
- US is useful for patients who present with localised symptoms. It can be used to assess the superficial pathologies of the foot and ankle whilst having an added benefit of being able to perform a dynamic assessment of these structures.
- MRI is a problem-solving tool that can be utilised to assess non-specific and generalised symptoms around the foot and ankle. It is used to assess the periarticular soft tissue structures, integrity of the articular cartilage and underlying BMO.

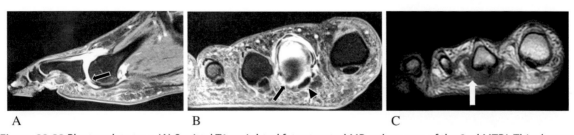

A B C

Figure 22.32 Plantar plate tear. (A) Sagittal T1-weighted fat saturated MR arthrogram of the 2nd MTPJ. This shows a defect through the plantar plate at its phalangeal insertion with contrast extravasating along the flexor tendon sheath (arrow). (B) Coronal T1-weighted fat saturated MR arthrogram of the same patient. The tear can be seen propagating towards the lateral accessory collateral ligament (arrow) with resultant medial subluxation of the flexor tendon (arrow head). (C) Coronal T1-weighted MRI showing thickening of the lateral accessory collateral ligament in keeping with the pseudoneuroma sign (arrow).

- Image-guided intervention of the foot and ankle is wide ranging and is an important step in the management of patients when the conservative treatment has failed and surgery is not yet indicated.

References

1. Hill CL, Gill TK, Menz HB, Taylor AW. Prevalence and correlates of foot pain in a population-based study: The North West Adelaide health study. J Foot Ankle Res. 2008; 28(1):2.

2. Saifuddin A. Musculoskeletal MRI (1st ed). London: Hodder Arnold; 2008. p. 484.

3. Orr JD, Dutton JR, Fowler JT. Anatomic location and morphology of symptomatic, operatively treated osteochondral lesions of the talus. Foot Ankle Int. 2012; 33(12):1051–1057.

4. Hepple S, Winson IG, Glew D. Osteochondral lesions of the talus: A revised classification. Foot Ankle Int. 1999; 20(12): 789–793.

5. Donovan A, Rosenberg ZS. MRI of ankle and lateral hindfoot impingement syndromes. AJR Am J Roentgenol. 2010; 195(3):595–604.

6. Grasel RP, Schweitzer ME, Kovalovich AM, Karasick D, Wapner K, Hecht P, Wander D. MR imaging of plantar fasciitis: Edema, tears, and occult marrow abnormalities correlated with outcome. AJR. 1999; 173:699–701.

7. Gerster JC, Vischer TL, Bennani A, Fallet GL. The painful heel: Comparative study in rheumatoid arthritis, ankylosing spondylitis, Reiter's syndrome, and generalized osteoarthritis. Ann Rheum Dis. 1977; 36:343–348.

8. Lee TH, Wapner KL, Hecht PJ. Plantar fibromatosis. J Bone Joint Surg Am. 1993; 75:1080–1084.

9. Hougeir FG, Elston DM, Plantar Fibromatosis Clinical Presentation. Medscape. updated 14th May 2014.

10. Lawrence DA, Rolen MF, Morshed KA, Moukaddam H. MRI of heel pain. AJR. 2013; 200:845–855.

11. Kong A, Van Der Vliet A. Imaging of tibialis posterior dysfunction. Br J Radiol. 2008; 81(970):826–836.

12. Lee S, Oliveira I, Li Y, Welck M, Saifuddin A. Fluid around the distal tibialis posterior tendon on ankle MRI: Prevalence and clinical relevance. Br J Radiol [Internet]. 2019; 92(1104):20190722. Available from: https://doi.org/10.1259/bjr.20190722

13. Sobel M, Levy ME, Bohne WH. Congenital variations of the peroneus quartus muscle: An anatomic study. Foot Ankle. 1990; 11:81–89.

14. Yu JS, Resnick D. MR imaging of the accessory soleus muscle appearance in six patients and a review of the literature. Skeletal Radiol. 1994; 23:525–528.

15. Kjaersgaard-Andersen P, Andersen K, Soballe K, Pilgaard S. Sinus tarsi syndrome: Presentation of seven cases and review of the literature. J Foot Surg. 1989; 28:3–6.

16. Donovan A, Rosenberg ZS, Cavalcanti CF. MR imaging of entrapment neuropathies of the lower extremity. Part 2. The knee, leg, ankle, and foot. Radiographics. 2010; 30(4): 1001–1019.

17. Erickson SJ, Quinn SF, Kneeland JB Smith JW, Johnson JE, Carrera GF, Shereff MJ, Hyde JS, Jesmanowicz A. MR imaging of the tarsal tunnel and related spaces: Normal and abnormal findings with anatomic correlation. AJR Am J Roentgenol. 1990; 155(2):323–328.

18. Schoots IG, Slim FJ, Busch-Westbroek TE, Maas M. Neuro-osteoarthropathy of the foot-radiologist: Friend or foe? Semin Musculoskelet Radiol. 2010; 14:365–376.

19. Ahmadi ME, Morrison WB, Carrino JA Schweitzer ME, Raikin SM, Ledermann HP. Neuropathic arthropathy of the foot with and without superimposed osteomyelitis: MR imaging characteristics. Radiology. 2006; 238(2):622–631.

20. Narvaez JA, Narvaez J, De Lama E, De Albert M. MR imaging of early rheumatoid arthritis. Radiographics. 2010; 30(1): 143–145.

21. Bencardino J, Rosenberg ZS, Beltran J, Liu X, Marty-Delfaut E. Morton's neuroma. Am J Roentgenol [Internet]. 2000; 175(3):649–653. Available from: https://doi.org/10.2214/ajr.175.3.1750649

22. Bignotti B, Signori A, Sormani MP, Molfetta L, Martinoli C, Tagliafico A. Ultrasound versus magnetic resonance imaging for Morton neuroma: Systematic review and meta-analysis. Eur Radiol. 2015; 25(8):2254–2262.

23. Cohen SL, Miller TT, Ellis SJ, Roberts MM, DiCarlo EF. Sonography of Morton neuromas. J Ultrasound Med [Internet]. 2016; 35(10):2191–2195. Available from: https://doi.org/10.7863/ultra.15.11022

24. Duan X, Li L, Wei D-Q, Liu M, Yu X, Xu Z, Long Y, Xiang Z. Role of magnetic resonance imaging versus ultrasound for detection of plantar plate tear. J Orthop Surg Res. 2017; 12(1):14.

25. Yamada AF, Crema MD, Nery C, Baumfeld D, Mann TS, Skaf AY, Fernandes ARC. Second and third metatarsophalangeal plantar plate tears: Diagnostic performance of direct and indirect MRI features using surgical findings as the reference standard. AJR Am J Roentgenol. 2017; 209(2): W100–108.

Further resources

1. https://radsource.us

2. https://radiopaedia.org

3. https://radiologyassistant.nl

4. Rosenberg ZS, Beltran J, Bencardino JT; Radiological Society of North America. From the RSNA refresher courses: MR imaging of the ankle and foot. RadioGraphics. 2000;20(spec no):S153–S179.

Index

Note: Locators in *italics* represent figures and **bold** indicate tables in the text.